S0-BTA-634

ACLS
STUDY GUIDE

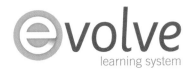

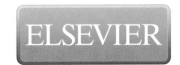

YOU'VE JUST PURCHASED
MORE THAN
A TEXTBOOK

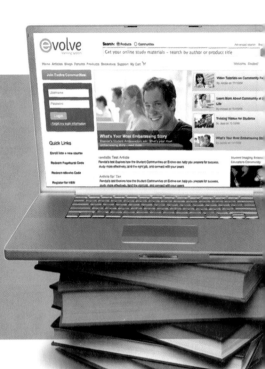

ACTIVATE THE COMPLETE LEARNING EXPERIENCE THAT COMES WITH YOUR BOOK BY REGISTERING AT

http://evolve.elsevier.com/Aehlert/ACLS/

Once you register, you will have access to your
FREE STUDY TOOLS:

Student:

- Stop and Review Quizzes

Instructor:

- Lesson Plans

- PowerPoint Presentations

- Test Banks

- Case Studies

REGISTER TODAY!

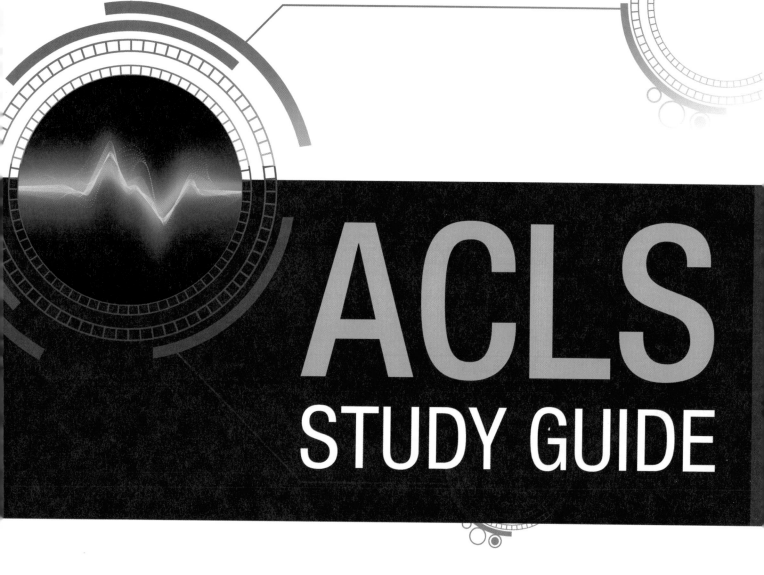

ACLS
STUDY GUIDE

FOURTH EDITION

Barbara Aehlert, RN, BSPA

Southwest EMS Education, Inc.

Phoenix, AZ/Pursley, TX

ELSEVIER

MOSBY

3251 Riverport Lane
St. Louis, Missouri 63043

ACLS STUDY GUIDE, FOURTH EDITION   ISBN: 978-0-323-08449-9

Copyright © 2012 by Mosby, an imprint of Elsevier Inc.
Copyright © 2007, 2002, 1994 by Mosby, Inc., an affiliate of Elsevier Inc.

No part of this publication may be reproduced or transmitted in any form or by any means, electronic or mechanical, including photocopying, recording, or any information storage and retrieval system, without permission in writing from the publisher. Details on how to seek permission, further information about the Publisher's permissions policies and our arrangements with organizations such as the Copyright Clearance Center and the Copyright Licensing Agency, can be found at our website: www.elsevier.com/permissions.

This book and the individual contributions contained in it are protected under copyright by the Publisher (other than as may be noted herein).

Notices

Knowledge and best practice in this field are constantly changing. As new research and experience broaden our understanding, changes in research methods, professional practices, or medical treatment may become necessary.

Practitioners and researchers must always rely on their own experience and knowledge in evaluating and using any information, methods, compounds, or experiments described herein. In using such information or methods they should be mindful of their own safety and the safety of others, including parties for whom they have a professional responsibility.

With respect to any drug or pharmaceutical products identified, readers are advised to check the most current information provided (i) on procedures featured or (ii) by the manufacturer of each product to be administered, to verify the recommended dose or formula, the method and duration of administration, and contraindications. It is the responsibility of practitioners, relying on their own experience and knowledge of their patients, to make diagnoses, to determine dosages and the best treatment for each individual patient, and to take all appropriate safety precautions.

To the fullest extent of the law, neither the Publisher nor the authors, contributors, or editors, assume any liability for any injury and/or damage to persons or property as a matter of products liability, negligence or otherwise, or from any use or operation of any methods, products, instructions, or ideas contained in the material herein.

ISBN: 978-0-323-08449-9

Via President and Publisher: Andrew Allen
Acquisitions Editor: Laura Bayless
Publishing Services Manager: Julie Eddy
Senior Project Manager: Andrea Campbell
Design Direction: Karen Pauls

Working together to grow
libraries in developing countries

www.elsevier.com | www.bookaid.org | www.sabre.org

ELSEVIER   BOOK AID International   Sabre Foundation

Printed in the United States of America

Last digit is the print number: 9 8 7 6 5 4 3 2 1

PREFACE TO THE FOURTH EDITION

I took my first Advanced Cardiac Life Support (ACLS) class many years ago. I was terrified (and lost) throughout the entire course. Although I spent weeks studying before the course, the information I read seemed to me to be written in a foreign language. I could find no resources to "translate" the information into something that was useful to me. The course consisted of very long lectures by instructors that read slides and offered little useful insight. The most memorable part of the course was the "Patient Management" station in which each course participant was evaluated one-on-one by an instructor. (For those of you who have been around a while, you are probably having flashbacks to those days). I will *never* forget that experience.

Despite the time spent studying, as soon as the door closed behind me I was a mental wreck. The instructor proceeded to methodically strip away any self-confidence I might have had in treating a patient who had a cardiac-related emergency. I was able to answer the questions asked of me until I was presented with a patient who had a symptomatic bradycardia. Atropine had not worked (transcutaneous pacing was not a readily available option that many years ago) and the next drug that was recommended at that time was isoproterenol. I knew that. What I could not recall was whether isoproterenol was given in mcg/min (correct) or mg/min. I took a "50/50" guess and said mg/min. Because that was the wrong decision, I was told I had failed the course and would need to schedule myself to attend another 2-day class.

Before driving home, I sat outside for a few minutes contemplating what had happened and what I could have done to change the outcome. On that day, I made a promise to myself that I would become an ACLS instructor someday and find a way to teach the information in a more user-friendly atmosphere. I promised myself that I would be a part of teaching courses that were useful to practicing health care professionals and that were delivered in an environment in which the participants looked forward to the class—instead of dreading it.

As the years passed, I did become an ACLS instructor and loved it. At the conclusion of each course, participants would often write on their course evaluations that a study guide would have been helpful in preparing for class. Those suggestions resulted in writing a few pages of information, which ultimately became a book—*this* book.

The *ACLS Study Guide* is designed for use by paramedic, nursing, and medical students, ECG monitor technicians, nurses, and other allied health personnel working in emergency departments, critical care units, postanesthesia care units, operating rooms, and telemetry units who are preparing for an ACLS Student Course. The fourth edition of this book is based on the following science, treatment recommendations, and guidelines:

- 2010 American Heart Association Guidelines for Cardiopulmonary Resuscitation and Emergency Cardiovascular Care
- 2010 International Consensus on Cardiopulmonary Resuscitation and Emergency Cardiovascular Care Science With Treatment Recommendations
- Other evidence-based treatment recommendations or sources are cited in the reference section of relevant chapters.

This book is designed for use with the American Safety and Health Institute (ASHI) ACLS Student Course. This book may be used as supplemental material by participants of ACLS courses offered by other organizations.

The ACLS Study Guide consists of two primary sections. Chapters 1 through 6 in the first section of this book provide the "why," "when," and "how" for the case studies in the second section. In addition to the 50-question pre- and post-tests, each chapter contains learning objectives and a chapter quiz. Answers and rationales are provided for all questions in this text.

It has been proved that to learn how to do something, you must actually *do* it. The opportunity to "do" the skills taught in an ACLS course and make decisions regarding patient care is provided during ten "core" case studies in an ACLS course. A sample case study has been provided for each of the standard "core" cases presented in an ACLS course. The case studies are not intended to cover every possible dysrhythmia that may be presented in an actual ACLS course. Rather, they are provided as examples to help you understand the information presented in the preparatory section of the text. To help you prepare for the ACLS course, each case study includes a scenario sheet that represents dialogue between an ACLS "Coach" and team leader. This has been done to simulate the interaction between an ACLS instructor and student (team leader) in an ACLS course. After you have read each of the case studies, ask another person to assist you by assuming the role of the "Coach."

Every attempt has been made to provide information that is consistent with current literature, including current resuscitation guidelines. However, medicine is a dynamic field. Resuscitation guidelines change, new medications and technology are being developed, and medical research is ongoing. As a result, be sure to learn and follow local protocols as defined by your medical advisors. The author and publisher assume no responsibility or liability for loss or damage resulting from the use of information contained within.

I genuinely hope you find the information contained in the pages that follow helpful and I wish you success in your ACLS course and clinical practice.

Sincerely,
Barbara Aehlert

To
My father, Bobby R. Mahoney
For your inspiration, guidance, love, and support

and

In loving memory of:
My grandfather, John Dallas Mahoney
and uncles
William Jarrell Mahoney and Donald C. Mahoney

ACKNOWLEDGMENTS

The transformation of manuscript pages into a textbook is a formidable task, but it is one that is undertaken every day by the Editorial and Production teams at Elsevier. My sincerest thanks to Laura Bayless and Andrea Campbell for their suggestions, guidance, and patience throughout the development and production of this text. A special thanks to the manuscript reviewers who provided insightful comments and suggestions.

A special thanks to these instructors who share the same philosophy about teaching ACLS as I do: Andrew Baird, CEP; Eileen Blackstone, CEP; Lynn Browne-Wagner, RN; Randy Budd, CEP; Joanna Burgan, CEP; Thomas Cole, CEP; Mike Connor, CEP; Paul Honeywell, CEP; James Johnson, CEP; Stephen Knox, CEP; Justin Lawrence, CEP; Bill Loughran, RN; Terence Mason, RN; Sean Newton, CEP; Anthony Pino; Jan Post, RN; Greg Ruiz, CEP; Gary Smith, MD; David Stockton, CEP; Kevin Taussig, CEP; Ed Tirone, CEP; Nicky Treece, RN; and Maryalice Witzel, RN.

PUBLISHER ACKNOWLEDGMENTS

The editors wish to acknowledge and thank the many reviewers of this book who devoted countless hours to intensive review. Their comments were invaluable in helping develop and fine-tune the manuscript.

Peter Connick, EMT-P, EMT I/C
Captain-Chatham Fire Rescue
Chatham, Massachusetts
Adjunct Faculty
Cape Cod Community College
West Barnestable, Massachusetts

Jon S. Cooper, Paramedic, NCEE
Lieutenant
Baltimore City Fire Department
Baltimore, Maryland

Janet Fitts, RN, BSN, CEN, TNS, EMT-P
Training Officer
New Haven Ambulance District
New Haven, Missouri

Mark Goldstein, RN, MSN, EMT-P I/C
Emergency Services Clinical Nurse Specialist
    and EMS Coordinator
William Beaumont Hospital
Grosse Pointe, Michigan

Terry L. Horrocks, BS, NREMT-P
Captain
Baltimore City Fire Department
Baltimore, Maryland

Reylon Meeks, RN, PhD
Clinical Nurse Specialist/Fire Chief
Blank Children's Hospital/Pleasant Hill Fire
    Department
Pleasant Hill, Iowa

Jeff Messerole, PS
Clinical Instructor
Spencer Hospital
Spencer, Iowa

Deborah L. Petty, BS, CICP, EMT-P I/C
Paramedic Training Officer
St. Charles County Ambulance District
St. Peters, Missouri

Warren J. Porter, MS, BA LP NREMTP
Director, Clinical and Education
American Medical Response- South Region
Arlington, Texas

Erik J. Usher, RN, BS, CEN, CPEN, EMT-P, CFRN
Flight Nurse
Bayflite
St. Petersburg, Florida

ABOUT THE AUTHOR

Barbara Aehlert, RN, BSPA, is the President of Southwest EMS Education, Inc., in Phoenix, Arizona and Pursley, Texas. She has been a registered nurse for more than 35 years with clinical experience in medical/surgical and critical care nursing and prehospital education. Barbara is an active CPR, First Aid, Paramedic, ACLS, and PALS instructor and takes a special interest in teaching basic dysrhythmia recognition and ACLS to nurses and paramedics.

TABLE OF CONTENTS

3 Rhythms and Management

PART II CASE STUDIES

Multiple Choice

Identify the choice that best completes the statement or answers the question.

a 1.   An oral airway:
   a. May result in an airway obstruction if improperly inserted
   b. Is usually well tolerated in the responsive or semi-responsive patient
   c. Should be lubricated with a petroleum-based lubricant before insertion
   d. Is of proper size if it extends from the tip of the nose to the tip of the ear

b 2.   A patient who presents with a possible acute coronary syndrome should receive a targeted history and physical examination and an initial 12-lead electrocardiogram (ECG) within _____ minutes of patient contact (prehospital) or arrival in the emergency department.
   a. 5
   b. 10
   c. 30
   d. 60

a 3.   During cardiopulmonary resuscitation (CPR):
   a. The adult sternum should be depressed 1.5 to 2 inches
   b. No more than 30 seconds should be spent checking for a pulse
   c. Cardiac output is approximately 25% to 33% of normal
   d. Chest compressions should be interrupted every 10 minutes to allow team members to change positions

b 4.   A 50-year-old woman is complaining of substernal chest discomfort and nausea. She rates her discomfort 8/10 and states her symptoms began about 3 hours ago. Her BP is 162/94, P 122, R 16. Breath sounds are clear. The cardiac monitor shows a sinus tachycardia with ST depression in lead II. Her SpO_2 on room air is 98%. An IV line has been started and a 12-lead ECG has been ordered. Which of the following reflects the most appropriate treatment for this patient?
   a. Oxygen, atropine 1 mg IV, sublingual nitroglycerin, and morphine IV
   b. Aspirin 162 to 325 mg (chewed), sublingual nitroglycerin, and morphine IV
   c. Sublingual nitroglycerin, adenosine 6 mg IV, and a 250-mL IV fluid challenge
   d. Oxygen, aspirin 162 to 325 mg (chewed), vasopressin 20 U IV, and lidocaine 1.5 mg/kg IV

d 5.   Shockable cardiac arrest rhythms include:
   a. Asystole and pulseless electrical activity
   b. Pulseless ventricular tachycardia and asystole
   c. Pulseless electrical activity and ventricular fibrillation
   d. Ventricular fibrillation and pulseless ventricular tachycardia

_b_ ✓6.   With an oxygen flow rate of 0.25 to 8 L/min, a nasal cannula can deliver an estimated oxygen concentration of:
a. 17% to 21%
b. 22% to 45%
c. 40% to 60%
d. 60% to 100%

_b_ 7✗   An 84-year-old man is in cardiac arrest. Which of the following statements is correct?
a. Begin single rescuer bag-mask ventilation as soon as possible.
b. The ratio of chest compressions to ventilations that should be delivered is 15:2.
c. If an advanced airway is inserted, the patient should be ventilated at a rate of 8 to 10 breaths/min.
d. After insertion of an advanced airway, briefly pause chest compressions (about 3 to 4 seconds) to deliver 2 ventilations after every 30 chest compressions.

_d_ 8✗   Establishing vascular access is part of:
a. "A" in the primary survey
b. "B" in the secondary survey
c. "C" in the secondary survey
d. "D" in the primary survey

_C_ 9✗   When ACLS medications are administered via a tracheal tube, the dose generally is __ the IV dose.
a. 2 to 2.5 times
b. 3 to 3.5 times
c. 5 to 5.5 times
d. 10 times

_C_ 10.   Which of the following may be used in the management of a stable patient with monomorphic ventricular tachycardia (VT)?
a. Adenosine, diltiazem, and verapamil
b. Atropine, adenosine, and amiodarone
c. Procainamide, amiodarone, and sotalol
d. Lidocaine, atropine, and isoproterenol

_b_ 11.   Mouth-to-mask breathing combined with supplemental oxygen at a minimum flow rate of 10 L/min can deliver an oxygen concentration of approximately

_____.
a. 25%
b. 50%
c. 65%
d. 90%

_a_ 12.   The first *antiarrhythmic* administered in the management of the patient in pulseless ventricular tachycardia or ventricular fibrillation is:
a. Amiodarone or lidocaine
b. Epinephrine or lidocaine
c. Procainamide or amiodarone
d. Vasopressin or procainamide

_a_ 13.   Which of the following is a common cause of excessive intrathoracic pressure during cardiopulmonary resuscitation?
a. Hyperventilation
b. Inability to open the victim's airway
c. Inadequate rate of chest compressions
d. Frequent interruptions for rhythm/pulse checks

d **14.** An anxious 44-year-old woman is complaining of difficulty breathing and substernal chest discomfort that radiates to her left shoulder. She states her symptoms have been present for about 40 minutes. Her oxygen saturation level on room air is 90%. Which of the following statements is correct?

a. Supplemental oxygen therapy is indicated only if the patient has obvious signs of heart failure or shock.

b. Supplemental oxygen therapy is indicated and should be titrated to maintain her SpO$_2$ at 94% or greater.

c. High-concentration supplemental oxygen is indicated for all patients with a suspected acute coronary syndrome.

d. Supplemental oxygen therapy is indicated and should be continued for at least 24 hours after symptom onset for all patients with a suspected acute coronary syndrome.

a **15.** A 78-year-old woman has suffered a respiratory arrest. A tracheal tube has been placed. You note that you are encountering no resistance but there is an absence of chest wall movement when ventilating with a bag-valve device. You are unable to auscultate breath sounds on either side of the chest. What is the most likely cause of this situation?

a. Esophageal intubation

b. A mucus plug in the tracheal tube

c. Left primary bronchus intubation

d. Right primary bronchus intubation

  16. Which of the following statements is INCORRECT regarding transcutaneous pacing (TCP)?

a. TCP is painful in conscious patients, particularly with the use of 50 mA or more.

b. TCP has been shown to be no more effective than drug therapy in survival to hospital discharge.

c. TCP is a reasonable temporizing measure that may be useful in the treatment of symptomatic bradycardia.

d. TCP is beneficial in the management of cardiac arrest rhythms such as asystole and pulseless electrical activity.

b **17.** Drugs given during cardiac arrest that __ blood vessels may improve perfusion pressures.

a. Constrict

b. Dilate

c **18.** Which of the following memory aids may be used when evaluating a patient's level of responsiveness?

a. ABCD

b. OPQRST

c. AVPU

d. CAB

d **19.** A patient is unresponsive with spontaneous ventilations at a rate of 4/min. Chest movement is barely visible with each breath. A pulse is present. Which of the following oxygen delivery devices would be most appropriate to use in this situation?

a. A nasal cannula at 4 L/min

b. A simple face mask at 4 L/min

c. A nonrebreather mask at 15 L/min

d. A bag-mask device with a reservoir at 15 L/min

_d_ In acute stroke management, which of the following phrases reflects the need for rapid assessment and intervention?
a. Golden Hour
 b. Time is Brain
c. Time is Tissue
d. Time is Muscle

_b_ 21. You have defibrillated a pulseless patient in monomorphic VT. The shock resulted in a return of a pulse. A few minutes later, the patient is once again unresponsive, apneic, and without a pulse. The monitor shows VF. You should:
a. Start over again using a lower energy level
b. Defibrillate with the last successful energy level
c. Charge the defibrillator to its maximum energy setting and deliver 3 shocks in rapid succession
d. Set the defibrillator at its lowest energy setting and deliver 3 shocks in rapid succession

_d_ 22. A 55-year-old woman is complaining of severe chest discomfort that has persisted after three doses of sublingual nitroglycerin. Moments after administration of morphine IV, her blood pressure dropped from 114/66 to 76/42 and her heart rate increased from 88 to 104 beats/min. The patient's breath sounds are clear and her ECG shows a sinus tachycardia. Your next action should be to:
a. Give another dose of sublingual nitroglycerin
b. Perform immediate synchronized cardioversion with 50 J
c. Perform vagal maneuvers and give adenosine 6 mg rapid IV push
d. Give a fluid challenge of 250 to 500 mL of normal saline and reassess

_d_ 23. Which of the following is preferred for confirmation and monitoring of tracheal tube placement?
a. Pulse oximetry
 b. Waveform capnography
c. Presence of water vapor in the tube
d. Gastric insufflation sounds over the stomach

_b_ 24. The initial treatment of any patient with a symptomatic bradycardia should focus on:
 a. Support of airway and breathing
b. Preparations for transcutaneous pacing
c. Preparations for synchronized cardioversion
d. Assessing oxygen saturation and establishing IV access

_b_ 25. Which of the following correctly reflects the priorities of care during cardiac arrest?
a. CPR and establishing IV access
b. CPR and defibrillation (if indicated)
c. Establishing IV access and drug administration
d. Defibrillation (if indicated) and drug administration

_c_ 26. Vasopressin:
a. Is given every 3 to 5 minutes during cardiac arrest
b. Is given as a continuous IV infusion at a rate of 40 U/hr in cardiac arrest
c. May replace either the first or second dose of epinephrine in the treatment of cardiac arrest
d. Can be used in cardiac arrest due to pulseless ventricular tachycardia or ventricular fibrillation, but not in cardiac arrest due to asystole or pulseless electrical activity

_b_   27.
A 48-year-old man has had chest discomfort for 2 hours. He has been diagnosed with an acute ST-elevation myocardial infarction (STEMI). When providing care to this patient, it is important to make sure that a defibrillator is readily available because his susceptibility to dysrhythmias is greatest during the first ____ since his onset of symptoms.
a. 4 to 6 minutes
b. 4 hours
c. 3 days
d. 2 weeks

_b_   28.
Identify the correct initial energy settings for the management of an unstable patient with a pulse who is in monomorphic ventricular tachycardia.
a. Defibrillate using 360 J (monophasic energy)
b. Defibrillate using 120 to 200 J (biphasic energy)
c. Perform synchronized cardioversion using 50 J initially (biphasic)
d. Perform synchronized cardioversion using 100 J initially (biphasic)

_c_   29.
If a patient wakes from sleep or is found with symptoms of a stroke, the time of onset of symptoms is defined as the time:
a. Of awakening
b. The patient retired for sleep
c. The patient was last known to be symptom-free
d. The patient was last seen by his health care provider

_b_   30.
The most common adverse effects of giving amiodarone are:
a. Nausea and asystole
b. Bradycardia and hypotension
c. Tachycardia and hypertension
d. Blurred vision and abdominal pain

_b_   31.
During a cardiac arrest, multiple attempts to establish a peripheral IV have proved unsuccessful. Your best course of action at this time will be to:
a. Insert a central line
b. Attempt intraosseous access
c. Discontinue resuscitation efforts
d. Continue peripheral IV attempts until successful

_d_   32.
Clopidogrel:
a. Is given rapidly as a 2.5 to 5 mg IV bolus (over 1 to 3 seconds)
b. Is a potent antiarrhythmic used in the management of regular, narrow-QRS tachycardias
c. Administration is limited to patients younger than 75 years with ST-elevation myocardial infarction
d. May be administered to patients who are unable to take aspirin because of hypersensitivity or major gastrointestinal intolerance

_a_   33.
The most common cause of a stroke is:
a. A clot (thrombus)
b. A ruptured blood vessel
c. Spasm of a cerebral artery
d. An arteriovenous malformation

_C_ ✓ 34. Which of the following reflects correct operation of a transcutaneous pacemaker for a patient experiencing a symptomatic bradycardia?
a. The rate should be set between 20 and 60. The current (milliamps) should be increased slowly to maximum output.
b. The rate should be set between 40 and 100. The current should be increased rapidly to a maximum of 160 milliamps.
c. The rate should be set between 60 and 80. The current should be increased slowly until capture is achieved.
d. The rate should be set between 80 and 100. The current should be increased rapidly to maximum output.

Matching

Match each description below with its corresponding answer.

a. May be used to treat torsades de pointes
b. Beta-adrenergic agent that may be used in the treatment of symptomatic bradycardia
c. Indirect inhibitor of thrombin
d. Prevents the conversion of angiotensin I to angiotensin II
e. Calcium channel blocker
f. Drug of choice for most narrow-QRS tachycardias
g. Alternative antiarrhythmic used in the treatment of stable monomorphic VT
h. One reperfusion therapy option for patients with ST elevation MI
i. __ IIb/IIIa inhibitors prevent fibrinogen binding and platelet clumping
j. Although given IV bolus in cardiac arrest, this drug is given by IV infusion in symptomatic bradycardia
k. Can be used in place of the first or second dose of epinephrine in cardiac arrest
l. Vasodilator used in normotensive patients with ischemic chest discomfort
m. Catecholamine with alpha and beta-adrenergic dose-related actions; used in the treatment of symptomatic bradycardia
n. First-line drug used in the treatment of symptomatic bradycardia
o. Diuretic
p. May be used as an alternative to amiodarone in pulseless VT/VF arrest

O	~~b~~ O	35.	Furosemide	M	___	43. Dopamine _brady_
d	d	36.	Angiotensin-converting enzyme (ACE) inhibitor	j	___	44. Epinephrine _brady_
b	___	37.	Isoproterenol	f	f	45. Adenosine _QRS narrow TC_
n	b	38.	Atropine _brady_	K	___	46. Vasopressin
e	e	39.	Diltiazem	a	a	47. Magnesium sulfate
l	l	40.	Nitroglycerin	h	c	48. Fibrinolytics
i	___	41.	Glycoprotein	P	~~k~~	49. Lidocaine _alternative to amiodarone VT/VF_
g	g	42.	Sotalol _VT_	C	___	50. Heparin

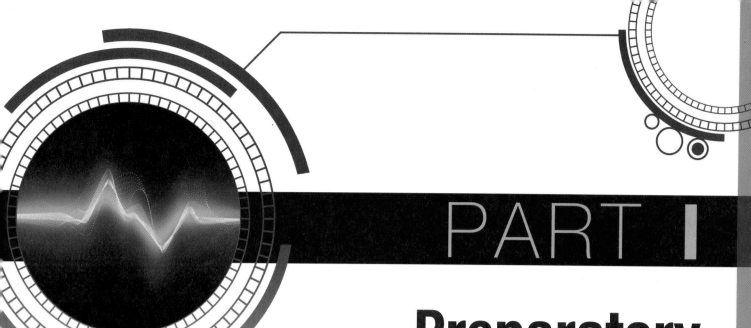

PART I

Preparatory

CHAPTER 1

The ABCDs of Emergency Cardiovascular Care

OBJECTIVES

Upon completion of this chapter, you will be able to:

1. Identify risk factors for coronary artery disease.
2. Define *cardiovascular collapse*, *cardiac arrest*, and *sudden cardiac death*.
3. Name four heart rhythms that are associated with cardiac arrest.
4. Differentiate between shockable and nonshockable cardiac arrest rhythms.
5. Describe the links in the Chain of Survival.
6. Identify possible reversible causes of a cardiac emergency.
7. Describe the phases of cardiopulmonary resuscitation.
8. List the purposes and components of the primary and secondary surveys.

INTRODUCTION

Heart disease is the leading cause of death for both men and women in the United States. In 2005, approximately 920,000 persons in the United States had a myocardial infarction (heart attack).[1] In the United States, someone has a heart attack every 34 seconds.[2] It has been estimated that about 300,000 individuals in the United States experience a cardiac arrest each year and fewer than 15% survive.[3-5]

As you can see from these statistics, the likelihood of encountering a patient who requires basic life support (BLS) or advanced cardiac life support (ACLS) care is high. In this chapter you will read about the essentials of ACLS. Just as BLS is a systematic way of providing care to a choking victim or to someone who needs cardiopulmonary resuscitation (CPR), ACLS is an orderly approach to providing advanced emergency care to a patient who is experiencing a cardiac-related problem.

This chapter discusses risk factors for coronary artery disease, sudden cardiac death, the Chain of Survival, the phases of CPR, and a systematic approach to patient assessment.

RISK FACTORS FOR CORONARY ARTERY DISEASE

[Objective 1]

Cardiovascular disease (CVD) is a collection of conditions that involve the circulatory system, which contains the heart (cardio) and blood vessels (vascular), and that include congenital CVDs. Approximately one in three American adults has one or more types of CVD.[2] **Heart disease** is a broad term that refers to conditions that affect the heart. **Coronary heart disease** (CHD) refers to disease of the coronary arteries and their resulting complications, such as angina pectoris and acute myocardial infarction. According to the Centers for Disease Control and Prevention, CHD is the most common type of heart disease.[6] **Coronary artery disease** (CAD) affects the arteries that supply the heart muscle with blood.

The prevention of CVD requires the management of risk factors. **Risk factors** are traits and lifestyle habits that may increase a person's chance of developing a disease. More than 300 risk factors have been associated with CHD and stroke. Major risk factors meet three criteria[7]:

1. They have a high frequency in many populations
2. They have a significant independent impact on the risk of CHD or stroke
3. The treatment and control of the risk factor results in reduced risk

Some risk factors can be modified, which means that they can be changed or treated. Risk factors that cannot be modified are called "nonmodifiable" or "fixed" risk factors. Contributing risk factors are thought to lead to an increased risk of heart disease, but their exact role has not been defined (Table 1-1).

SUDDEN CARDIAC DEATH

[Objectives 2, 3, 4]

Cardiovascular collapse is a sudden loss of effective blood flow that is caused by cardiac and/or peripheral vascular factors that may reverse spontaneously (such as syncope) or only with interventions (such as cardiac arrest).[8] **Cardiopulmonary (cardiac) arrest** is the absence of cardiac mechanical activity, which is confirmed by the absence of a detectable pulse, unresponsiveness, and apnea or agonal, gasping breathing. The term *cardiac arrest* is more commonly used than *cardiopulmonary arrest* when referring to a patient who is not breathing (or who is only gasping) and who has no pulse. Gasping is abnormal breathing and should not be interpreted as a sign of effective breathing.

Sudden cardiac death (SCD) is a natural death of cardiac cause that is preceded by an abrupt loss of consciousness within one hour of the onset of an acute change in cardiovascular status.[8] Approximately half of cardiac deaths occur before patients reach a hospital.[9,10] SCD is often the patient's first and only symptom of heart disease.[11-13] For others, warning signs may be present up to 1 hour before the actual arrest (Figure 1-1). Because of irreversible brain damage and dependence on life support, some patients may live days to weeks after resuscitation from the cardiac arrest before biologic death occurs. These factors influence the interpretation of the 1-hour definition of SCD.[8]

TABLE 1-1 Cardiovascular Disease Risk Factors		
Nonmodifiable (Fixed) Factors	**Modifiable Factors**	**Contributing Factors**
• Age • Gender • Heredity • Race	• Diabetes • Elevated serum cholesterol levels • High blood pressure • Metabolic syndrome • Obesity • Physical inactivity • Tobacco use	• Alcohol intake • Inflammatory markers • Psychosocial factors • Stress

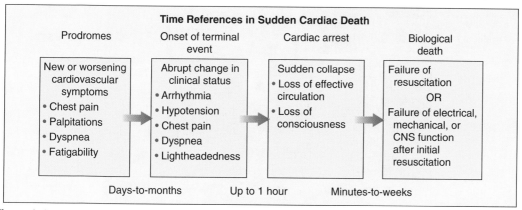

Figure 1-1 Sudden cardiac death viewed from four chronological perspectives: (1) warning signs (prodromes), (2) onset of the terminal event, (3) cardiac arrest, and (4) progression to biological death. CNS, Central nervous system.

Heart rhythms that may be observed in a cardiac arrest include the following:

1. Pulseless ventricular tachycardia (VT), in which the electrocardiogram (ECG) displays a wide, regular QRS complex at a rate faster than 120 beats/min
2. Ventricular fibrillation (VF), in which irregular chaotic deflections that vary in shape and height are observed on the ECG but there is no coordinated ventricular contraction
3. Asystole, in which no cardiac electrical activity is present
4. Pulseless electrical activity (PEA), in which electrical activity is visible on the ECG but central pulses are absent

VT and VF are *shockable* rhythms. This means that delivering a shock to the heart by means of a defibrillator may result in termination of the rhythm. Asystole and PEA are *nonshockable* rhythms.

Keeping It Simple

Cardiac Arrest Rhythms

Shockable rhythms
- Ventricular fibrillation
- Ventricular tachycardia

Nonshockable rhythms
- Asystole
- Pulseless electrical activity

CHAIN OF SURVIVAL

[Objective 5]

The **Chain of Survival** represents the ideal series of events that should take place immediately after the recognition of the onset of sudden cardiac illness. The Chain consists of five key steps that are interrelated. Following these steps gives the victim the best chance of surviving a heart attack or sudden cardiac arrest. The links in the Chain of Survival for adults include early recognition and activation, early CPR, early defibrillation, effective advanced life support (ALS), and integrated post–cardiac arrest care.[14] Because time is critical when dealing with a victim of SCD, a weak or missing link in the Chain of Survival can reduce the likelihood of a positive outcome.

YOU SHOULD KNOW   **Links in the Chain of Survival**
- Early recognition and activation
- Early CPR
- Early defibrillation
- Effective advanced life support
- Integration of post–cardiac arrest care

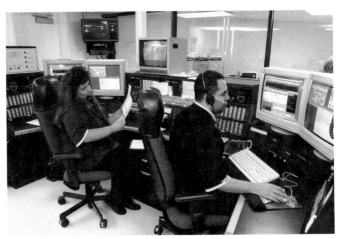

Figure 1-2 An appropriately trained dispatcher can provide telephone cardiopulmonary resuscitation (CPR) instruction, increasing the likelihood of bystander CPR performance and improved survival from cardiac arrest.

Early Recognition and Activation

The first link in the Chain of Survival is early recognition and activation. Although warning signs are often absent, the sudden onset of chest pain, difficulty breathing, or palpitations and other symptoms of abnormal heart rhythms may precede the onset of cardiac arrest.[8] In a 2005 study[1], a telephone survey of U.S. civilian adults was conducted and respondents were questioned about their awareness of the five major warning signs and symptoms of a heart attack. Respondent awareness of each of the warning signs varied: pain or discomfort in the jaw, neck, or back (48%); feeling weak, lightheaded, or faint (62%); chest pain or discomfort (92%); pain or discomfort in the arms or shoulder (85%); and shortness of breath (93%). Only 27% were aware of all major symptoms and knew to call 9-1-1 if they thought someone was having a heart attack. The results of this study emphasize the importance of teaching the public to recognize the early warning signs of a heart attack and the need for prompt attention, and to subsequently improve the rate of survival from cardiac arrest.

When a cardiac emergency occurs, the individual must identify his or her signs and symptoms, recognize that they are related to a heart condition, and seek medical assistance. Time delays occur from the call for assistance to the arrival of assistance and from the arrival of assistance to arrival at the hospital. Studies have found that about one third to one half of patients delay for more than 4 hours before calling for help, and that even greater delays in seeking help occur among female patients, older patients, nonwhite patients, and those who have a history of angina, heart failure, diabetes, and hypertension.[15]

Public education must include the early recognition of a patient's cardiac emergency and knowledge of how to gain rapid access to the emergency medical services (EMS) system (usually by telephone) via EMS dispatchers. When a call is placed to 9-1-1 (or similar emergency number), rapid recognition by EMS dispatchers of the bystander's description of a potential heart attack or cardiac arrest is important (Figure 1-2). Dispatchers quickly send appropriately trained and equipped EMS personnel to the scene. With appropriate training, EMS dispatchers provide telephone instructions to bystanders. They can ask bystanders to find out if the patient is unresponsive and if normal breathing is present. They can also provide telephone CPR instructions when needed until EMS personnel arrive.

Patients who experience a cardiac arrest in the hospital often show signs of deterioration several hours before the arrest.[16] Early recognition of the critically ill patient and activation of a Medical Emergency Team (MET) (also known as a Rapid Response Team) may prevent the development of cardiac arrest and improve patient outcome. A MET typically consists of a physician and nurse with critical care training who are available at all times. They are summoned by other hospital staff based on well-defined criteria for activation of the team.

Early Cardiopulmonary Resuscitation

[Objective 5]
Cardiopulmonary resuscitation is a part of BLS. BLS includes the recognition of signs of cardiac arrest, heart attack, stroke, and foreign body airway obstruction (FBAO); the relief of FBAO; CPR; and defibrillation with an automated external defibrillator (AED) (Box 1-1).

BOX 1-1 **Components of Basic Life Support**

- Recognition of signs of cardiac arrest, heart attack, stroke, and foreign body airway obstruction (FBAO)
- Relief of FBAO
- Cardiopulmonary resuscitation (CPR)
- Defibrillation with an automated external defibrillator (AED)

After recognizing that an emergency exists, the scene must be assessed to ensure that it is safe to enter. If the scene is safe, the patient must be quickly assessed for life-threatening conditions and the nature of the emergency determined. The emergency response system must be alerted for medical assistance (if not already done). BLS must be provided until advanced medical help arrives and assumes responsibility for the patient's care. Necessary care may include the following:

- Patient positioning
- CPR for victims of cardiac arrest
- Defibrillation with an AED
- Rescue breathing for victims of respiratory arrest
- Recognition and relief of FBAO

Blood flow through the vessels of the body (including the coronary vessels) is determined by driving pressure and vascular resistance to flow.[17] Aortic blood pressure and right atrial pressure determine the driving pressure through the coronary arteries. In the coronary arteries, vascular resistance is determined by the diameter of the coronary vessels and the degree of external compression caused by myocardial contraction (systole) and relaxation (diastole). Most coronary blood flow occurs during diastole because the coronary vessels are compressed as the myocardium contracts (systole). Under normal conditions, the coronary arteries can dilate or constrict to adjust (autoregulate) blood flow at the level of the arterioles in accordance with tissue needs. In the coronary circulation, autoregulation maintains constant blood flow at perfusion pressures (mean arterial pressure) between 60 and 180 mm Hg when other influencing factors are held constant.[18]

During cardiac arrest, compressing the chest compresses the heart and increases intrathoracic pressure, creating blood flow and enabling the delivery of oxygen to the brain and heart. When performing chest compressions, systole is the chest compression phase and diastole is the release phase.[19] Myocardial blood flow is dependent on coronary perfusion pressure, which is generated when performing external chest compressions. Coronary perfusion pressure is a key determinant of the success of resuscitation, and adequate cerebral and coronary perfusion pressures are critical to neurologically normal survival.[19] Because it takes time to build up cerebral and coronary perfusion pressures, the stopping of chest compressions for even a few seconds causes cerebral and coronary perfusion pressures to fall quickly and dramatically, thereby reducing blood flow to the brain and heart. When chest compressions are stopped during cardiac arrest, no blood flow is generated; this is referred to as *no flow time*. Even after compressions are resumed, several chest compressions are needed to restore coronary perfusion pressure.

Researchers have confirmed that when an adult develops VF and suddenly collapses, his or her lungs, pulmonary veins, left heart, aorta, and the arteries contain oxygenated blood.[19,20] The delivery of oxygen to tissues with CPR is limited more by blood flow and low cardiac output than by arterial oxygen content.[21,22] The low cardiac output associated with CPR results in low oxygen uptake from the lungs, which in turn reduces the need to ventilate the patient during this low-flow state.[23]

After a bystander or healthcare professional determines that CPR is indicated, chest compressions should be the initial action performed (instead of opening the airway or giving ventilations) when starting CPR in victims of sudden cardiac arrest (Figure 1-3).[24] Performing chest compressions before ventilations enables better delivery of the oxygen that is already present in the lungs and arterial circulation to the heart and brain.[25]

It has been estimated that cardiac output is approximately 25% to 33% of normal during CPR.[14] Therefore the quality of chest compressions is an important factor in the effectiveness of CPR (Figure 1-4).[22] High-quality chest compressions require the following[24]:

- Pushing hard on the victim's chest (a depth of at least 2 inches [5 cm] in adults, a depth of least one third the anterior-posterior diameter of the chest or about 1.5 inches [4 cm] in infants and about 2 inches [5 cm] in children)

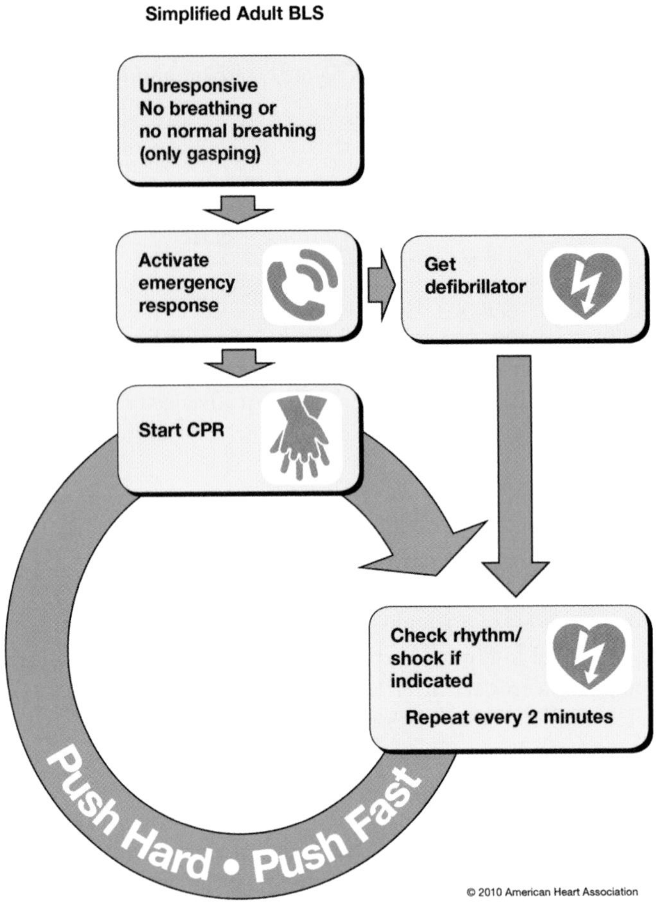

Simplified Adult BLS

Unresponsive
No breathing or
no normal breathing
(only gasping)

Activate
emergency
response

Get
defibrillator

Start CPR

Check rhythm/
shock if
indicated

Repeat every 2 minutes

Push Hard • Push Fast

© 2010 American Heart Association

Figure 1-3 The American Heart Association Basic Life Support algorithm.

- Compressing the chest at a rate of at least 100 compressions per minute, allowing full chest recoil after each compression (enabling the heart to refill with blood)
- Minimizing interruptions in chest compressions

YOU SHOULD KNOW   Key steps in basic life support include the following:
- Recognition of the emergency
- Activation of the emergency response system
- Early, high quality, CPR
- Rapid defibrillation

Early Defibrillation

When an individual experiences a cardiac arrest, the likelihood of successful resuscitation is affected by the speed with which CPR and defibrillation are performed. When a cardiac arrest is witnessed and the patient's heart rhythm is VF, the patient's survival rate decreases 7% to 10% per minute until defibrillation if no CPR is provided.[26,27] The decrease in survival rates is less rapid (averaging 3% to 4% per minute from collapse to defibrillation) when bystander CPR is provided.[27,28] Although early defibrillation can improve outcome,[29,30] most patients do not receive or are not candidates for early defibrillation.[5]

Since 1995, the American Heart Association has promoted the development of lay rescuer AED programs to improve survival from out-of-hospital sudden cardiac arrest. An **automated external defibrillator** is a machine with a sophisticated computer system that analyzes the patient's heart rhythm (Figure 1-5). The AED uses an algorithm to distinguish shockable rhythms from nonshockable rhythms. If the AED detects a shockable rhythm, it provides visual and auditory instructions to the rescuer to deliver an electrical shock. Defibrillation performed by citizens (such as flight attendants,

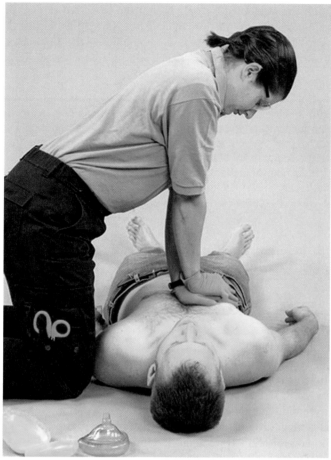

Figure 1-4 The delivery of high quality chest compressions is essential for effective cardiopulmonary resuscitation.

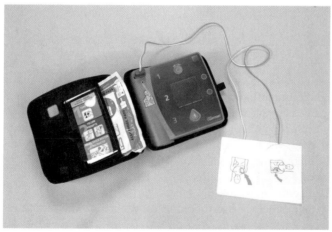

Figure 1-5 An automated external defibrillator (AED) uses an algorithm to distinguish shockable rhythms from nonshockable rhythms.

casino security officers, athletic or golf club employees, and ushers at sporting events) at the scene is called **public access defibrillation**. AEDs permit bystanders to perform three of the five links of the Chain of Survival. In the first few minutes after defibrillation, the cardiac rhythm may be slow and the pumping effectiveness of the patient's heart may be inadequate. CPR may be needed for several minutes after defibrillation until adequate heart function resumes.[28]

The American Heart Association has stated that AED programs will be most cost effective if they are present at sites where at least one witnessed cardiac arrest is likely to occur every few years.[28] In a

2004 study, resuscitation was attempted for only half of the witnessed cardiac arrest victims and the on-site AED was used for only about one third of cardiac arrest victims, despite the presence of rescuers trained to respond to cardiac arrest.[31] These findings emphasize the importance of recognizing that the mere presence of an AED does not ensure that it will be used when a cardiac arrest occurs.[28]

> **YOU SHOULD KNOW** Because 70% of cardiac arrests occur in the home, it has been supposed that providing CPR training for families and having an AED in the home might offer an opportunity to improve survival for patients at risk of cardiac arrest.[32] A 2008 study evaluated the role of home AED placement in 7001 survivors of anterior wall myocardial infarction (MI) who were not candidates for implantable cardioverter-defibrillators. The results of this study suggest that for high-risk patients, placement of home AEDs did not significantly improve overall survival from cardiac arrest.[33]

A summary of the treatment for adult, child, and infant CPR and choking can be found in Table 1-2.

Effective Advanced Life Support

Emergency situations that require lifesaving interventions necessitates the coordination of a series of tasks including chest compressions, airway management, ECG monitoring and defibrillation, and vascular access and drug administration. These tasks are performed by personnel who are part of a resuscitation team. In situations involving a cardiac arrest, the goals of the resuscitation team are to continue high-quality CPR, restore spontaneous breathing and circulation, and preserve vital organ function throughout the resuscitation effort.

In the prehospital setting, early advanced care is provided by paramedics (and/or nurses) arriving on the scene. Prehospital professionals work quickly to stabilize the patient by providing ventilation support, vascular access, and giving emergency medications, among other interventions. They then transfer the patient to the closest most appropriate ED where definitive care can be provided. In the hospital setting, healthcare professionals provide advanced care including advanced airway management, ventilation support, and possible surgical interventions (Box 1-2).

Integration of Post–Cardiac Arrest Care

[Objective 6]

After successful resuscitation from cardiac arrest, neurological impairment and other types of organ dysfunction cause significant morbidity and mortality. The ischemia-reperfusion response that occurs during cardiac arrest and subsequent return of spontaneous circulation (ROSC) results in a series of pathophysiological processes that have been termed the *post–cardiac arrest syndrome*. The components of post–cardiac arrest syndrome include the following[34]:

- Post–cardiac arrest brain injury
- Post–cardiac arrest myocardial dysfunction
- Systemic ischemia/reperfusion response
- Persistent precipitating pathology that caused or contributed to the cardiac arrest

---

BOX 1-2 **Components of Advanced Cardiac Care**

- Basic life support
- Advanced airway management
- Ventilation support
- Electrocardiogram (ECG)/dysrhythmia recognition
- 12-lead ECG interpretation
- Vascular access and fluid resuscitation
- Electrical therapy including defibrillation, synchronized cardioversion, and pacing
- Medication administration
- Coronary artery bypass, stent insertion, angioplasty, and intraaortic balloon pump therapy

TABLE 1-2 Summary of Treatment for Adult, Child, Infant CPR and Choking

Parameter	Infant	Child	Adult
Age	Younger than 1 year	1 year to puberty (about 12 to 14 years)	Older than 12 to 14 years

Cardiopulmonary Resuscitation (CPR)

Parameter	Infant	Child	Adult
Level of responsiveness	Establish unresponsiveness, tap and ask loudly, "Are you OK?"		
Check for breathing	If normal breathing is present, CPR is not needed. If the victim is unresponsive and not breathing (or only gasping), ask someone to activate the emergency response system and get a defibrillator.*		
C = Circulation	Check pulse for up to 10 sec		
Check pulse	Brachial	Carotid or femoral	Carotid
	Pulse present, support airway and breathing		
Chest compressions**	If there is no pulse or you are unsure if there is a pulse, begin chest compressions. If a pulse is present but slower than 60 beats/min with signs of poor perfusion (pallor, mottling, cyanosis) despite support of oxygenation and ventilation, begin chest compressions.		If there is no pulse or you are unsure if there is a pulse, begin chest compressions.
Compression rate	At least 100/min allowing for complete chest recoil after each compression		
Compress chest with	Two fingers (one rescuer) or two thumb-encircling hands (two rescuers)	Heel of one hand or as for adult	Heel of one hand, other hand on top
Chest landmarks	Just below nipple line; avoid pressing on xiphoid, ribs, or abdomen	Lower half of sternum; avoid pressing on xiphoid, ribs, or abdomen	Lower half of sternum; avoid pressing on xiphoid, ribs, or abdomen
Compression depth	At least 1/3 the depth of the chest (about 1.5 in [4 cm])	At least 1/3 the depth of the chest (about 2 in [5 cm])	At least 2 in (5 cm)
A = Airway***	Open the airway with a head tilt-chin lift. If trauma is suspected, use jaw-thrust without head tilt maneuver.		
B = Breathing	Deliver 2 breaths; each breath should take about 1 sec. Make sure the breaths are effective (the chest rises). If the chest does not rise, reposition the head, make a better seal, and try again.		
	Avoid excessive ventilation (too many breaths, too large a volume).		
Compression/ ventilation ratio	One rescuer = 30:2 Two rescuers = 15:2		One or two rescuers = 30:2
After advanced airway placement	Ventilate without pausing for chest compressions giving 1 breath every 6 to 8 sec (8 to 10 breaths/min). Avoid excessive ventilation.		
D = Defibrillation	Manual defibrillator preferred. If a manual defibrillator is not available, an AED equipped with a pediatric attenuator is desirable. If neither is available, use a standard AED.	Use AED equipped with a pediatric attenuator, if available, for children up to about 25 kg (approximately 8 years of age). If unavailable, use standard AED.	Use standard AED.
	If shock advised, clear victim, give 1 shock, immediately resume CPR for 5 cycles, then reanalyze rhythm. Shock delivery should ideally occur as soon as possible after compressions. If no shock advised, immediately resume CPR.		

Choking

Parameter	Infant	Child	Adult
Responsive victim	Five back blows (slaps), then five chest thrusts in rapid sequence until object is expelled or victim becomes unresponsive	Give abdominal thrusts in rapid sequence until object is expelled or victim becomes unresponsive	Give abdominal thrusts in rapid sequence until object is expelled or victim becomes unresponsive; use chest thrusts if patient obese or in late stages of pregnancy

Continued

TABLE 1-2	Summary of Treatment for Adult, Child, Infant CPR and Choking—cont'd		
Parameter	**Infant**	**Child**	**Adult**
Victim becomes unresponsive	Begin CPR with chest compressions (no pulse check). After 30 compressions, open the airway. Remove foreign body if visualized. Attempt two breaths. Continue cycles of chest compressions and ventilations until object expelled. After 2 min, activate emergency response system (if not already done).		
Rescue Breathing			
Ventilations/min	About 12 to 20 breaths/min, 1 breath every 3 to 5 sec		About 10 to 12 breaths/min 1 breath every 5 to 6 sec

*A lone rescuer should perform 5 cycles of CPR (about 30 compressions and 2 breaths for about 2 minutes) before leaving an infant or child victim (or adult victim of presumed asphyxial arrest, such as drowning) to activate the emergency response system and obtain an AED.
**Minimize delays in, and interruptions of, chest compressions; limit interruptions to less than 10 seconds. Rotate chest compressors at 2-minute intervals (ideally in less than 5 seconds) to avoid tiring. Recheck pulse every 2 minutes.
***CPR for drowning victims should use the traditional A-B-C approach because of the hypoxic nature of the arrest.
AED, Automated external defibrillator.

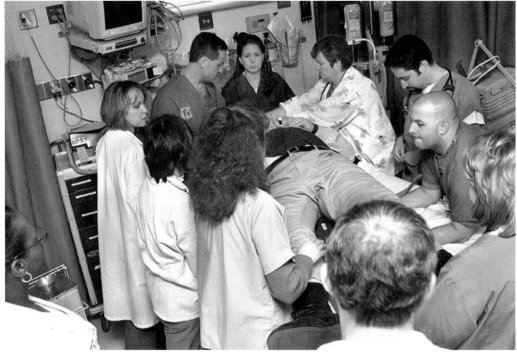

Figure 1-6 Post–cardiac arrest care includes transport of the out-of-hospital post–cardiac arrest patient to an appropriate facility capable of providing comprehensive post–cardiac arrest care.

The initial goals of post–cardiac arrest care include the following[35]:
- Provide cardiorespiratory support to optimize tissue perfusion—especially to the heart, brain, and lungs (the organs most affected by cardiac arrest).
- Transport of the out-of-hospital post–cardiac arrest patient to an appropriate facility capable of providing comprehensive post–cardiac arrest care including acute coronary interventions, neurological care, goal-directed critical care, and therapeutic hypothermia (Figure 1-6).
- Transport of the in-hospital post–cardiac arrest patient to a critical care unit capable of providing comprehensive post–cardiac arrest care.
- Attempt to identify the precipitating cause of the arrest, start specific treatment if necessary, and take actions to prevent recurrence.

The memory aids "PATCH-4-MD" and "The 5 H's and 5 T's" may be used to recall possible treatable causes of cardiac emergencies, including cardiac arrest (Boxes 1-3 and 1-4).

PHASES OF CARDIOPULMONARY RESUSCITATION

[Objective 7]

Research has shown that cardiac arrest due to VF occurs in a three-phase, time-dependent manner[36] (Table 1-3).

- *Phase 1 (electrical phase).* This phase extends from the time of VF cardiac arrest to about 5 minutes following the arrest. Prompt defibrillation is the most important treatment during this phase.
- *Phase 2 (circulatory phase or hemodynamic phase).* This phase varies in duration from about 5 to 15 minutes after the cardiac arrest. High-quality CPR is very important during this phase. Factors affecting perfusion pressures during cardiac arrest include the following[19]:
  - *Interruptions in the delivery of chest compressions.* When caring for a patient in cardiac arrest it is *essential* that interruptions for rhythm and pulse checks, ventilations, placing an advanced airway, establishing intravenous access, charging the defibrillator, or other procedures be kept to a minimum.[37] Interrupting chest compressions to obtain intravenous access also may be

---

BOX 1-3 PATCH-4-MD

Pulmonary embolism–anticoagulants? Surgery?
Acidosis–ventilation, correct acid-base disturbances
Tension pneumothorax–needle decompression
Cardiac tamponade–pericardiocentesis
Hypovolemia–replace intravascular volume
Hypoxia–ensure adequate oxygenation and ventilation
Heat/cold (hyperthermia/hypothermia)–cooling/warming methods
Hypo-/hyperkalemia (and other electrolytes)–monitor serum glucose levels closely in concert with correcting electrolyte disturbances
Myocardial infarction–reperfusion therapy
Drug overdose/accidents—antidote/specific therapy

BOX 1-4 Five H's and Five T's

Hypovolemia	Tamponade, cardiac
Hypoxia	Tension pneumothorax
Hypothermia	Thrombosis: lungs (massive pulmonary embolism)
Hypo-/Hyperkalemia	Thrombosis: heart (acute coronary syndromes)
Hydrogen ion (acidosis)	Tablets/toxins: drug overdose

TABLE 1-3 Phases of Cardiopulmonary Resuscitation

Phase	Phase Name	Time from VF arrest	Important intervention
1	Electrical phase	From time of arrest to about the first 5 min after arrest	Electrical therapy
2	Circulatory (hemodynamic) phase	About 5 min to 15 min after arrest	CPR before electrical therapy
3	Metabolic phase	After about 15 min	Therapeutic hypothermia

VF, Ventricular fibrillation.

counterproductive. Administering medications (such as epinephrine) via the intraosseous route can minimize the interruption and allow for quicker drug delivery.[38]

- *Vascular resistance.* Drugs given during cardiac arrest that constrict blood vessels (vasopressors) may improve perfusion pressures. Drugs given that dilate blood vessels (vasodilators) decrease perfusion pressures.
- *Vascular volume.* An adequate blood volume is necessary for adequate perfusion. An adequate perfusion pressure cannot be obtained and patients cannot be resuscitated if their blood volume is low (such as that due to blood loss or significant venous dilation).
- *Intrathoracic pressure.* During the release (diastolic) phase of chest compression, intrathoracic pressure is low. This helps increase the return of venous blood into the chest. If intrathoracic pressure is too high during this phase, venous return is inhibited. Hyperventilation is a common cause of excessive intrathoracic pressure during CPR. It is important to ventilate a patient in cardiac arrest at an age-appropriate rate and with just enough volume to see the patient's chest rise gently. Ventilating a cardiac arrest patient too fast or with too much volume results in excessive intrathoracic pressure, which results in decreased venous return into the chest, decreased coronary and cerebral perfusion pressures, diminished cardiac output, and decreased rates of survival.
- *Phase 3 (metabolic phase).* This phase extends beyond the first 15 minutes after cardiac arrest. During this phase, the effectiveness of immediate defibrillation and CPR followed by defibrillation decreases rapidly and survival rates appear to be poor.[36] Studies have shown the benefit of inducing therapeutic hypothermia within minutes to hours after the return of spontaneous circulation following resuscitation of adults from VF.[39,40] It is now recognized that therapeutic hypothermia should be part of a standardized treatment strategy for comatose survivors of cardiac arrest.[34] Therapeutic hypothermia appears to provide the following beneficial effects[41]:
- Suppression of many of the chemical reactions associated with reperfusion injury
- Possible improvement in oxygen delivery to the brain
- Decrease in heart rate and an increase in systemic vascular resistance, while maintaining stroke volume and arterial blood pressure

> **ACLS Pearl**
>
> The University of Arizona Sarver Heart Center developed an EMS protocol termed *cardiocerebral resuscitation* (CCR) that emphasizes high quality, minimally interrupted chest compressions, delayed active ventilation, and early epinephrine administration. Using this protocol, defibrillator pad electrodes are applied and the patient is given 200 chest compressions and then a single defibrillation shock that is immediately followed by 200 more chest compressions before the rhythm and pulse are analyzed. Epinephrine (1 mg intravenous or intraosseous) is given as soon as possible or with each 200 compression cycle. Tracheal intubation is delayed until after three cycles of chest compressions. Studies have shown that use of the CCR protocol has resulted in an overall improved survival to hospital discharge, especially in patients with witnessed VF.[42,43,44]

PATIENT ASSESSMENT

The interval preceding a cardiac arrest is called the **prearrest period**. The **periarrest period** is considered 1 hour before and 1 hour after a cardiac arrest. Recognizing and promptly treating critical conditions in the "prearrest" or "periarrest" period may prevent a full cardiac arrest. Recognition of critical conditions requires good patient assessment skills.

Scene Safety

Before approaching the patient, make sure that the scene is safe. Note any hazards or potential hazards and any visible mechanism or injury or illness. Always use appropriate personal protective equipment.

General Impression

Once you come into view of the patient, immediately begin to form a general impression, which is an impression of the severity of the patient's condition. Your general impression should initially focus on three main areas that can be remembered by the mnemonic ABC: **A**ppearance, (work of) **B**reathing, and **C**irculation. As you finish forming your general impression, you will have a good idea if the patient is sick (unstable) or not sick (stable).

- *Appearance.* The patient's appearance reflects the adequacy of oxygenation, ventilation, brain perfusion, homeostasis, and central nervous system function. When forming a general impression, appearance refers to the patient's mental status, muscle tone, and body position. Is the patient's condition life threatening? Can you tell if the patient is in severe distress, moderate distress, mild distress, or no apparent distress? Normal findings include a patient who is aware of your approach and has normal muscle tone and equal movement of all extremities.
- *Breathing.* When forming a general impression, breathing refers to the presence or absence of visible movement of the chest or abdomen, signs of breathing effort, and the presence of audible airway sounds. Breathing reflects the adequacy of the patient's airway, oxygenation, and ventilation. Normal findings include breathing that is quiet and unlabored with equal rise and fall of the chest and a ventilatory rate within the normal range for the patient's age. Abnormal findings include nasal flaring; retractions; muffled or hoarse speech; a ventilatory rate outside the normal range for the patient's age; use of accessory muscles to breathe; and abnormal breathing sounds such as stridor, grunting, gasping, gurgling, or wheezing.
- *Circulation.* Circulation reflects the adequacy of cardiac output and perfusion of vital organs (core perfusion). When forming a general impression, circulation refers to skin color. Skin color normally is some shade of pink. Even patients who have heavy pigmentation have an underlying pink color to the skin. Abnormal findings include pallor, mottling, and cyanosis.

If the patient appears sick (abnormal findings are present), move quickly. Proceed *immediately* to the primary survey. If the patient's condition does not appear to be urgent, proceed systematically starting with the primary survey and then the secondary survey.

Primary Survey

[Objective 8]

Approach the patient and perform a primary survey only after making sure that the scene is safe. The primary survey is a rapid hands-on assessment of the patient that usually requires less than 60 seconds to complete, but may take longer if you must provide emergency care at any point. The purpose of the primary survey is to detect the presence of life-threatening problems and immediately correct them (Table 1-4). During this phase of patient assessment, assessment and management occur at the same time—"Treat as you find."

The ABCDE sequence of the primary survey is taught to physicians, nurses, and prehospital personnel in many types of educational courses. In programs other than cardiac-related courses, the primary survey sequence stands for **A**irway, **B**reathing, **C**irculation, **D**isability (referring to a brief neurological exam), and **E**xposure. In cardiac-related courses, the "D" stands for **D**efibrillation. Both terms appear in Table 1-4 for completeness.

Repeat the primary survey:
- With any sudden change in the patient's condition
- When interventions do not appear to be working
- When vital signs are unstable
- Before any procedures
- When a change in rhythm is observed on the cardiac monitor

Secondary Survey

[Objective 8]

The purpose of the physical examination in the secondary survey is to detect potentially life-threatening conditions and provide care for those conditions. The secondary survey focuses on *advanced* life support interventions and management (Table 1-5).

TABLE 1-4 Primary Survey

Action Steps	Necessary Tasks	Notes
Assess responsiveness	Start by asking, "Are you all right?" or "Can you hear me?" If there is no response, then gently tap or squeeze the victim's shoulder while repeating verbal cues.	Use the AVPU acronym: • A = Alert • V = Responds to verbal stimuli • P = Responds to painful stimuli • U = Unresponsive
RESPONSIVE PATIENT		
Airway	Determine if the patient has an open airway.	If the patient is responsive, ask him or her questions to determine his or her level of responsiveness and the adequacy of his or her airway and breathing. If the airway is not clear, clear it with suctioning or positioning as indicated.
Breathing	Assess the rate and quality of breathing.	If breathing is inadequate, assist ventilations with an appropriate device and oxygen.
Circulation	Assess the pulse rate and quality. Assess perfusion.	Estimate the rate and determine the quality of the pulse (i.e., fast or slow, regular or irregular, weak or strong). Evaluate the patient's skin temperature, color, and condition (moisture) to assess perfusion.
Defibrillation and disability	Assess the need for a defibrillator. Perform a brief neurological evaluation.	Obtain a Glasgow Coma Scale score.
Exposure	Expose the patient as necessary.	Remove clothing as necessary to facilitate examination.
UNRESPONSIVE PATIENT*		
Circulation	If the patient is not breathing (or only gasping), assess a pulse for up to 10 sec. If there is no pulse or you are unsure if there is a pulse, begin chest compressions.	Ask someone to activate the emergency response system and get a defibrillator while you continue patient care. Minimize delays in, and interruptions of, chest compressions; limit interruptions to less than 10 seconds. Rotate chest compressors at 2-minute intervals (ideally in less than 5 seconds) to avoid tiring. Recheck pulse every 2 minutes.
Airway	After 30 compressions (15 compressions if two rescuers), open the airway.	Use a head tilt-chin lift to open the airway. If trauma is suspected, use the jaw-thrust without head tilt maneuver.
Breathing	Deliver two breaths; each breath should take about 1 sec.	Make sure the breaths are effective (the chest rises). If the chest does not rise, reposition the head, make a better seal, and try again. Avoid excessive ventilation (too many breaths, too large a volume).
Defibrillation and disability	Apply an AED. If a shock is advised, clear the victim, give 1 shock, immediately resume CPR for 5 cycles, and then reanalyze the rhythm. If no shock is advised, immediately resume CPR.	Refer to specific operating instructions of the AED model being used as models may vary. Obtain a Glasgow Coma Scale score.

*If the patient is unresponsive but has normal breathing, CPR is not needed. Perform a primary survey as you would for a responsive patient.

TABLE 1-5 | **Secondary Survey**

Action Steps	Necessary Tasks	Notes
Obtain vital signs, SAMPLE history	Obtain vital signs, attach a pulse oximeter, ECG, and blood pressure monitor. Obtain a focused history.	The history is often obtained while the physical examination is being performed and emergency care is being given.
Reassess airway	Reassess the effectiveness of initial airway maneuvers and interventions. If needed, insert an advanced airway.	Examples of advanced airways include the tracheal tube, Combitube, laryngeal mask airway, and laryngeal tube (Laryngeal Tube or King LT).
Reassess breathing	Assess the adequacy of oxygenation and ventilation.	Reassess chest rise, oxygen saturation, and capnography or capnometry. If an advanced airway has been inserted, confirm proper placement using clinical assessment and waveform capnography. Provide positive-pressure ventilation with supplemental oxygen and assess the effectiveness of ventilations. Make sure the tube is adequately secured.
Reassess circulation	If the patient has a pulse, check its rate and quality often. If not already done, attach ECG electrodes and connect the patient to an ECG monitor. Obtain a 12-lead ECG if appropriate. Establish vascular access (intravenous or intraosseous). Give medications appropriate for the cardiac rhythm/clinical situation.	ECG monitoring allows continuous recording and reassessment of the cardiac rhythm. Vascular access is usually established via a peripheral IV; however, intraosseous access in cardiac arrest is safe, effective, and appropriate for patients of all ages. During cardiac arrest, establishing vascular access is important, but it should not interfere with CPR and the delivery of shocks. Each drug given in a cardiac arrest should be followed with a 20-mL IV fluid bolus and elevation of the extremity. During a cardiac arrest, drugs should be given at the time of the rhythm check.
Differential diagnosis/ Diagnostic procedures	Search for, find, and treat reversible causes of the cardiac arrest, rhythm, or clinical situation.	Use PATCH-4-MD or the 5 H's and 5 T's to help recall possible reversible causes.
Evaluate interventions, pain management	Reassess the effectiveness of the care given thus far. Troubleshoot as needed. If the patient is responsive and complaining of discomfort, begin appropriate pain management if his or her blood pressure and other vital signs will tolerate it.	The safe and effective relief of pain should be a priority in the management of a patient of any age.
Facilitate family presence	Facilitate family presence for invasive and resuscitative procedures.	Explain what is being done for the patient to family members who are present. Studies have demonstrated that the presence of family members during resuscitation helped them cope with the grief following the death of a loved one.[45,46]

STOP AND REVIEW

Matching

Indicate the cardiac rhythms that are most likely to be terminated by a shock and those that are not.

a. Shockable rhythm
b. Nonshockable rhythm

b 1. Asystole

a 2. Pulseless ventricular tachycardia

b 3. Pulseless electrical activity

a 4. Ventricular fibrillation

Match the components of patient assessment with their descriptions.

a. General impression
b. Primary survey
c. Secondary survey

c **b** 5. Focuses on advanced life support assessment and interventions

b **b** 6. Apply pads to the patient's bare chest and defibrillate, if indicated

a **a** 7. Purpose is to develop a sense if the patient is sick (unstable) or not sick (stable)

c **c** 8. Evaluate interventions, pain management

b **a** 9. Purpose is to detect the presence of life-threatening problems and immediately correct them

b **a** 10. Determine if breathing is adequate or inadequate

c **a** 11. Purpose is to detect potentially life-threatening conditions and provide care for those conditions

a **a** 12. From a distance, assess for visible movement of the chest or abdomen, signs of breathing effort, and the presence of audible airway sounds

b **b** 13. Focuses on basic life support assessment and interventions

c **c** 14. Ask the patient, family, bystanders, or others questions regarding the patient's history

c **b** 15. Insert an advanced airway, if needed

a **a** 16. From a distance, assess mental status, muscle tone, and body position

c **c** 17. Obtain vital signs, attach a pulse oximeter, ECG, and blood pressure monitor

b **b** 18. Begin chest compressions, if indicated

c **b** 19. Establish vascular access

a **a** 20. From a distance, assess skin color

b   b   21. Open the airway if the patient is unresponsive

C   b   22. Search for, find, and treat reversible causes of the cardiac arrest, rhythm, or clinical situation

Match each of the following terms with their descriptions.

a. Metabolic phase
b. Chain of Survival
c. Post–cardiac arrest care
d. At least 2 inches (5 cm)
e. Cardiovascular collapse
f. Ventricular fibrillation
g. AVPU
h. Circulatory (hemodynamic) phase
i. Cardiac arrest
j. At least 100 per minute
k. Diastole
l. Early recognition and access

m. About 1.5 inches (4 cm)
n. Post–cardiac arrest syndrome
o. Risk factors
p. Apnea or agonal, gasping breathing
q. Electrical phase
r. Cerebral and coronary perfusion pressures
s. Vascular resistance
t. Appearance
u. Therapeutic hypothermia
v. Pulseless electrical activity
w. Differential diagnosis
x. Early defibrillation (if indicated)

P   p   23. Examples of breathing that may be evident in the first few minutes of cardiac arrest

L   I   24. First link in the adult Chain of Survival

H   ___   25. Second phase of CPR

S   S   26. One of the factors affecting perfusion pressures during cardiac arrest

W   w   27. The "D" in the secondary survey

J   j   28. Chest compression rate for adults, children, and infants

V   v   29. Cardiac rhythm in which electrical activity is visible on the ECG but central pulses are absent

I   i   30. The absence of cardiac mechanical activity, confirmed by the absence of a detectable pulse, unresponsiveness, and apnea or agonal, gasping breathing

T   t   31. The "A" assessed when you form a general impression of a patient

O   o   32. Traits and lifestyle habits that may increase a person's chance of developing a disease

A   q   33. Phase of CPR during which the effectiveness of immediate defibrillation and CPR followed by defibrillation decreases rapidly and survival rates appear to be poor

X   X   34. Third link in the adult Chain of Survival

K   k   35. Period of the cardiac cycle during which most coronary blood flow occurs

D   d   36. Chest compression depth for adults

Q   ___   37. First phase of CPR

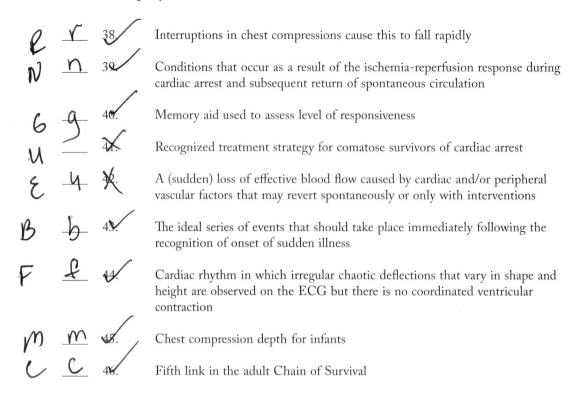

ℓ	r	38.	Interruptions in chest compressions cause this to fall rapidly
N	n	39.	Conditions that occur as a result of the ischemia-reperfusion response during cardiac arrest and subsequent return of spontaneous circulation
6	g	40.	Memory aid used to assess level of responsiveness
U		41.	Recognized treatment strategy for comatose survivors of cardiac arrest
E	4	42.	A (sudden) loss of effective blood flow caused by cardiac and/or peripheral vascular factors that may revert spontaneously or only with interventions
B	b	43.	The ideal series of events that should take place immediately following the recognition of onset of sudden illness
F	f	44.	Cardiac rhythm in which irregular chaotic deflections that vary in shape and height are observed on the ECG but there is no coordinated ventricular contraction
m	m	45.	Chest compression depth for infants
C	C	46.	Fifth link in the adult Chain of Survival

REFERENCES

1. Centers for Disease Control and Prevention: Disparities in adult awareness of heart attack warning signs and symptoms—14 states, 2005, *Morb Mortal Wkly Rep* 57(07):175–179, 2008.
2. Lloyd-Jones D, Adams RJ, Brown TM, et al: Heart disease and stroke statistics—2009 update. A report from the American Heart Association Statistics Committee and Stroke Statistics Subcommittee, *Circulation* 119:e1–e161, 2009.
3. Abella BS, Alvarado JP, Myklebust H, et al: Quality of cardiopulmonary resuscitation during in-hospital cardiac arrest, *JAMA* 293:305–310, 2005.
4. Nadkarni VM, Larkin GL, Peberdy MA, et al: First documented rhythm and clinical outcome from in-hospital cardiac arrest among children and adults, *JAMA* 295:50–57, 2006.
5. Halperin HR, Lee K, Zviman M, et al: Outcomes from low versus high-flow cardiopulmonary resuscitation in a swine model of cardiac arrest, *Am J Emerg Med* 28(2):195–202, 2010.
6. Centers for Disease Control and Prevention: *Heart disease facts*, www.cdc.gov/heartdisease/facts.htm. Page last updated January 25, 2010. Accessed August 7, 2010.
7. Mackay J, Mensah GA: *Atlas of heart disease and stroke*, Hong Kong, 2009, World Health Organization. pp. 1-16.
8. Myerburg RJ, Castellanos A: Cardiac arrest and sudden cardiac death. In Bonow RO, Mann DL, Zipes DP, et al, editors: *Braunwald's heart disease: a textbook of cardiovascular medicine*, ed 9, Philadelphia, Saunders, 2012.
9. Zheng ZJ, Croft JB, Giles WH, et al: Sudden cardiac death in the United States, 1989 to 1998, *Circulation* 104(18):2158–2163, 2001.
10. O'Connor RE, Brady W, Brooks SC, et al: Part 10: acute coronary syndromes: 2010 American Heart Association guidelines for cardiopulmonary resuscitation and emergency cardiovascular care, *Circulation* 122(Suppl 3):S787–S817, 2010.
11. Kuller L, Lilienfeld A, Fisher R: Epidemiological study of sudden and unexpected deaths due to arteriosclerotic heart disease, *Circulation* 34:1056–1068, 1966.
12. Doyle JT, Kannel WB, McNamara PM, et al: Factors related to suddenness of death from coronary disease: combined Albany-Framingham studies, *Am J Cardiol* 37(7):1073–1078, 1976.
13. Kannel WB, Schatzkin A: Sudden death: lessons from subsets in population studies, *J Am Coll Cardiol* 5(6 Suppl):141B–149B, 1985.
14. Berg RA, Hemphill R, Abella BS, et al: Part 5: adult basic life support: 2010 American Heart Association guidelines for cardiopulmonary resuscitation and emergency cardiovascular care, *Circulation* 122(Suppl 3):S685–S705, 2010.
15. Hankins DG, Luke A: Emergency medical service aspects of emergency cardiac care, *Emerg Med Clin North Am* 23(4):1219–1231, 2005.

16. International Liaison Committee on Resuscitation: 2005 International consensus on cardiopulmonary resuscitation and emergency cardiovascular care science with treatment recommendations. Part 4: advanced life support, *Resuscitation* 67(Suppl 1):213–247, 2005.

17. Levy MN, Pappano AJ: Hemodynamics. In Levy MN, Pappano AJ, editors: *Cardiovascular physiology,* ed 9, St Louis, 2007, Mosby, pp 107–124.

18. Brashers VL, McCance KL: Structure and function of the cardiovascular and lymphatic systems. In McCance, KL, Huether SE, Brashers VL, Rote NS, editors: *Pathophysiology: the biologic basis for disease in adults and children,* ed 9, St. Loius, 2009, Mosby. p. 131.

19. Ewy GA: Cardiocerebral resuscitation: the new cardiopulmonary resuscitation, *Circulation* 111(16):2134–2142, 2005.

20. Meursing BT, Wulterkens DW, van Kesteren RG: The ABC of resuscitation and the Dutch (re)treat, *Resuscitation* 64:279–286, 2005.

21. Ornato JP, Garnett AR, Glauser FL: Relationship between cardiac output and the end-tidal carbon dioxide tension, *Ann Emerg Med* 19:1104–1106, 1990.

22. Chandra NC, Gruben KG, Tsitlik JE, et al: Observations of ventilation during resuscitation in a canine model, *Circulation* 90:3070–3075, 1994.

23. McGlinch BP, White RD: Cardiopulmonary resuscitation: basic and advanced life support. In Miller RD, editor: *Miller's Anesthesia,* ed 7, St. Loius, 2009, Churchill Livingstone, p. 2972.

24. Travers AH, Rea TD, Bobrow BJ, et al: Part 4: CPR overview: 2010 American Heart Association guidelines for cardiopulmonary resuscitation and emergency cardiovascular care, *Circulation* 122(suppl 3):S676–S684, 2010.

25. Kern KB, Mostafizi K: A hands-on approach. What compression-only CPR means for EMS, *JEMS* Suppl:suppl 8–11, 2009 Sep.

26. Larsen MP, Eisenberg MS, Cummins RO, et al: Predicting survival from out-of-hospital cardiac arrest: a graphic model, *Ann Emerg Med* 22(11):1652–1658, 1993.

27. Link MS, Atkins DL, Passman RS, et al: Part 6: electrical therapies: automated external defibrillators, defibrillation, cardioversion, and pacing: 2010 American Heart Association guidelines for cardiopulmonary resuscitation and emergency cardiovascular care, *Circulation* 122(Suppl 3):S706–S719, 2010.

28. Hazinski MF, Idris AH, Kerber RE, et al; American Heart Association Emergency Cardiovascular Committee; Council on Cardiopulmonary, Perioperative, and Critical Care; Council on Clinical Cardiology: Lay rescuer automated external defibrillator ("public access defibrillation") programs: lessons learned from an international multicenter trial: advisory statement from the American Heart Association Emergency Cardiovascular Committee; the Council on Cardiopulmonary, Perioperative, and Critical Care; and the Council on Clinical Cardiology, *Circulation* 111(24):3336–3340, 2005.

29. Sandroni C, Nolan J, Cavallaro F, et al: In-hospital cardiac arrest: incidence, prognosis and possible measures to improve survival, *Intensive Care Med* 33:237–245, 2007.

30. Weaver WD, Copass MK, Bufi D, et al: Improved neurologic recovery and survival after early defibrillation, *Circulation* 69:943–948, 1984.

31. PAD Trial Investigators: Public-access defibrillation and survival after out-of-hospital cardiac arrest, *N Engl J Med* 351:637- 646, 2004.

32. Weisfeldt ML: Public access defibrillation: good or great? *BMJ* 328(7438):E271–E272, 2004.

33. Bardy GH, Lee KL, Mark DB, et al; HAT Investigators: Home use of automated external defibrillators for sudden cardiac arrest, *N Engl J Med* 358(17):1793–1804. Epub April 1, 2008, 2008 24.

34. Neumar RW, Nolan JP, Adrie C, et al: Post–cardiac arrest syndrome: epidemiology, pathophysiology, treatment, and prognostication: a consensus statement from the International Liaison Committee on Resuscitation (American Heart Association, Australian and New Zealand Council on Resuscitation, European Resuscitation Council, Heart and Stroke Foundation of Canada, InterAmerican Heart Foundation, Resuscitation Council of Asia, and the Resuscitation Council of Southern Africa); the American Heart Association Emergency Cardiovascular Care Committee; the Council on Cardiovascular Surgery and Anesthesia; the Council on Cardiopulmonary, Perioperative, and Critical Care; the Council on Clinical Cardiology; and the Stroke Council, *Circulation* 118:2452–2483, 2008.

35. Peberdy MA, Callaway CW, Neumar RW, et al: Part 9: post–cardiac arrest care: 2010 American Heart Association guidelines for cardiopulmonary resuscitation and emergency cardiovascular care, *Circulation* 122(Suppl 3):S768–S786, 2010.

36. Weisfeldt ML, Becker LB: Resuscitation after cardiac arrest: a 3-phase time-sensitive model, *JAMA* 288(23):3035–3038, 2002.

37. Eftestol T, Wik L, Sunde K, et al: Effects of cardiopulmonary resuscitation on predictors of ventricular fibrillation defibrillation success during out-of-hospital cardiac arrest, *Circulation* 110(1):10–15, 2004.

38. Attaran RR, Ewy GA: Epinephrine in resuscitation: curse or cure? *Future Cardiol* 6(4):473–482, 2010.

39. Bernard SA, Gray TW, Buist MD, et al: Treatment of comatose survivors of out-of-hospital cardiac arrest with induced hypothermia, *N Engl J Med* 346(8):557–563, 2002.

40. Hypothermia after Cardiac Arrest Study Group: Mild therapeutic hypothermia to improve the neurologic outcome after cardiac arrest, *N Engl J Med* 346(8):549–556, 2002.

41. Bernard S: Therapeutic hypothermia after cardiac arrest, *Neurol Clin* 24(1):61–71, 2006.

42. Bobrow BJ, Clark LL, Ewy GA, et al. Minimally interrupted cardiac resuscitation by emergency medical services for out-of-hospital cardiac arrest, *JAMA* 299:1158–1165, 2008.

43. Kellum MJ, Kennedy KW, Barney R, et al: Cardiocerebral resuscitation improves neurologically intact survival of patients with out-of-hospital cardiac arrest, *Ann Emerg Med* 52(3):244–252. Epub March 28, 2008, 2008.

44. Kellum MJ, Kennedy KW, Ewy GA: Cardiocerebral resuscitation improves survival of patients with out-of-hospital cardiac arrest, *Am J Med* 119:335–340, 2006.

45. Barratt F, Wallis DN: Relatives in the resuscitation room: their point of view, *J Accid Emerg Med* 15:109–111, 1998.

46. Beckman AW, Sloan BK, Moore GP, et al: Should parents be present during emergency department procedures on children, and who should make that decision? A survey of emergency physician and nurse attitudes, *Acad Emerg Med* 9:154–158, 2002.

CHAPTER 2

Airway Management: Oxygenation and Ventilation

OBJECTIVES

Upon completion of this chapter, you will be able to:

1. Discuss the evaluation of oxygenation and ventilation with the use of pulse oximetry and capnography.
2. Describe the advantages, disadvantages, oxygen liter flow per minute, and estimated oxygen percentage delivered with each of the following devices:
   - Nasal cannula
   - Simple face mask
   - Partial nonrebreather mask
   - Nonrebreather mask
3. Describe and demonstrate the steps needed to perform the head tilt–chin lift, jaw thrust, and jaw thrust without head tilt maneuvers and relate the mechanism of injury to the opening of the airway.
4. Describe and demonstrate the procedure for suctioning the upper airway and discuss possible complications associated with this procedure.
5. Discuss the indications, contraindications, advantages, and disadvantages of oral and nasal airways and demonstrate how to correctly size and insert each of these airway adjuncts.
6. Describe the indications for positive pressure ventilation and demonstrate how to provide positive pressure ventilation with a barrier device and a pocket face mask.
7. Describe the oxygen liter flow per minute and the estimated inspired oxygen concentration delivered with a pocket face mask and a bag-mask device.
8. Describe how to ventilate a patient with a bag-mask and two rescuers.
9. Recognize the signs of adequate and inadequate bag-mask ventilation.
10. Describe methods that are used to confirm the correct placement of an advanced airway and describe the ventilation of a patient who has an advanced airway in place.

ANATOMY OF THE RESPIRATORY SYSTEM

Upper Airway

The upper airway extends from the mouth and nose to the trachea (Figure 2-1). The upper airway functions as a passageway for gas flow; for filtering, warming, and humidifying the air; and for protecting the surfaces of the lower respiratory tract. The upper airway also functions in phonation and in the senses of smell and taste.

The nasal cavity and the mouth meet at the pharynx (i.e., throat). The pharynx extends from the nasal cavities to the larynx and includes three parts: the nasopharynx, the oropharynx, and the laryngopharynx or hypopharynx. The pharynx is a passageway that is common to both the respiratory and digestive systems. The separation of the respiratory and digestive tracts occurs immediately below the laryngopharynx.

The nasopharynx is located at the posterior end of the nasal cavity, and it extends to the tip of the uvula. The mucous lining of the nasopharynx filters, warms, and moistens the air. The nasopharynx contains two pharyngeal tonsils (also called adenoids) and the eustachian tube openings. Tissues of the nasopharynx are extremely delicate and vascular. The improper or overly aggressive placement of tubes or airways may result in significant bleeding.

The oropharynx begins at the **uvula**, which is fleshy tissue that hangs down from the soft palate and into the posterior portion of the oral cavity. The posterior portion of the oral cavity opens into the oropharynx. The oropharynx extends to the upper rim of the epiglottis. The **epiglottis** is a small, leaf-shaped piece of cartilage located at the top of the larynx that prevents foreign material from entering the trachea during swallowing. The oropharynx functions in respiration and digestion. The anterior oropharynx opens into the oral cavity, which is comprised of the lips, cheeks, teeth, tongue, and hard and soft palates (Figure 2-2). The anterior roof of the oral cavity is formed by the maxillary bone and is called the **hard palate**. The posterior portion of the roof of the mouth is called the **soft palate** because it is made up of mucous membrane, muscular fibers, and mucous glands. The cheeks form the walls

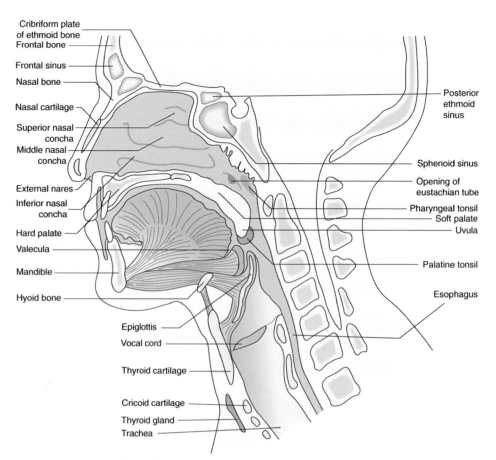

Figure 2-1 Midsagittal section through the upper airway.

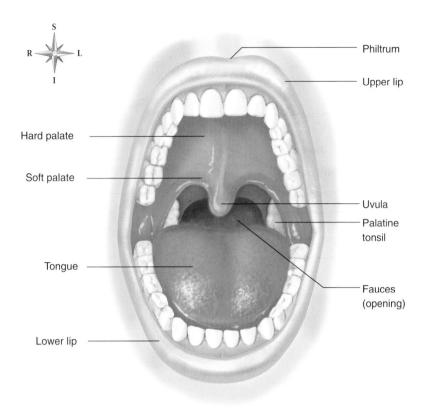

Figure 2-2 Frontal view into the open mouth showing the major structures within.

and the tongue dominates the floor of the oral cavity. Located on the lateral walls of the oropharynx are a pair of palatine tonsils that can cause a partial airway obstruction if they become excessively swollen. The space (or "pocket") between the base of the tongue and the epiglottis is called the **vallecula**. When performing orotracheal intubation, the epiglottis is lifted out of the way to visualize the area during the passage of the tracheal tube between the vocal cords. The vallecula is an important anatomical landmark to identify when intubating a patient with the use of a curved laryngoscope blade.

The laryngopharynx extends from the upper rim of the epiglottis to the **glottis**, which encompasses the true vocal cords and the space between them (i.e., the glottis opening). The glottis is the narrowest part of the adult larynx. The laryngopharynx is connected to the esophagus. The esophagus and the laryngopharynx functions in respiration and digestion.

> **ACLS Pearl**
> In the unresponsive patient, a partial or complete airway obstruction can result when the muscles of the tongue and laryngopharynx relax, thus allowing the tongue and other soft tissues to block the opening of the laryngopharynx.

The larynx (voice box) connects the pharynx to the trachea at the level of the cervical vertebrae (Figure 2-3). It conducts air between the pharynx and the lungs; it prevents food and foreign substances from entering the trachea; and it houses the vocal cords, which are involved in speech production. The larynx is a tubular structure made up of muscles, ligaments, and nine cartilages (Figure 2-4). The thyroid cartilage (Adam's apple) is the largest and most superior cartilage of the larynx. It is more pronounced in adult males than adult females. The thyroid gland lies over the outer surface of the thyroid cartilage. The pyramid-shaped arytenoid cartilages of the larynx serve as a point of attachment for the vocal cords. The arytenoid cartilages often serve as an important landmark during intubation.

The cricoid cartilage lies inferior to the thyroid cartilage. It is considered the first tracheal ring, and it is the only complete ring of cartilage in the larynx. The other cartilages of the larynx are incomplete C-shaped rings on the posterior surface. The C-shaped rings are open to permit the esophagus, which

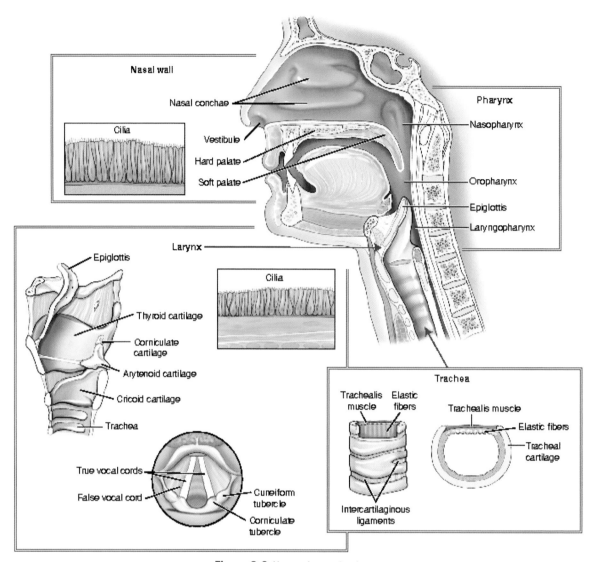

Figure 2-3 Upper airway structures.

lies behind the trachea, to bulge forward as food moves to the stomach. The narrowest diameter of the airway in infants and children who are less than 10 years old is at the cricoid cartilage. The **cricothyroid membrane** is a fibrous membrane that is located between the cricoid and thyroid cartilages. This site may be used for surgical and alternative airway placement.

> **ACLS Pearl**
> Most of the larynx is innervated with nerve endings from the vagus nerves. Because bradycardia, hypotension, and decreased ventilatory rate can result from the stimulation of the larynx by a laryngoscope blade, tracheal tube, or suction catheter, it is important to monitor the patient closely for these effects and to discontinue the treatment that is causing them to appear.

Lower Airway

The lower airway extends from the larynx to the alveoli, and it functions in the exchange of oxygen and carbon dioxide. Air moves from the larynx through the glottic opening and into the trachea. The adult trachea is about 12 cm in length and has an inner diameter of about 2 cm. It divides (bifurcates) into two separate tubes called the *left* and *right primary bronchi* (Figure 2-5). The point where the trachea divides into the right and left primary bronchi is called the **carina**. The right bronchus serves three lobes of the lung and the left bronchus serves two.

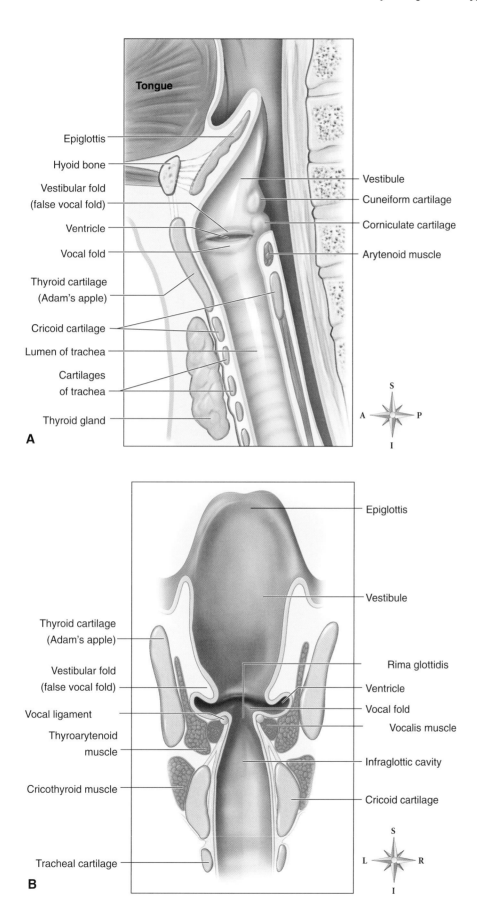

Figure 2-4 Anatomy of the larynx. **A,** Anterior view. **B,** Posterior view.

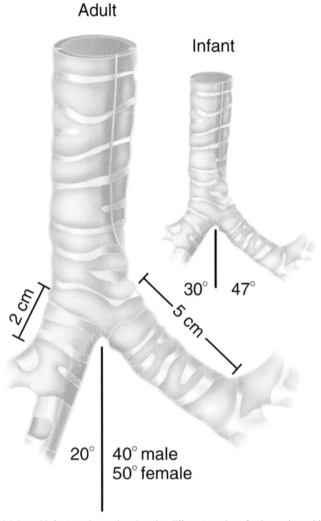

Figure 2-5 Adult and infant tracheas showing the different angles of primary bronchi bifurcation.

The right primary bronchus is straighter or less angled than the left, because the heart occupies space in the left chest cavity. These angles become important for several reasons. First, when intubating, if the tip of the tracheal tube is inserted too deeply, it will most likely lie within the right primary bronchus. When this occurs, your assessment of tube placement when auscultating the chest will reveal good lung sounds on the right and diminished or absent sounds over the left chest. In this situation, withdraw the tracheal tube a few centimeters and then reassess. In addition, foreign bodies tend to make their way into the right primary bronchus more often than they do into the left.[1]

The walls of the trachea are supported and held open by a series of 16 to 20 C-shaped cartilaginous rings. The area between the tracheal cartilages is composed of connective tissue and smooth muscle, which allow for changes in the diameter of the trachea. Tracheal smooth muscle is innervated by the parasympathetic division of the autonomic nervous system.

Internally, the trachea is lined with a mucous membrane that contains cilia as well as mucus-producing cells. The cilia sweep foreign materials out of the airway and the mucus can also trap particulate matter that is then expelled during coughing.

ACLS Pearl

Obstruction of the trachea will result in death if not corrected within minutes.

The primary bronchi branch into narrowing secondary and tertiary bronchi, which then branch into bronchioles (Figure 2-6). As the bronchi continue to divide into the lung tissue and become smaller

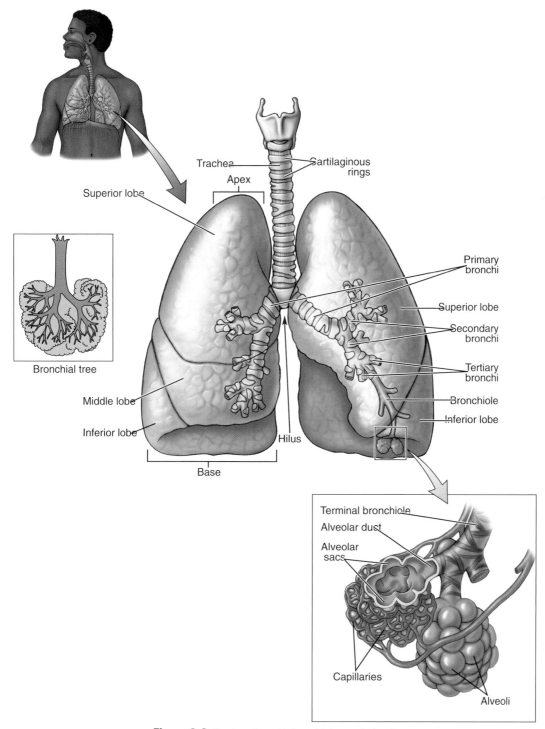

Figure 2-6 Trachea, bronchi, bronchioles, and alveoli.

passageways, they become bronchioles. Bronchioles are composed entirely of smooth muscle that is supported by connective tissue. Bronchioles are responsible for regulating the flow of air to the alveoli. The stimulation of beta-2 receptor sites in the bronchioles results in relaxation of bronchial smooth muscle. After multiple subdivisions, the bronchioles divide into tiny tubes called alveolar ducts, where gas exchange first becomes possible. These ducts end in alveoli, which are tiny, hollow air sacs. Each lung of an average adult contains about 300 million alveoli, and each alveolus is surrounded by a pulmonary capillary. Oxygen diffuses through the thin walls of the alveoli to the capillaries, and carbon dioxide diffuses from the capillaries to the alveoli.

LUNG VOLUMES AND CAPACITIES

Lung Volumes

During normal, quiet breathing, an adult male moves an average of 500 mL (5-7 mL/kg)[2,3] of air into and out of the respiratory tract; this amount is called the **tidal volume** (Figure 2-7). Tidal volume can be indirectly evaluated by observing the rise and fall of a patient's chest.

During forceful breathing (such as during and after heavy exercise), an additional 3000 mL[2,3] can be inspired (this is the inspiratory reserve volume), and an extra 1200 mL[2,3] or so can be expired (this is the expiratory reserve volume).

Residual volume is the amount of air that remains in the respiratory tract after a forceful expiration. In the average adult the residual volume is 1200 mL.[2,3]

Lung Capacities

Lung capacities include two or more lung volumes. The inspiratory capacity is comprised of the tidal volume plus the inspiratory reserve volume, and it is approximately 3500 mL (500 mL + 3000 mL).[2,3]

The functional residual capacity is composed of the expiratory reserve volume plus the residual volume, which is approximately 2400 mL (1200 mL + 1200 mL).[2,3] Functional residual capacity is the volume of air that remains in the lungs at the end of a normal expiration.

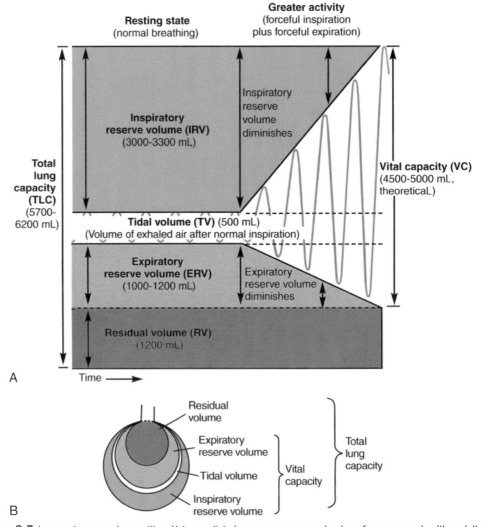

Figure 2-7 Lung volumes and capacities. Volumes listed are average normal values for a young, healthy adult male. **A,** A tracing like that produced with a spirometer. **B,** The pulmonary volumes as relative proportions of an inflated balloon.

The vital capacity is the amount of air that can be forcibly expired after a maximal inspiration. It is composed of the inspiratory capacity plus the expiratory reserve volume, and it is about 4700 mL (3500 mL + 1200 mL).[2,3] Its value increases with body size, male gender, and physical conditioning, and it decreases with age. Vital capacity reflects the largest volume of air that can be moved in and out during ventilation.

The total lung capacity includes all of the lung volumes: It is the vital capacity plus the residual volume, which is about 5900 mL (4700 mL + 1200 mL).[2,3]

> **ACLS Pearl**
> - Evaluation of a patient's breathing should include assessment of the patient's depth of breathing (estimation of tidal volume) and ventilation rate.
> - Ventilation (which is often misnamed respiration) is the mechanical movement of gas or air into and out of the lungs. Respiration is the exchange of oxygen and carbon dioxide during cellular metabolism.[4]

Ventilation Rates

Minute volume is the amount of air that is moved in and out of the respiratory tract over the course of 1 minute. It is determined by multiplying the tidal volume by the ventilatory rate (breaths/min).

A change in either the tidal volume *or* the ventilation rate will affect minute volume. For example, as the tidal volume decreases, the patient's ventilatory rate must increase to provide adequate ventilation. Respiratory failure can result when an increased ventilatory rate can no longer make up for the lack of tidal volume. Alternatively, tidal volume must increase to maintain adequate ventilation when the ventilatory rate slows. Respiratory failure can result when an increased tidal volume cannot increase sufficiently to make up for the decreased ventilatory rate.

DEVICES FOR ASSESSING OXYGENATION AND VENTILATION

Pulse Oximetry

[Objective 1]

Oxygenation is the process of getting oxygen into the body and to its tissues for metabolism. **Pulse oximetry** is a noninvasive method of measuring oxygen saturation of functional hemoglobin. A pulse oximeter, which is commonly called a *pulse ox*, is a small instrument with a light sensor. The sensor is typically applied to a finger, but the forehead, an earlobe, or a toe can also be used with the selection of a sensor that is appropriate for the chosen site. For example, an adhesive or clip-on sensor can be used for a finger, while a forehead sensor is usually adhesive. The placement of a sensor in a central location such as the earlobe may reflect the most rapid oximeter response (i.e., within about 10 seconds) to a drop in the saturation of peripheral oxygen (SpO_2). With finger placement, the response delay may take 30 to 60 seconds, and with toe placement, the delay may take up to 90 seconds.[5]

Pulse oximetry sensors may be disposable or reusable. Disposable foam-wrap or adhesive sensors are recommended when the patient is active, when monitoring continuously for more than 10 minutes, and when a risk for cross-contamination with microbial pathogens exists.[6] When using a disposable sensor, the American Association of Critical-Care Nurses (AACN) recommends assessing the site every 2 to 4 hours and replacing the sensor every 24 hours.[7] Assess the site for decreased temperature, decreased peripheral pulse, cyanosis, and tissue integrity. Reusable clip-on sensors are generally used when spot-checking oximetry values, when monitoring continuously for less than 10 minutes, and when monitoring patients who are immobile (Figure 2-8). When a reusable sensor is applied, the AACN recommends assessing the site every 2 hours and changing the site every 4 hours.[7]

The instrument sensor emits two light frequencies: one is a red beam that is the approximate color of oxygenated hemoglobin, and the other is an infrared beam that is the approximate wavelength of deoxygenated hemoglobin (Figure 2-9). By measuring the absorption of the two frequencies, the oximeter quickly and accurately calculates the percentage of hemoglobin that is saturated with oxygen in a pulsating capillary bed. This calculation is called the *saturation of peripheral oxygen* or SpO_2. The

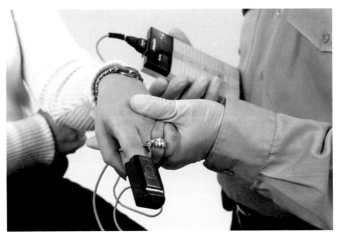

Figure 2-8 Because it can provide a continuous measurement of oxygenation, use of pulse oximetry provides healthcare professionals with an early warning of decreased oxygenation.

Figure 2-9 Schematic block diagram of a pulse oximeter.

oximeter displays this value as a percentage and the patient's pulse rate on its screen. The SpO_2 is a generally reliable indicator of the status of the partial pressure of oxygen in the arterial blood or PaO_2.[1] A healthy adult who is breathing room air at sea level generally has an SpO_2 in the range of 96% to 100%. Patients with SpO_2 values that are significantly lower than normal are likely to be hypoxic.

> **YOU SHOULD KNOW** After hyperoxygenation, the oxyhemoglobin saturation detected by pulse oximetry may not decline for as long as 3 minutes, even when ventilation is ineffective.[8-10]

Possible indications for continuous pulse oximetry monitoring include the following:
- A patient with a critical or unstable airway.
- A patient who requires oxygen therapy.
- During the intrahospital and interhospital transfer of a critically ill patient.
- A patient who is undergoing hemodialysis.
- A patient who has a condition or who is undergoing a procedure that alters oxygen saturation or a patient who has a condition or history that suggests a risk for significant desaturation.
  - A patient who requires oxygenation monitoring during emergency airway management.
  - A patient who is undergoing ventilator and oxygen therapy changes.
  - A patient who is being evaluated for the adequacy of preoxygenation before tracheal intubation.
  - A patient who is being monitored during the delivery of and recovery from conscious sedation or after surgery.
  - A patient who has acute respiratory distress or a chronic respiratory condition.
  - A patient with a chest wall injury or chest pain.

BOX 2-1 Factors Affecting the Accuracy of Pulse Oximetry Readings

- Anemia (conflicting evidence)
- Artificial acrylic nails (conflicting evidence)
- Bright ambient light (such as sunlight or surgical, fluorescent, or heating lamps) (conflicting evidence)
- Carbon monoxide or cyanide poisoning or other molecules that bind to hemoglobin
- Dark or metallic nail polish (conflicting evidence)
- Dark skin pigmentation[11,12]
- Medications (such as vasoconstrictors)
- Motion artifact
- Poor peripheral perfusion as a result of cardiac arrest, shock, hypotension, or hypothermia

- A patient who is morbidly obese.
- A patient who has obstructive sleep apnea.
- A patient who is receiving analgesics at a dose or by a route of administration that is likely to produce ventilatory depression.

Pulse oximetry may be inaccurate in situations that involve poor capillary blood flow, an abnormal hemoglobin concentration, or an abnormal shape of the hemoglobin molecule. Examples of conditions that may give misleading results are listed in Box 2-1.

> **ACLS Pearl**
>
> A pulse oximeter is an adjunct to—not a replacement of—vigilant patient assessment. You must correlate your assessment findings with pulse oximeter readings to determine appropriate treatment interventions for the patient.

Carbon Dioxide Monitoring

[Objective 1]

Carbon dioxide is produced during cellular metabolism, carried to the lungs by the circulatory system, and excreted by the lungs during ventilation. **Capnography** is the continuous analysis and recording of CO_2 concentrations in respiratory gases. Capnography-related terms appear in Table 2-1. Capnography provides healthcare professionals with breath-to-breath patient information, thereby enabling the early recognition of hypoventilation, apnea, or airway obstruction and thus preventing hypoxic episodes. The monitoring of exhaled carbon dioxide with either capnometry or capnography can detect changes in metabolism, circulation, respiration, the airway, or respiratory system.

Exhaled carbon dioxide detection devices are used in conjunction with the history and clinical assessment of the patient, which may include mental status, lung sounds, pulse rate, and skin color. An example of a combination handheld capnograph and pulse oximeter is shown in Figure 2-10. Examples of situations in which exhaled CO_2 monitoring is commonly used include the following:

- Verification of tracheal tube placement (capnography should not be used as the only means of assessing tracheal tube placement)
- Performance of procedural sedation and analgesia
- Evaluation of mechanical ventilation and resuscitation efforts
- Continuous monitoring of tracheal tube position (including during patient transport)
- Monitoring of exhaled CO_2 levels in patients with suspected increased intracranial pressure
- Assessment of the adequacy of ventilation in patients with altered mental status, bronchospasm, asthma, chronic obstructive pulmonary disease, anaphylaxis, heart failure, drug overdose, stroke, shock, or circulatory compromise

Alveolar CO_2 and arterial CO_2 ($PaCO_2$) values are closely related in patients with normal cardiopulmonary function, and they usually range between 35 and 45 mm Hg. In patients with normal lung and cardiac function, end-tidal carbon dioxide ($EtCO_2$) is usually 2 to 5 mm Hg less than the $PaCO_2$ because of the contribution of physiologic dead space gas to the end-tidal gases.[13] The normal values for $Etco_2$ range between 33 mm Hg and 43 mm Hg. This is dependent upon adequate ventilation and adequate perfusion: a change in either factor will increase or decrease the amount of exhaled CO_2.

TABLE 2-1	Capnography-Related Terms
Term	**Description**
Capnography	Continuous analysis and recording of CO_2 concentrations in respiratory gases
	Output displayed as a waveform
	Graphic display of the CO_2 concentration vs. time during a respiratory cycle
	CO_2 concentration may also be plotted vs. expiratory volume
	Most reliable method for confirmation and monitoring of tracheal tube placement
Capnometer	Device used to measure the concentration of CO_2 at the end of exhalation
Capnometry	A numeric reading of exhaled CO_2 concentrations without a continuous written record or waveform
	Output is a numerical value
	Numeric display of CO_2 on a monitor
Capnograph	A device that provides a numeric reading of exhaled CO_2 concentrations and a waveform (tracing)
Colorimetric $EtCO_2$ detector	A device that provides CO_2 readings by chemical reaction on pH-sensitive litmus paper housed in the detector
	The presence of CO_2 (evidenced by a color change on the colorimetric device) suggests tracheal tube placement
$EtCO_2$ detector	A capnometer that provides a noninvasive estimate of alveolar ventilation, the concentration of exhaled CO_2 from the lungs, and arterial carbon dioxide content
Qualitative $EtCO_2$ monitor	A device that uses a light to indicate the presence of $EtCO_2$

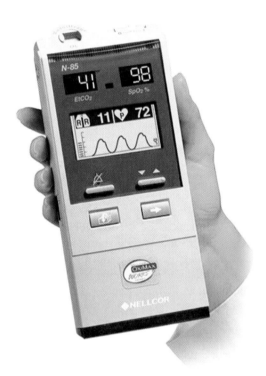

Figure 2-10 A combination handheld capnograph and pulse oximeter.

Digital capnometers use infrared technology to analyze exhaled gas. These devices provide a quantitative measurement of the exhaled CO_2, in that they provide the exact amount of CO_2 exhaled. This is beneficial because trends in CO_2 levels can be monitored and the effectiveness of treatment can be determined.

Capnography devices function through infrared technology. In addition to providing quantitative data as do digital capnometers, they also provide information about air movement in and out of the

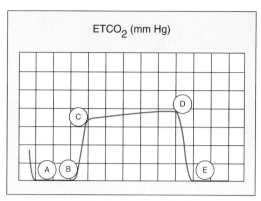

Figure 2-11 Phases of a normal capnogram. A-B of the waveform is the baseline. B-C represents the transition from inspiration to expiration and the mixing of dead space and alveolar gas. C-D is the alveolar plateau, representing alveolar gas rich in carbon dioxide passing the sensor. D-E represents the change to the inspiratory portion of the respiratory cycle. D reflects the point at which expiration ends and inspiration begins and is the end-tidal CO_2 (Etco$_2$) value.

lungs with a graphical waveform. The process of CO_2 elimination produces a characteristic waveform called the *capnogram*. An example of a normal capnogram is shown in Figure 2-11. A and B of the waveform show the baseline and represent the beginning of expiration, when air from the anatomic dead space is being exhaled. Because this air contains undetectable amounts of CO_2 there is no movement of the wave from the baseline. B and C (expiratory upstroke) reflect the rapid upstroke of the curve and represent the transition from inspiration to expiration and the mixing of dead space and alveolar gas. C and D (expiratory plateau) show the alveolar plateau, which represents alveolar gas that is rich in carbon dioxide passing the sensor. The plateau tends to slope gently upward with the uneven emptying of the alveoli. D and E (inspiratory downstroke) demonstrate a rapid, sharp downstroke that represents the change to the inspiratory portion of the respiratory cycle. The downstroke is a nearly vertical drop to the baseline that reflects the rapid decrease in the levels of carbon dioxide passing the sensor. D reflects the point at which expiration ends and inspiration begins, and it is the end-tidal CO_2 (EtCO$_2$) value. It is this number that is reported by most capnometers. The space that occurs between waveforms is the result of the pause between ventilations. Changes in the Etco$_2$ generally result from changes in perfusion or ventilation rates. Changes in the morphology of the waveform indicate a change in air movement through the lower airways caused by alterations in metabolism, circulation, ventilation, or equipment function. During cardiac arrest, waveform capnography appears to demonstrate high sensitivity and specificity for proper tracheal tube placement.

> **ACLS Pearl**
> Interpreting capnograms should be done with the use of a systematic approach that includes the evaluation of height, contour, baseline, frequency, and rhythm. Capnogram interpretation is beyond the scope of this text and the Advanced Cardiac Life Support course.

A colorimetric capnometer functions through a pH change that occurs with the breath of a patient (Figure 2-12). The patient's breath causes a chemical reaction on pH-sensitive litmus paper housed in the detector. The capnometer is placed between a tracheal tube or advanced airway device and a ventilation device (Figure 2-13). The presence of CO_2, which is evidenced by a color change on the colorimetric device, suggests placement of the tube in the trachea. A colorimetric capnometer is qualitative in that it simply shows the presence of CO_2. It has no ability to provide an actual CO_2 reading or to indicate the presence of hypercarbia, and it provides no opportunity for ongoing monitoring to ensure that the tube remains in the trachea. A lack of CO_2 (i.e., no color change) suggests tube placement in the esophagus, particularly in patients with a perfusing rhythm (not in cardiac arrest).

Some manufacturers of colorimetric capnometers recommend ventilating the patient at least six times before attempting to use an exhaled CO_2 detector to assess tracheal tube placement. The rationale for this action is to quickly wash out any retained CO_2 that is present in the stomach or esophagus as a result of bag-mask ventilation. CO_2 that is detected after six positive pressure ventilations can be presumed to be from the lungs.[14,15]

In animals, false-positive results (i.e., CO_2 is detected despite tube placement in the esophagus) have been reported when large amounts of carbonated beverages were ingested before a cardiac arrest.[15]

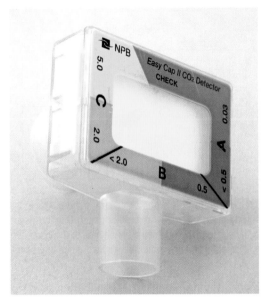

Figure 2-12 Colorimetric exhaled carbon dioxide detector.

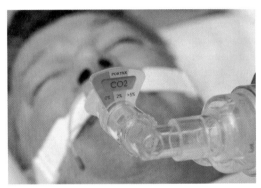

Figure 2-13 Colorimetric exhaled carbon dioxide detector connected to a tracheal tube.

False-negative results (i.e., a lack of CO_2 detection despite tube placement in the trachea) may occur because of poor pulmonary blood flow, such as in patients with cardiac arrest, severe airway obstruction (e.g., status asthmaticus), pulmonary edema, or significant pulmonary embolus.[16] Colorimetric capnometers are susceptible to inaccurate results as result of the age of the paper and exposure of the paper to the environment. A colorimetric capnometer may not change color if the paper is contaminated with patient secretions (e.g., vomitus) or acidic drugs (e.g., tracheally administered epinephrine).[17] When CO_2 is not detected, an alternative method should be used to confirm tracheal tube placement, such as direct visualization or the use of an esophageal detector device.[18]

YOU SHOULD KNOW Pulse oximetry provides important information about oxygenation, but does not provide information about the effectiveness of a patient's ventilation. Capnography provides information about the effectiveness of ventilation, but does not measure oxygenation.

OXYGEN DELIVERY DEVICES

The fraction of inspired gas that is oxygen is abbreviated as FIO_2 and is often expressed as a percentage. Supplemental oxygen administration is indicated if the patient is cyanotic; if he or she is having difficulty breathing or having obvious signs of heart failure or shock, or if his or her oxygen saturation level declines to less than 94%. Titrate oxygen therapy to maintain the patient's SpO_2 at 94% or more.[19]

Nasal Cannula

[Objective 2]

A nasal cannula, which is also called *nasal prongs*, is a piece of plastic tubing with two soft prongs that project from the tubing. The prongs are inserted into the patient's nostrils and the tubing is then secured to the patient's face (Figure 2-14). Oxygen flows from the cannula into the patient's nasopharynx, which acts as an anatomic reservoir.

Although the actual inspired oxygen concentration depends on the patient's ventilatory rate and depth, a nasal cannula can deliver oxygen concentrations of about 22% to 45% at 0.25 to 8 L/min flow.[20,21] Flow rates of more than 6 L/min do not enhance delivered oxygen concentration; they dry the mucous membranes of the nasal cavity, and they often cause discomfort (e.g., headaches). Advantages and disadvantages of using a nasal cannula are shown in Box 2-2.

Simple Face Mask

[Objective 2]

A **simple face mask,** which is also called a *standard mask*, is a plastic reservoir that has been designed to fit over the nose and mouth of a spontaneously breathing patient. The mask is secured around the patient's head by means of an elastic strap. The internal capacity of the mask produces a reservoir effect. Small holes on each side of the mask allow for the passage of inspired and expired air. Supplemental oxygen is delivered through a small-diameter tube connected to the base of the mask (Figure 2-15).

At 5 to 10 L/min, the simple face mask can deliver an inspired oxygen concentration of approximately 35% to 60%. The patient's actual inspired oxygen concentration will vary, because the amount of air that mixes with supplemental oxygen is dependent on the patient's inspiratory flow rate. Advantages and disadvantages of using a simple face mask are shown in Box 2-3.

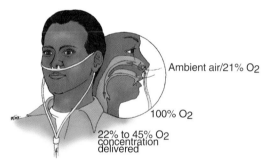

Ambient air/21% O_2

100% O_2

22% to 45% O_2 concentration delivered

Figure 2-14 At flow rates of 0.25 to 8 L/min, a nasal cannula can deliver an oxygen concentration of 22% to 45%.

BOX 2-2   **Nasal Cannula—Advantages and Disadvantages**

Advantages
- Comfortable and well tolerated by most patients
- Does not interfere with patient assessment or impede patient communication with healthcare personnel
- Allows for talking and eating
- No rebreathing of expired air
- Can be used with mouth breathers
- Useful for patients who are predisposed to carbon dioxide retention
- Can be used for patients who require oxygen but who cannot tolerate a nonrebreather mask

Disadvantages
- Can only be used in a spontaneously breathing patient
- Easily displaced
- Nasal passages must be open
- Involves a drying of mucosa that may cause sinus pain
- Tubing may cause skin breakdown above the ears
- Deviated septum and mouth breathing may reduce FIO_2
- Oxygen flow rates of more than 6 L/min do not enhance delivered oxygen concentration

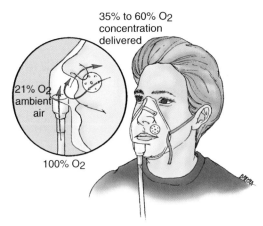

35% to 60% O2 concentration delivered

21% O2 ambient air

100% O2

Figure 2-15 The simple face mask can deliver an oxygen concentration of approximately 35% to 60% with an oxygen flow rate of 5 to 10 L/min.

BOX 2-3	**Simple Face Mask—Advantages and Disadvantages**

Advantages
- Higher oxygen concentration delivered than by nasal cannula

Disadvantages
- Can be used only in a spontaneously breathing patient
- Not tolerated well by severely dyspneic patients
- Can be uncomfortable
- Difficult to hear the patient speaking when the device is in place
- Must be removed at meals
- Requires a tight face seal to prevent the leakage of oxygen
- Oxygen flow rates of more than 10 L/min do not enhance delivered oxygen concentration

ACLS Pearl

When using a simple face mask, the oxygen flow rate must be higher than 5 L/min to flush the buildup of the patient's exhaled carbon dioxide from the mask.

Partial Rebreather Mask

[Objective 2]

A partial rebreather mask is similar to a simple face mask, but it has an attached oxygen-collecting device (i.e., reservoir) at the base of the mask that is filled before patient use. One hundred percent oxygen is delivered through oxygen tubing to the reservoir bag. The reservoir collects the oxygen and allows some of the patient's exhaled air (i.e., an amount that is approximately equal to the volume of the patient's anatomic dead space) to enter the reservoir bag and be reused (Figure 2-16).

The oxygen concentration of the patient's exhaled air, in combination with the supply of 100% oxygen, allows for the use of oxygen flow rates that are lower than those that are necessary for a non-rebreather mask. Depending on the patient's breathing pattern, the mask fit, and the oxygen flowmeter setting, oxygen concentrations of 35% to 60% can be delivered when an oxygen flow rate is used that prevents the reservoir bag from completely collapsing on inspiration (i.e., typically 6-10 L/min).[20] Advantages and disadvantages of using a partial rebreather mask are shown in Box 2-4.

Nonrebreather Mask

[Objective 2]

A nonrebreather mask is similar to a partial rebreather mask, but it does not permit the mixing of the patient's exhaled air with 100% oxygen. A one-way valve between the mask and the reservoir bag and a flap over one of the exhalation ports on the side of the mask prevent the inhalation of room air.

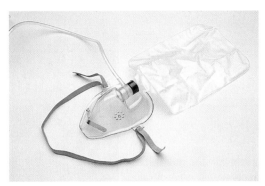

Figure 2-16 The partial rebreather mask has an attached oxygen-collecting device (reservoir) at the base of the mask. The reservoir collects oxygen and allows some of the patient's exhaled air to enter the reservoir bag and be reused.

BOX 2-4	Partial Rebreather Mask—Advantages and Disadvantages

Advantages
- Higher oxygen concentration delivered than by nasal cannula

Disadvantages
- Can only be used in a spontaneously breathing patient
- Not tolerated well in severely dyspneic patients
- Can be uncomfortable
- Difficult to hear the patient speaking when the device is in place
- Must be removed at meals
- Requires a tight face seal to prevent the leakage of oxygen
- Potential suffocation hazard
- Oxygen flow rates of more than 10 L/min do not enhance delivered oxygen concentration

When the patient breathes in, oxygen is drawn into the mask from the reservoir (bag) through the one-way valve that separates the bag from the mask. When the patient breathes out, the exhaled air exits through the open side port on the mask. The one-way valve prevents the patient's exhaled air from returning to the reservoir bag (thus the name *nonrebreather*). This ensures a supply of 100% oxygen to the patient with minimal dilution from the entrainment of room air.

A nonrebreather mask is the delivery device of choice when high concentrations of oxygen are needed for the spontaneously breathing patient. Depending on the patient's breathing pattern, the fit of the mask, and the oxygen flowmeter setting, oxygen concentrations of 60% to 80%[21] can be delivered when an oxygen flow rate (typically a minimum of 10 L/min) is used that prevents the reservoir bag from collapsing completely on inspiration. Inflate the reservoir bag with oxygen *before* placing the nonrebreather mask on the patient (Figure 2-17). Advantages and disadvantages of using a nonrebreather mask are shown in Box 2-5. A summary of oxygen percentages by device is shown in Table 2-2.

ACLS Pearl

When using a partial rebreather or nonrebreather mask, make sure that the bag does not collapse when the patient inhales. Should the bag collapse, increase the delivered oxygen by 2-liter increments until the bag remains inflated. The reservoir bag must remain at least two-thirds full so that sufficient supplemental oxygen is available for each breath.

MANUAL AIRWAY MANEUVERS

Basic to any type of airway management procedure is the ability to open a patient's airway manually. Manual maneuvers require no special equipment, they are noninvasive, and they must not be ignored in lieu of advanced procedures. The first step in every airway procedure, whether basic or advanced, is to manually open the airway.

The purpose of a manual maneuver is to position the anatomic structures of the patient's airway so that the airway passages are open to the flow of air. Each method helps lift the tongue off of the back

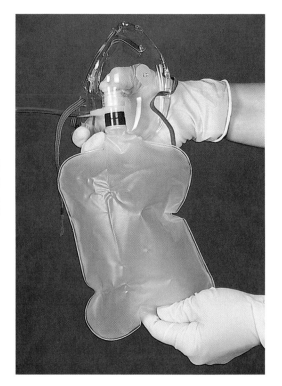

Figure 2-17 Be sure to fill the reservoir bag of a partial rebreather or nonrebreather mask with oxygen before placing the mask on the patient. After placing the mask on the patient, adjust the flow rate so that the bag does not completely deflate when the patient inhales.

BOX 2-5 Nonrebreather Mask—Advantages and Disadvantages

Advantages
- Higher oxygen concentration delivered than by nasal cannula, simple face mask, and partial rebreather mask
- Inspired oxygen is not mixed with room air

Disadvantages
- Can only be used with a spontaneously breathing patient
- Not tolerated well in severely dyspneic patients
- Can be uncomfortable
- Difficult to hear the patient speaking when the device is in place
- Must be removed at meals
- Mask must fit snugly on the patient's face to prevent room air from mixing with oxygen inhaled from the reservoir bag

TABLE 2-2 Oxygen Percentage Delivery by Device

Device	Approximate Inspired Oxygen Concentration	Liter Flow (Liters/Minute)
Nasal cannula	22% to 45%	0.25 to 8
Simple face mask	35% to 60%	5 to 10
Partial rebreather mask	35% to 60%	Typically 6 to 10 to prevent bag collapse on inspiration
Nonrebreather mask	60% to 80%	Typically a minimum of 10 to prevent bag collapse on inspiration

of the throat, which is the most common cause of a partial airway obstruction in an unresponsive patient. If the patient is breathing, snoring sounds are a sign of airway obstruction from displacement of the tongue. If the patient is not breathing, airway obstruction from the tongue may go undetected until positive pressure ventilation is attempted. Ventilating an apneic patient with an airway obstruction is difficult. If the airway obstruction is caused by the tongue, repositioning the patient's head and jaw may be all that is needed to open the airway.

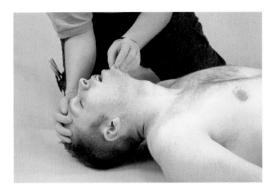

Figure 2-18 Opening the airway with a head tilt–chin lift maneuver.

An important consideration when determining which maneuver to perform is the possible presence of spinal trauma. Because manual maneuvers manipulate the cervical spine, a modification is required to minimize spinal movement and to maintain a neutral spinal position. When opening a patient's airway, the fact that you are doing so means that your patient is unable to maintain his or her own airway. You must be prepared with additional equipment (e.g., airway adjuncts, a ventilation device) and anticipate the need for suction.[1]

Head Tilt–Chin Lift

[Objective 3]
The head tilt–chin lift is the preferred technique for opening the airway of an unresponsive patient without suspected cervical spine injury (Figure 2-18). Follow these steps to perform a head tilt–chin lift:
1. Place the patient in a supine position.
2. Place one hand on the patient's forehead and apply firm pressure with your palm to tilt the patient's head back.
3. Place the tips of the fingers of your other hand under the bony part of the patient's chin and gently lift up and pull the jaw forward. Positioning your fingers under the bony part of the patient's chin is important because compression of the soft tissue under the patient's chin can obstruct the airway.
4. If needed, open the patient's mouth by pulling down on the patient's lower lip using the thumb of the same hand used to lift the chin.

Jaw Thrust

[Objective 3]
A jaw thrust maneuver may be performed with or without an accompanying head tilt. For patients who are unresponsive without any risk of spinal injury, perform the following technique:
1. With the patient supine, position yourself above the patient's head or at his or her side, looking at the face.
2. Place your fingers on each side of the lower jaw at the angle of the jaw near the bottom of the patient's ears.
3. Lift the jaw forward toward the patient's face and gently open the mouth.
4. Gently tilt the patient's head while maintaining displacement of the lower jaw.

Jaw Thrust without Head Tilt

[Objective 3]
The jaw thrust without head tilt maneuver (also called the *modified jaw thrust*) is the technique that is recommended for opening the airway when cervical spine injury is suspected (Figure 2-19). Perform the following for a jaw thrust without head tilt maneuver:
1. Ensure that the patient is in a supine position (log roll, if necessary).
2. While stabilizing the patient's head in a neutral position, grasp the angles of the patient's lower jaw with your fingertips.
3. Displace the lower jaw forward.
   Manual airway maneuvers are summarized in Table 2-3.

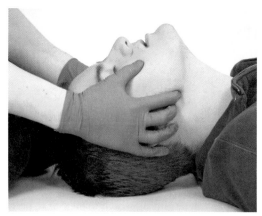

Figure 2-19 Opening the airway with the jaw thrust without head tilt maneuver.

TABLE 2-3	**Manual Airway Maneuvers**	
Considerations	**Head Tilt–Chin Lift**	**Jaw Thrust without Head Tilt**
Indications	• Unresponsive patient • No mechanism for cervical spine injury • Unable to protect own airway	• Unresponsive patient • Possible cervical spine injury • Unable to protect own airway
Contraindications	• Awake patient • Possible cervical spine injury	• Awake patient
Advantages	• Simple to perform • No equipment required • Noninvasive	• No equipment required • Noninvasive
Disadvantages	• Does not protect the lower airway from aspiration • May cause spinal movement	• Difficult to maintain • Second rescuer needed for bag-mask ventilation • Does not protect the lower airway from aspiration • May cause spinal movement

ACLS Pearl

The jaw thrust without head tilt maneuver is a difficult technique for one person to manage. In most cases, one rescuer is needed to displace the patient's lower jaw forward while a second rescuer ventilates the patient.

SUCTIONING

Purpose of Suctioning

Suctioning is performed for the following reasons:
• To remove vomitus, saliva, blood, or other material from the patient's airway
• To improve gas exchange by allowing air to pass through to the lower airway
• To prevent atelectasis
• To obtain secretions for diagnosis

Suction Catheters

Suction catheters are essentially one of two types: rigid or soft (Figure 2-20). Rigid catheters are also called *hard, tonsil tip*, or *Yankauer* catheters. They are made of hard plastic and angled to help with the removal of secretions from the mouth and throat. Because of its size, a rigid suction catheter is not used to suction the nares, except externally. The catheter typically has one large and several small holes at the distal end through which particles may be suctioned.

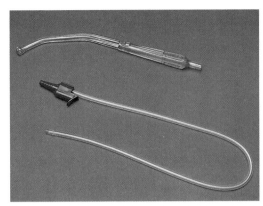

Figure 2-20 Suction catheters. Rigid suction catheter (*top*) and soft suction catheter (*bottom*).

Soft suction catheters are also called *whistle tip, flexible,* or *French* catheters. They are long, narrow, flexible pieces of plastic that are primarily used to clear blood or mucus from a tracheal tube or the nasopharynx. A soft suction catheter can be inserted into the nares, oropharynx, or nasopharynx; through an oral or nasal airway; or through a tracheal tube or a tracheostomy tube.

A side opening is present at the proximal end of most catheters that is covered with the thumb to produce suction. (In some cases, suctioning is initiated when a button is pushed on the suction device itself.)

Upper Airway Suctioning

[Objective 4]

Skill 2-1 shows and explains the steps necessary for suctioning the upper airway.

Lower Airway Suctioning[1]

A patient who has a tracheal or tracheostomy tube in place may require suctioning to remove secretions or mucus plugs. In some instances the mucus can be large and thick, leading to respiratory distress. Only soft catheters are used when suctioning the lower airway, using sterile technique. Skill 2-2 shows and explains the steps necessary for this procedure.

> **ACLS Pearl**
> If a patient is intubated and requires suctioning, perform tracheal suction before suctioning the mouth and throat. The mouth and throat contain more bacteria than the trachea. Suctioning the trachea first leads to less potential for the bacterial contamination of the lungs.

SKILL 2-1 | Upper Airway Suctioning

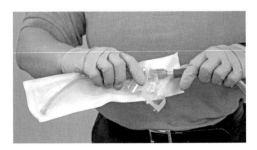

Step 1 Put on appropriate personal protective equipment, including gloves, eye protection, and a face shield. Assemble the necessary equipment, including the suction unit, tubing, and suction catheter. Preoxygenate the patient before suctioning, if possible.

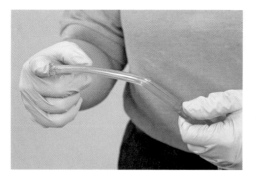

Step 2 Turn on the power to the suction unit. Test for adequate suction by sealing the side port on the catheter with one finger. After confirming that adequate suction is present, remove the finger from the port or turn off the suction unit.

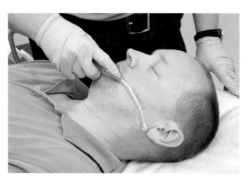

Step 3 To determine the appropriate depth for catheter insertion, measure the catheter from the corner of the patient's mouth to the earlobe or the angle of the jam.

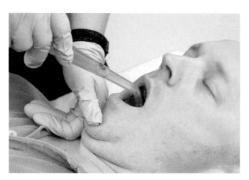

Step 4 Insert the catheter into the patient's mouth to the proper depth *without* applying suction.

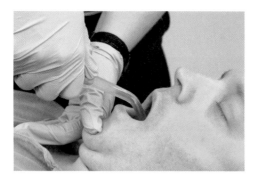

Step 5 To begin suctioning, turn on the power to the suction unit or cover the catheter side port with one finger.

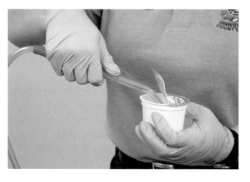

Step 6 Withdraw the catheter while applying suction. In adults, suction should not be applied for more than 10 seconds. Before repeating the procedure, ventilate the lungs with 100% oxygen for approximately 30 seconds and flush the suction catheter and tubing with saline. Document the amount, color, and consistency of the secretions that are obtained.

SKILL 2-2 Lower Airway Suctioning

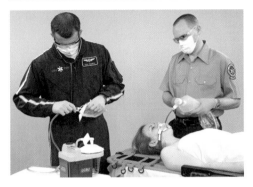

Step 1 Put on appropriate personal protective equipment including gloves, eye protection, and a face shield. Assemble the necessary equipment including the suction unit, tubing, and suction catheter. Preoxygenate the patient before suctioning if possible.

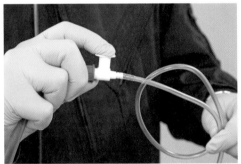

Step 2 Turn on the power to the suction unit. Test for adequate suction by sealing the side port on the catheter with one finger. After confirming that adequate suction is present, remove the finger from the port or turn off the suction unit.

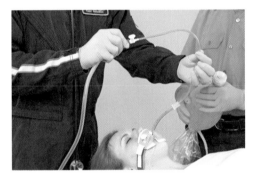

Step 3 Insert the catheter into the tracheal or tracheostomy tube to the proper depth *without* applying suction. To minimize the risk of atelectasis and hypoxemia when suction is applied, the diameter of the suction catheter should be no more than half the internal diameter of the tracheal tube.[22]

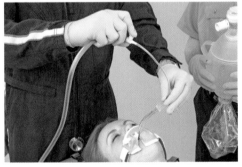

Step 4 To begin suctioning, turn on the power to the suction unit or cover the catheter side port with one finger.

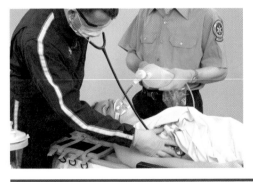

Step 5 Withdraw the catheter while applying suction. In adults, suction should not be applied for more than 10 seconds. Reevaluate airway patency and auscultate lung sounds. Before repeating the procedure, ventilate the patient with 100% oxygen for approximately 30 seconds and flush the suction catheter and tubing with saline. Document the amount, color, and consistency of the secretions that are obtained. Possible complications of suctioning are shown in Box 2-6.

BOX 2-6 **Suctioning—Possible Complications**

- Arrhythmias
- Bradycardia and hypotension from vagal stimulation
- Bronchospasm
- Hemorrhage
- Hypertension
- Hypoxia
- Increased intracranial pressure
- Local swelling
- Tachycardia
- Tracheal infection
- Tracheal trauma

AIRWAY ADJUNCTS

Manual maneuvers facilitate the opening of an airway, and several devices can assist with keeping it open. Airway adjuncts are devices that assist with the maintenance of an open passageway in the respiratory tract, thereby allowing air movement to reach the lower airways and facilitating gas exchange.

As evidenced by the many devices that are available for maintaining an open airway, a positive patient outcome often hinges on your knowledge and skill with regard to selecting appropriate adjuncts for each patient. You must consider the potential risks and benefits of each option available and use the most appropriate adjunct for the specific patient circumstances. Two options that have been specifically designed to prevent the tongue from falling back into the airway and blocking the flow of air are oral and nasal airways.[1]

Oral Airways

[Objective 5]

An oral airway is also called an *oropharyngeal airway* or *OPA*. Indications for insertion include patients who are unresponsive and have no gag reflex. An oral airway may be used as a bite block after the insertion of a tracheal tube or an orogastric tube.

An oral airway is a J-shaped plastic device that is used to create an air passage between the patient's mouth and the posterior wall of the pharynx (Figure 2-21). When correctly positioned, the flange of the device rests on the patient's lips or teeth. The distal tip lies between the base of the tongue and the back of the throat, thereby preventing the tongue from blocking the airway (Figure 2-22). Air passes around and through the device.

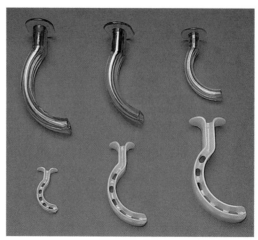

Figure 2-21 A sampling of oral airways.

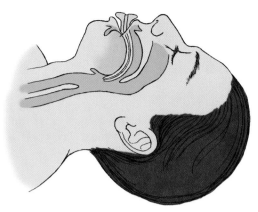

Figure 2-22 An oral airway in proper position.

Oral airways are available in a variety of sizes that range from 0 for neonates up to 6 for large adults. The size of the airway is based on the distance, in millimeters, from the flange to the distal tip. Skill 2-3 explains the steps for insertion of an oral airway.

SKILL 2-3   Oral Airway Insertion

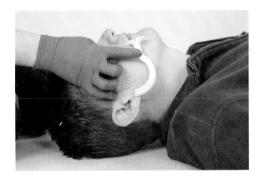

Step 1 Take appropriate standard precautions. Select an oral airway of appropriate size by measuring from the corner of the mouth to the tip of the earlobe or the angle of the jaw.

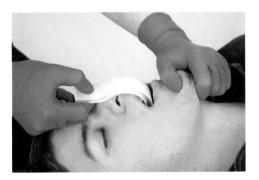

Step 2 Open the patient's mouth. Make sure the patient's mouth and throat are clear of secretions, blood, and vomitus. Suction the patient if needed. Hold the oral airway at its flange end and insert it into the patient's mouth, with the tip pointing toward the roof of the mouth.

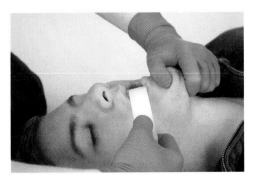

Step 3 Slide the airway along the roof of the patient's mouth. When the distal end nears the back of the throat, rotate the airway 180 degrees so that it is positioned over the tongue. Alternatively, the airway can be inserted sideways and rotated 90 degrees into position.

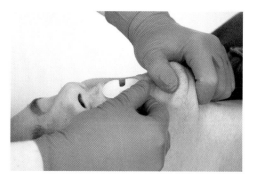

Step 4 When the oral airway is inserted properly, the flange of the device should rest comfortably on the patient's lips or teeth. The proper placement of the device is confirmed by ventilating the patient. If the airway is placed correctly, chest rise should be visible and breath sounds should be present on auscultation of the lungs during ventilation. If the patient is not breathing or if his or her breathing is inadequate, begin positive pressure ventilation.

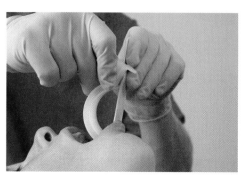

Step 5 Another method of oral airway insertion requires the use of a tongue blade to depress the tongue. If this method is used, the airway is inserted with its tip facing the floor of the patient's mouth (i.e., curved side down). With the use of the tongue blade to depress the tongue, the oral airway is advanced gently into place over the tongue.

Proper oral airway size is important. If the airway is too long, it may press the epiglottis against the entrance of the larynx, which may result in a complete airway obstruction (Figure 2-23). If the airway is too short, it will not displace the tongue, and it may advance out of the mouth (Figure 2-24).

Care during insertion is necessary to ensure that the tongue is not forced farther back in the pharynx, which can result in obstruction. When inserting any device into the airway, never force the device because trauma may result. When inserting an oral airway in pediatric patients, a tongue depressor is recommended to avoid any trauma to the palate.

Although the oral airway is easily inserted and considered noninvasive, it is not without potential complications, which are as follows:

* The insertion of an oral airway in a patient with an intact gag reflex may stimulate vomiting and thus increase the risk of aspiration.

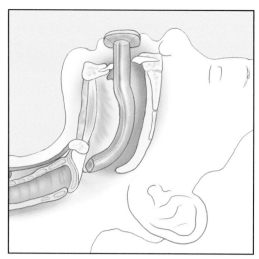

Figure 2-23 If an oral airway is too long, it may press the epiglottis against the entrance of the larynx, resulting in a complete airway obstruction.

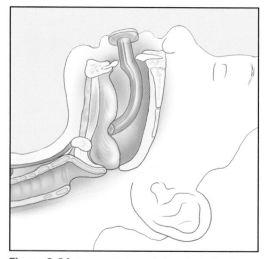

Figure 2-24 If an oral airway is too short, the tongue may be pushed back into the throat resulting in an airway obstruction, or the airway may advance out of the mouth.

- The oral airway does not definitively protect from aspiration. Vigilance on your part is necessary to ensure that the oral airway is keeping the tongue off the posterior pharynx.
- If the patient's gag reflex returns or if he or she spontaneously attempts to displace the airway, remove the airway to minimize the risk of aspiration.

Nasal Airways

[Objective 5]

A nasal airway (also called a *nasopharyngeal airway, NPA,* or *nasal trumpet*) is a soft, uncuffed rubber or plastic tube that is designed to keep the tongue away from the back of the throat. Nasal airways are available in many sizes varying in length and internal diameter (Figures 2-25 and 2-26). Distally, the tube is beveled to help facilitate advancement into the airway. Proximally, the tube takes on a trumpet-shaped appearance that comes to rest on the external surface of the nostril.

A nasal airway is used to help in the maintenance of an airway when the use of an oral airway is contraindicated or when it is difficult to place (e.g., when the patient's jaw is clenched during a seizure, or if oral trauma is present). Indications for the use of a nasal airway include unresponsive patients or those with an altered level of consciousness who continue to have an intact gag reflex but who need assistance with maintaining an open airway.

The determination of the proper nasal airway size is important. A nasal airway that is too long may stimulate the gag reflex; one that is too short may not be inserted far enough to keep the tongue away from the back of the throat. Skill 2-4 explains the steps for insertion of a nasal airway.

As with any device that is inserted into the nose, you must be extremely cautious when working with patients who have sustained any type of facial or head trauma. Such injuries may compromise the bony structures behind the nose and lead to the inadvertent placement of the nasal airway in the cranial vault.[23,24] Patients with known or suspected nasal obstruction or those who are prone to epistaxis (e.g., patients who are receiving anticoagulant therapy) are not acceptable candidates for a nasal airway. Indications, contraindications, sizing, advantages, and disadvantages of oral and nasal airways are shown in Table 2-4.

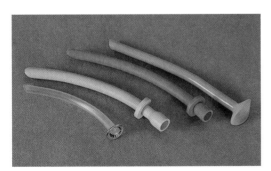

Figure 2-25 Nasal airways are available in many sizes varying in length and internal diameter.

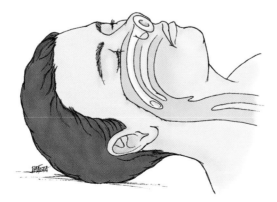

Figure 2-26 A nasal airway in proper position.

SKILL 2-4 **Nasal Airway Insertion**

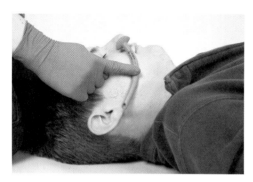

Step 1 Take proper standard precautions. Determine proper airway size by holding the nasal airway against the side of the patient's face. An airway of proper size extends from the tip of the patient's nose to the angle of the jaw or to the tip of the ear.

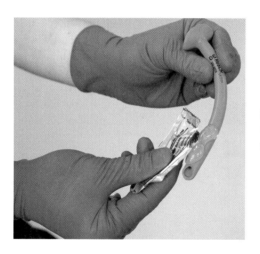

Step 2 Lubricate the distal tip of the device liberally with a water-soluble lubricant to minimize resistance and to decrease the irritation of the nasal passage.

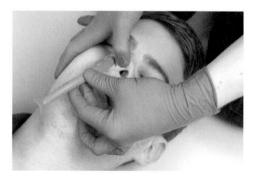

Step 3 Hold the nasal airway at its flange end like a pencil, and slowly insert it into the larger of the patient's two nares, with the bevel pointing toward the nasal septum. The nasal cavity is very vascular. During insertion, do not force the airway, because it may cut or scrape the nasal mucosa; this may result in significant bleeding, which increases the risk of aspiration. Use of a vasoconstricting nasal spray before insertion may facilitate placement. If resistance is encountered, a gentle back-and-forth rotation of the device between your fingers may ease insertion. If resistance continues, withdraw the nasal airway, reapply lubricant, and attempt insertion in the patient's other nostril.

Generally the right nostril is the preferred nostril for nasal airway adjuncts; this is because, in most patients, it is larger and straighter. If the procedure is unsuccessful the left nostril may be used, or a smaller-diameter device may be tried.

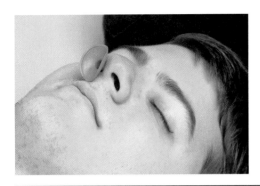

Step 4 Advance the airway along the floor of the nostril, following the natural curvature of the nasal passage until the flange is flush with the nostril. The proper placement of the device is confirmed by ventilating the patient. If the nasal airway is correctly placed, chest rise should be visible, and breath sounds should be present on auscultation of the lungs during ventilation. If the patient is not breathing or if breathing is inadequate, begin positive pressure ventilation.

TABLE 2-4	Oral and Nasal Airways	
Considerations	**Oral Airway**	**Nasal Airway**
Indications	• Helps maintain an open airway in an unresponsive patient who is not intubated • Helps maintain an open airway in an unresponsive patient with no gag reflex who is being ventilated with a bag-mask or other positive pressure device • May be used as a bite block after insertion of a tracheal tube or orogastric tube	• To aid in maintaining an airway when use of an oral airway is contraindicated or difficult to place, such as when the patient's jaw is clenched during a seizure or if oral trauma is present
Contraindications	• Responsive patient	• Severe craniofacial trauma • Patient intolerance
Sizing	• Corner of mouth to tip of earlobe or angle of the jaw	• Tip of nose to angle of the jaw or the tip of the ear
Advantages	• Positions the tongue forward and away from the back of the throat • Easily placed	• Provides a patent airway • Tolerated by responsive patients • Does not require mouth to be open
Disadvantages	• Does not protect the lower airway from aspiration • May produce vomiting if used in a responsive or semi-responsive patient with a gag reflex	• Does not protect the lower airway from aspiration • Improper technique may result in severe bleeding, resulting epistaxis may be difficult to control • Suctioning through the device is difficult • Although tolerated by most responsive and semi-responsive patients, can stimulate the gag reflex in sensitive patients, precipitating vomiting, gagging, or laryngospasm
Precautions	• Use of the device does not eliminate the need for maintaining proper head position	• Use of the device does not eliminate the need for maintaining proper head position

ACLS Pearl

Some nasal airways have a slide at the flange end of the device to adjust for proper length. If present, this slide should *not* be removed. Incidents have occurred during which nasal airways that were improperly sized to be too small and which had their adjustable slides removed were subsequently "sucked" into the patients' lower airways, thus necessitating removal by bronchoscopy.

TECHNIQUES OF POSITIVE PRESSURE VENTILATION

[Objective 6]

Adequate oxygenation requires an open airway *and* adequate air exchange. After the airway has been opened, determine if the patient's breathing is adequate or inadequate. If respiratory efforts are inadequate, the patient's breathing may be assisted by forcing air into the lungs (i.e., delivering positive pressure ventilations). Mouth-to-mouth, mouth-to-mask, and bag-mask ventilation are methods that may be used to deliver positive pressure ventilation.

Mouth-to-Mouth Ventilation

Mouth-to-mouth ventilation is a basic method for providing positive pressure ventilation to apneic patients, and it requires no special equipment to perform. Mouth-to-mouth ventilation is capable of delivering excellent tidal volumes. Because expired air from the lungs contains approximately 16% oxygen, it will also deliver an adequate level of oxygen to the patient.

To provide mouth-to-mouth ventilation, open the victim's airway, pinch the victim's nose, place your mouth over the victim's mouth and create an airtight seal. Give two breaths, with each breath given over the course of 1 second, and give enough air to make the victim's chest visibly rise. Take a regular breath before ventilating the victim. Taking deep breaths is unnecessary and may cause hyperventilation. If you experience difficulty when ventilating the victim (e.g., his or her chest does not rise with the first rescue breath), reposition the head and lift the chin, because an improperly opened airway is the most common cause of an inability to ventilate. If the victim has a mouth injury, if the mouth cannot be opened, or if you have difficulty maintaining a good seal, mouth-to-nose ventilation can be performed.

Although it has been said that the risk of disease transmission with mouth-to-mouth ventilation is very low,[25] in this day of heightened awareness of communicable diseases, an issue of concern with the use of this ventilation method is direct contact with oral secretions, possibly including blood. The U.S. Occupational Safety and Health Administration (OSHA) requires that healthcare professionals use standard precautions (such as a barrier device, pocket face mask, or bag-mask device) in the workplace, including during CPR.

Mouth-to-Barrier Device Ventilation

[Objective 6]

A barrier device is a thin film of material, usually plastic or silicone, that is placed on the patient's face and used to prevent direct contact with the patient's mouth during positive pressure ventilation. One common type of barrier device is a face shield. Face shields are compact and portable; they are sometimes equipped with a short tube (i.e., 1 to 2 inches) that is inserted into the patient's mouth. A one-way valve or filter is present in the center of most face shields to divert the patient's exhaled air away from you when you lift your mouth off of the shield between breaths, thereby reducing the risk of infection. Skill 2-5 shows the steps for mouth-to-barrier device ventilation.

Keeping It Simple

Regardless of the method used, effective positive pressure ventilation requires the delivery of an adequate volume of air at an appropriate rate.

Mouth-to-Mask Ventilation

[Objective 6]

The device used for mouth-to-mask ventilation is commonly called a **pocket face mask, ventilation face mask,** or **resuscitation mask** (Box 2-7). A pocket face mask is a clear, semirigid mask that is sealed around the mouth and nose of an adult, child, or infant. Masks used for ventilation should have the following characteristics:

SKILL 2-5 | Mouth-to-Barrier Device Ventilation

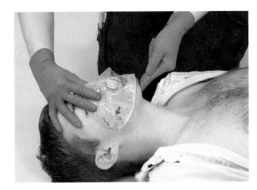

Step 1 Put on appropriate personal protective equipment. Open the patient's airway and place the barrier device over the patient's mouth.

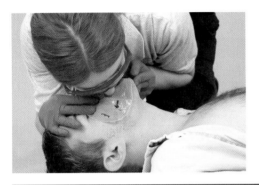

Step 2 Place your mouth over the mouthpiece of the barrier device. Take a normal breath and then breathe into the device with enough force to cause the patient's chest to rise gently.

BOX 2-7 | Mouth-to-Mask Ventilation

Inspired Oxygen Concentration
- Without supplemental oxygen equals about 16% to 17% (exhaled air)
- Mouth-to-mask breathing combined with supplemental oxygen at a minimum flow rate of 10 L/min equals about 50%

Advantages
- Aesthetically more acceptable than mouth-to-mouth ventilation
- Easy to teach and learn
- Physical barrier between the rescuer and the patient's nose, mouth, and secretions
- Reduces (but does not prevent) the risk of exposure to infectious diseases
- Use of a one-way valve at the ventilation port decreases exposure to the patient's exhaled air
- If the patient resumes spontaneous breathing, the mask can be used as a simple face mask to deliver 40% to 60% oxygen by giving supplemental oxygen through the oxygen inlet on the mask (if so equipped)
- Can deliver a greater tidal volume as compared with a bag-mask device
- Rescuer can feel the compliance of the patient's lungs (compliance refers to the resistance of the patient's lung tissue to ventilation)

Disadvantages
- Rescuer fatigue
- Possible gastric distention

- Made of transparent material to allow assessment of the patient's lip color and detection of vomitus, secretions, or other substances.
- Capable of a tight seal on the face, covering the mouth and nose.
- Fitted with a standard 15-/22-mm connector that enables connection to a bag-mask (or other ventilation) device.
- Available in one average size for adults, with additional sizes for infants and children.
- Fitted with an oxygen (insufflation) inlet to allow the delivery of increased oxygen concentrations to the patient.

The selection of a mask of proper size is necessary to ensure a good seal between the patient's face and the mask. A mask of correct size should extend from the bridge of the nose to the groove between the lower lip and chin. If the mask is not properly positioned and a tight seal maintained, air will leak from between the mask and the patient's face, thereby resulting in the delivery of less tidal volume delivery to the patient. Less tidal volume results in less lung inflation, which means less oxygenation. If you do not have a mask of the proper size available, use a larger mask, and turn it upside down. Remember that adequate ventilation is present if you ventilate with just enough volume to see gentle chest rise. Skill 2-6 shows the steps necessary to perform mouth-to-mask ventilation.

> ### ACLS Pearl
> Gastric distention is a complication of positive pressure ventilation that can lead to vomiting and subsequent aspiration. Gastric distention also restricts movement of the diaphragm, impeding ventilation, and decreases the effectiveness of cardiopulmonary resuscitation (CPR) if the patient is in cardiac arrest.

> ### ACLS Pearl
> If a good seal is maintained between the patient's mouth and the mask, you can deliver a greater tidal volume to the patient with mouth-to-mask ventilation than with a bag-mask device because both of your hands can be used to secure the mask in place while simultaneously maintaining proper head position. Your vital capacity can also compensate for leaks between the mask and the patient's face, thereby resulting in greater lung ventilation.

SKILL 2-6 | Mouth-to-Mask Ventilation

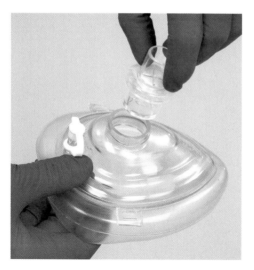

Step 1 Put on appropriate personal protective equipment. Connect a one-way valve to the ventilation port on the mask. If an oxygen inlet is present on the mask and oxygen is available, connect oxygen tubing to the oxygen inlet and set the flow rate at 10 to 12 L/min.

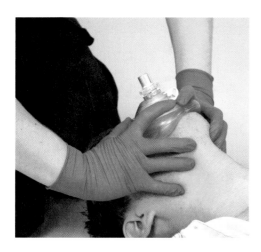

Step 2 Position yourself at the patient's head or side. Positioning yourself directly above the patient's head allows you to watch the patient's chest while delivering ventilations. This position is used if the patient is in respiratory arrest (but not cardiac arrest) or when two-rescuer CPR is being performed. If you are by yourself, positioning yourself at the patient's side allows you to maintain the same position for both rescue breathing and chest compressions.

Open the patient's airway. If needed, clear the patient's airway of secretions or vomitus. If the patient is unresponsive, insert an oral airway. Select a mask of appropriate size and place it on the patient's face. Apply the narrow portion (apex) of the mask over the bridge of the patient's nose and stabilize it in place with your thumbs. Lower the mask over the patient's face and mouth. Use your index fingers to stabilize the wide end (base) of the mask over the groove between the patient's lower lip and chin. When in proper position, your thumb and index finger create a C. Use your remaining fingers to maintain proper head position. Your remaining fingers create an E.

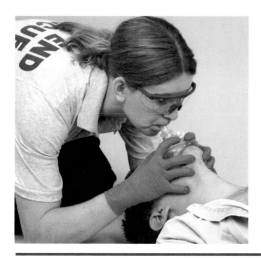

Step 3 Ventilate the lungs through the one-way valve on the top of the mask at an age-appropriate rate. Give each breath over 1 second, and watch for gentle chest rise. Stop ventilation when adequate chest rise is observed. Allow the patient to exhale between breaths. Adequate ventilation is being provided if you see the chest rise and fall gently with each breath and if you hear and feel air escape during exhalation.

Bag-Mask Ventilation

[Objective 6]

A bag-mask device consists of a self-inflating bag; a nonrebreathing valve with an adapter that can be attached to a mask, a tracheal tube, or another invasive airway device; and an oxygen inlet valve (Figure 2-27). A bag-mask device may also be referred to as a *bag-mask, bag-valve-mask device*, or as *bag-mask resuscitator* (when the mask is used), or as a *bag-valve device* (when the mask is not used, i.e., when ventilating a patient with a tracheal tube or tracheostomy tube in place). The bag-mask device should have the following features[25]:

- A nonjam inlet valve
- Either no pop-off valve (pressure-release valve) or a pop-off valve that can be bypassed during resuscitation
- Standard 15-/22-mm fittings to allow for attachment of the device to a standard mask, tracheal tube, or other ventilation device
- An oxygen reservoir to allow delivery of high concentrations of oxygen

- A nonrebreathing outlet valve that cannot be obstructed by foreign material and will not jam with an oxygen flow of 30 L/min
- Capability to perform satisfactorily under common environmental conditions and temperature extremes

Oxygen Delivery
[Objective 7]

When using a bag-mask device, the amount of delivered O_2 is dependent on the ventilatory rate, the volume delivered during each breath, the O_2 flow rate into the ventilating bag, the filling time for the reservoir bag, and the type of reservoir used.[26] Delivered tidal volumes vary with bag type, hand size, and patient body characteristics.[27]

A bag-mask device that is used without supplemental oxygen will deliver 21% oxygen (i.e., room air) to the patient (Figure 2-28). The bag-mask device should be connected to an oxygen source. To do this, attach one end of a piece of oxygen connecting tubing to the oxygen inlet on the bag-mask device and the other end to an oxygen regulator. A bag-mask that is used with supplemental oxygen set at a flow rate of 10 to 15 L/min delivers about 40% to 60% oxygen to the patient when an oxygen collection device (i.e., reservoir) is not used (Figure 2-29).

Ideally, an oxygen reservoir should be attached to the bag-mask to deliver a high concentration of oxygen. The reservoir collects a volume of 100% oxygen that is equal to the capacity of the bag. After the bag is squeezed, it re-expands and draws in 100% oxygen from the reservoir into the bag. A bag-mask device that is used with supplemental oxygen set at a flow rate of 10 to 15 L/min and with an attached reservoir delivers about 90% to 100% oxygen to the patient (Figure 2-30). Advantages and disadvantages of bag-mask ventilation are shown in Box 2-8.

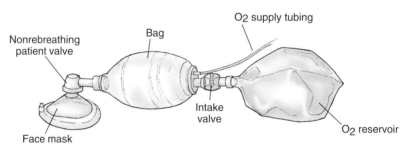

Figure 2-27 Components of a bag-mask device.

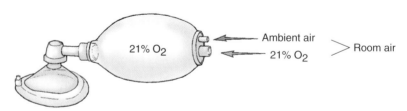

Figure 2-28 A bag-mask used without supplemental oxygen will deliver 21% oxygen (room air).

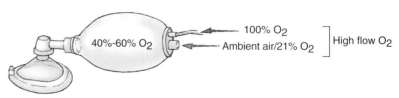

Figure 2-29 A bag-mask used with supplemental oxygen set at a flow rate of 15 L/min will deliver approximately 40% to 60% oxygen to the patient.

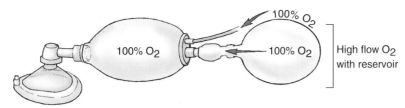

Figure 2-30 A bag-mask used with supplemental oxygen set at a flow rate of 15 L/min and a reservoir will deliver approximately 90% to 100% oxygen to the patient.

BOX 2-8   Bag-Mask Ventilation

Advantages
- Provides a means for delivery of an oxygen enriched mixture to the patient
- Conveys a sense of compliance of the patient's lungs to the bag-mask device operator
- Provides a means for immediate ventilatory support
- Can be used with the spontaneously breathing patient as well as with the nonbreathing patient

Disadvantages
- Requires practice to be used effectively
- Delivers inadequate tidal volume
- Causes rescuer fatigue
- Leads to possible gastric distention

Bag-Mask Ventilation
[Objective 8]

Performing positive pressure ventilation with a bag-mask device can be quite difficult. Risk factors for difficult mask ventilation are listed in Box 2-9. Several reasons contribute to this, but none as much as the inability to create a good seal with the mask while simultaneously generating an adequate tidal volume by squeezing the bag. Thus as a lone rescuer, mastering the technique of bag-mask ventilation may be difficult.

BOX 2-9   Risk Factors for Difficult Mask Ventilation[28-30]

- Age older than 55 years
- Body mass index of more than 26 kg/m^2
- Edentulousness (i.e., absence of natural teeth)
- History of snoring
- Limited protrusion of the lower jaw
- Presence of a beard

YOU SHOULD KNOW   Current resuscitation guidelines do not recommend bag-mask ventilation by a single rescuer during CPR. Instead, the single rescuer is encouraged to use the mouth-to-mouth or mouth-to-mask methods of ventilation because they are more efficient.[18]

Bag-mask ventilation should be a two-rescuer operation. With two people, one is assigned the responsibility of opening and maintaining the airway while creating a good seal with the mask. That frees a second person to squeeze the bag, thereby ensuring the delivery of an adequate tidal volume. As with any form of positive pressure ventilation, you must remain cognizant of not causing gastric distention or hyperinflation of the lungs. Skill 2-7 shows the steps for bag-mask ventilation. Keep in mind that this sequence of steps illustrates only one of many possible methods of ensuring an adequate seal between a patient's face and a mask.

ACLS Pearl

If an adult has a pulse but requires ventilatory support, provide positive pressure ventilation and deliver 1 breath every 5 to 6 seconds (i.e., about 10-12 breaths/min). Each ventilation should be given over 1 second and deliver a tidal volume of about 600 mL (a volume that is usually adequate to cause visible chest rise).[25]

| SKILL 2-7 | Bag-Mask Ventilation |

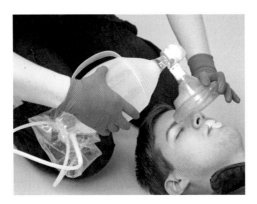

Step 1 Put on personal protective equipment and position yourself at the top of the supine patient's head. Open the patient's airway. If needed, clear the patient's airway of secretions or vomitus. If the patient is unresponsive, insert an oral airway.

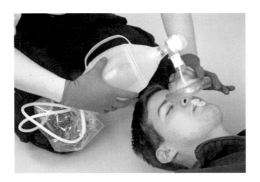

Step 2 Select a mask of appropriate size for the patient. Connect the bag to the mask if this has not already been done. Connect the bag to oxygen at a flow rate of 15 L/min and attach a reservoir.

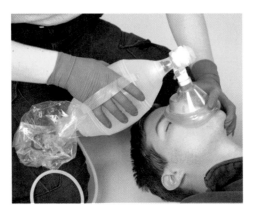

Step 3 Place the mask on the patient's face. Apply the narrow portion (apex) of the mask over the bridge of the patient's nose and the wide end (base) of the mask over the groove between the patient's lower lip and chin. If the mask has a large, round cuff that surrounds the ventilation port, center the port over the patient's mouth. Create a good seal using the *E and C* techniques described previously with the mask seated over the patient's mouth and nose. The *E* serves to control the lower jaw with the small, ring, and middle fingers, and the thumb and index finger serve to create a *C* on the mask itself.

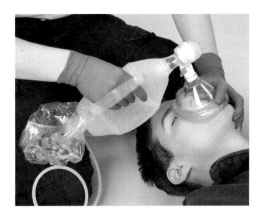

Step 4 Although single-rescuer bag-mask ventilation is not recommended during CPR, if you find yourself in this situation, press the mask firmly against the patient's face with one hand (and simultaneously use it to maintain the patient's proper head position) and then squeeze the bag with the other hand. Alternatively, use a pocket face mask with an oxygen inlet that is attached to oxygen, and perform mouth-to-mask ventilation.

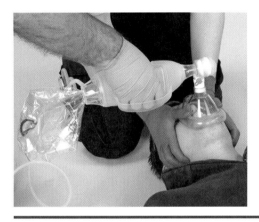

Step 5 If you have an assistant available, ask him or her to squeeze the bag until the patient's chest rises while you press the mask firmly against the patient's face with both hands and simultaneously maintain the patient's proper head position. Observe the rise and fall of the patient's chest with each ventilation. Stop ventilations when you see gentle chest rise. Allow for adequate exhalation after each ventilation. Ventilate the patient at an age-appropriate rate.

Troubleshooting Bag-Mask Ventilation
[Objective 9]

During bag-mask ventilation, remember to avoid overinflation and to allow adequate time for exhalation to occur. Also, while ventilating, feel for compliance when ventilating the patient's lungs. The lungs are normally pliable and expand easily. If the lungs feel stiff or inflexible, lung compliance is said to be poor. Upper airway obstruction, lower airway obstruction, severe bronchospasm, and tension pneumothorax are examples of conditions that can cause poor lung compliance and an inability to ventilate. If at any time you sense poor compliance, reassess the patient to ensure that the airway remains unobstructed and that lung sounds are clear and equal. Another indication that the patient is being well ventilated is an improvement of the patient's condition as evidenced by improvements in color, pulse oximeter readings, and responsiveness.

The most frequent problems with bag-mask ventilation are the inability to deliver adequate ventilatory volumes and gastric inflation. The delivery of an inadequate ventilatory volume may be the result of difficulty with providing a leak-proof seal to the face while simultaneously maintaining an open airway, incomplete bag compression, or both. Gastric inflation may result if excessive force and volume are used during ventilation.

If the chest does not rise and fall with bag-mask ventilation, reassess the patient in the following manner:

- Begin by reassessing the patient's head position. Reposition the airway and try to ventilate again.
- Inadequate tidal volume delivery may be the result of an improper mask seal or incomplete bag compression. If air is escaping from under the mask, reposition your fingers and the mask, and reevaluate the effectiveness of bag compression.
- Check for an airway obstruction. Lift the jaw and suction the airway as needed. If the chest still does not rise, select an alternative method of positive pressure ventilation.

> **ACLS Pearl**
>
> The presence of a beard can interfere with sealing the mask to the patient's face, presenting a challenge to effective mask ventilation. Some experts have noted that the use of a water-soluble lubricant liberally applied to the mask area in contact with the beard surprisingly gives a much better seal in these patients.[27]

Cricoid Pressure

With the use of magnetic resonance imaging, a 2009 study demonstrated that the laryngopharynx is the structure that lies behind the cricoid ring and is compressed by cricoid pressure (this is also called the *Sellick maneuver*).[31] The distal laryngopharynx, which is the portion of the alimentary canal at the cricoid level, is fixed with respect to the cricoid ring and not mobile. In this study, the mean antero-posterior diameter of the laryngopharynx was reduced by 35% with cricoid pressure and the lumen was likely obliterated (see Figure 2-31).

Studies suggest that cricoid pressure is frequently applied incorrectly. In some studies participants applied too little pressure, which placed patients at risk of regurgitation; in other studies, excessive pressure was used.[32-37]

Although some studies have not found cricoid pressure to cause a barrier to advanced airway insertion,[38] most have shown that cricoid pressure impedes placement, impairs the rate of successful ventilation, and hinders ventilation.[25,39-42] Aspiration can occur despite the application of pressure. The use of cricoid pressure in adult cardiac arrest is not recommended.[18,25] If the decision is made to use cricoid pressure during cardiac arrest, the pressure should be adjusted, relaxed, or released if it impedes ventilation or advanced airway placement.[18]

Complications of cricoid pressure include laryngeal trauma when excessive force is applied and esophageal rupture from unrelieved high gastric pressures. Excessive pressure may obstruct the trachea in small children.

ADVANCED AIRWAYS

[Objective 10]

Advanced airways include the esophageal-tracheal Combitube (ETC), the King laryngeal tube airway, the laryngeal mask airway (LMA), and the tracheal tube. The Combitube, the King laryngeal tube, and the LMA may be used in areas where tracheal intubation is not permitted, or in communities in which healthcare providers have little opportunity to obtain experience with the technique of orotracheal intubation as a result of having few patients. They may also be used by anesthesiologists for short, low-risk procedures.

Advanced airway insertion requires a high degree of skill and knowledge as well as regular practice to maintain proficiency. Regular practice, continuing education programs, and an effective quality management program to monitor skill performance are essential for all healthcare professionals who perform this skill. Although the techniques used for the insertion of advanced airways is beyond the

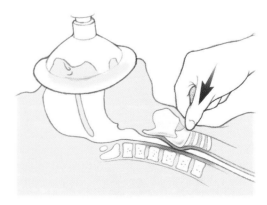

Figure 2-31 Cricoid pressure is applied by applying firm pressure to the cricoid cartilage with the thumb and index finger, just lateral to the midline.

scope of this text and the Advanced Cardiac Life Support (ACLS) course, a short description of the types of advanced airways, equipment needed for their insertion, and methods of confirming their placement is provided below.

The Esophageal-Tracheal Combitube[1]

The esophageal-tracheal Combitube, which is commonly called the Combitube, allows for the ventilation of the lungs and it reduces the risk of the aspiration of the gastric contents. It does not require the visualization of the vocal cords (i.e., blind insertion) to ventilate the trachea. The Combitube is available in 41- and 37-French (Fr) diameter sizes. The 37-Fr size is used for patients who are between 4 and 5 feet tall and the 41-Fr size is used for patients more than 5 feet tall. Healthcare professionals who have been trained to use a Combitube can use it as an acceptable alternative to bag-mask ventilation or a tracheal tube for airway management during cardiac arrest.[18]

The Combitube is called a *dual-lumen airway* because two separate tubes have been joined together with separate airflow passages. An examination of the tube reveals several key features (Figure 2-32). Proximally, there are two tubes with universal adapters; one is longer, blue, and clearly labeled "#1"; the second tube is shorter, clear, and labeled "#2." Each tube has a pilot balloon labeled #1 or #2 that contains the corresponding amount of air that is inserted to fill one of two cuffs. As you progress toward the distal end of the tube, you will see an area that has two solid black rings encircling the device. The black rings become important that indicate the proper depth of tube insertion when the teeth and gum line are located between the black lines. Near the center of the tube is a large latex cuff encircling the device called the *pharyngeal cuff*. When inflated, this cuff anchors the Combitube in place, and it occludes the nasopharynx and the oropharynx; this prevents air leaks once the device is properly placed. Toward the distal tip of the tube, a second cuff accomplishes one of two functions. The first function is the occlusion of the esophagus (in most cases) to prevent gastric insufflation and to minimize the risk of aspiration. Second, if the tube is blindly placed in the trachea, this cuff protects and isolates the lower airway as a tracheal tube does (Figure 2-33). Between the cuffs on one side of the tube you will note several small holes. These holes facilitate the passage of air into and out of the lungs with an esophageal placement of the Combitube.

Combitube kits also come with a large syringe that is capable of inflating the pharyngeal cuff, a smaller syringe that is used to inflate the distal cuff, a flexible suction catheter, and an emesis deflection elbow. The pharyngeal cuff on the small adult tube (37 Fr) is inflated with 80 mL of air, whereas the pharyngeal cuff on the large adult tube (41 Fr) is inflated with 100 mL of air. The distal cuff is inflated with 15 mL of air on both tubes.

After the insertion of the Combitube, the patient is initially ventilated through the longer blue tube (Figure 2-34). Confirm placement by assessing for chest rise, the presence of bilateral breath sounds, and the absence of gastric sounds, and the use of waveform capnography. In addition, assess placement by monitoring for adequate SpO_2 levels. If chest rise and bilateral breath sounds are present, then the tube is in the esophagus. Continue to ventilate the patient through the blue tube. Secure the tube in place with a commercial tube holder or tape.

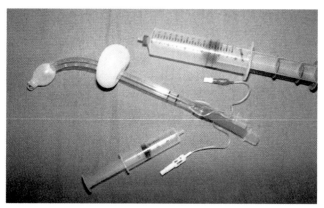

Figure 2-32 The esophageal-tracheal Combitube.

> **ACLS** Pearl
>
> Measure exhaled carbon dioxide through the tube that is used for ventilation. Because the stomach may house residual carbon dioxide from the esophageal ventilation of expired air into the stomach during bag-mask ventilation, ventilate the patient between 6 and 12 times before relying on capnography to confirm proper tube position.

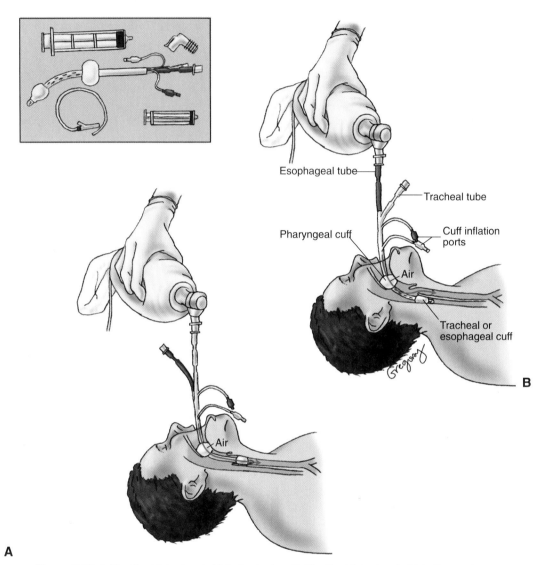

Esophageal tube

Tracheal tube

Pharyngeal cuff

Cuff inflation ports

Air

Tracheal or esophageal cuff

A

B

Figure 2-33 A, The Combitube inserted into the trachea. **B,** The Combitube inserted into the esophagus.

Figure 2-34 After the insertion of the Combitube, the patient is initially ventilated through the longer blue tube.

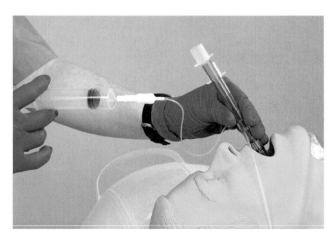

If there is no chest rise or if bilateral breath sounds are absent, place the bag-valve device on the clear tube, and ventilate the patient. Reassess for placement. If chest rise and bilateral breath sounds are present, then the tube is in the trachea. Confirm placement by assessing for adequate chest rise, the presence of bilateral breath sounds, the absence of gastric sounds, and the use of waveform capnography. If the patient has a perfusing rhythm, also assess for adequate SpO_2 levels. Secure the device in place after confirming appropriate placement.

If your assessment of the patient reveals that breath sounds *and* epigastric sounds are both absent, immediately deflate the cuffs (blue first). Slightly withdraw the tube and then reinflate the cuffs (blue first). Ventilate the patient and reassess tube placement. If breath sounds and epigastric sounds are still absent, immediately deflate the cuffs and remove the tube. Suction as necessary, insert an oral or nasal airway, ventilate the patient with a bag-mask device, and reassess. Indications, contraindications, advantages, and disadvantages of Combitubes are shown in Box 2-10.

The King Laryngeal Tube Airway[1]

The King LT-D airway is a single lumen supraglottic airway device. It consists of a curved tube with a proximal cuff and a distal cuff. Along the tube is an orientation/radiograph line that is used when inserting the device and for locating the device on a radiograph. The proximal cuff occludes the oropharynx, whereas the distal tube occludes the esophagus. Both cuffs are inflated with the use of a single pilot balloon. Unlike dual lumen devices, this device is designed to be placed in the esophagus only. Therefore, you must ensure that there is not inadvertent tracheal placement. Ventilations are delivered via a bag-valve device attached to the proximal end of the tube and air escapes through holes in the tube that are located between the two cuffs. An alternate version of the King LT-D airway, the King LTS-D, allows for the passage of a flexible suction catheter for gastric decompression. The same principles apply as described for the Combitube. Healthcare professionals who have been trained to use a laryngeal tube can use the device as an acceptable alternative to bag-mask ventilation or a tracheal tube for airway management in cardiac arrest.[18]

The insertion of the device begins with selection of the appropriate size. The King airway devices are available in three adult sizes and two sizes for children (Figure 2-35). Size 3 is for patients who

---

BOX 2-10 Combitube

Indications
- Difficult face mask fit (beards, absence of teeth)
- Patient in whom intubation has been unsuccessful and ventilation is difficult
- Patient in whom airway management is necessary but the healthcare provider is untrained in the technique of visualized orotracheal intubation

Contraindications
- Patient with an intact gag reflex
- Patient with known or suspected esophageal disease
- Patient known to have ingested a caustic substance
- Suspected upper airway obstruction due to laryngeal foreign body or pathology
- Patient shorter than 4 feet tall

Advantages
- Minimal training and retraining is required
- Visualization of the upper airway or use of special equipment is not required for insertion
- Reasonable technique for use in suspected neck injury because the head does not need to be hyperextended
- Because of the oropharyngeal balloon, the need for a face mask is eliminated
- Can provide adequate ventilation with either esophageal or tracheal placement
- If placed in the esophagus, allows suctioning of gastric contents without interruption of ventilation
- Reduces risk of aspiration of gastric contents

Disadvantages
- Proximal port may be occluded with secretions
- Proper identification of tube location may be difficult, leading to ventilation through the wrong lumen
- Soft tissue trauma may be caused by rigidity of tube
- Impossible to suction the trachea when the tube is in the esophagus
- Esophageal or tracheal trauma due to poor insertion technique or use of wrong size device
- Damage to the cuffs by the patient's teeth during insertion
- Inability to insert because of limited mouth opening

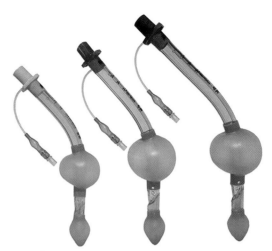

Figure 2-35 The King laryngeal tube airway.

are between 4 and 5 feet tall, and the cuffs are inflated with 45 to 60 mL of air. Size 4 is for patients who are between 5 and 6 feet tall, and the cuffs are inflated with 60 to 80 mL of air. Finally, size 5 is for patients who are more than 6 feet tall, and the cuffs are inflated with 70 to 90 mL of air.

Before the insertion of the device, test the cuffs for integrity, remove all of the air, and lubricate the tube. Lubricate only the posterior side of the device so that the lubricant does not clog the holes from which air escapes. After the King airway has been inserted and the cuffs are inflated, ventilate the lungs while gently withdrawing the device to achieve minimal ventilation pressures. Continue attempts to ventilate while pulling the tube gently and slowly out of the mouth. You will observe chest rise when the tube slides into place. Confirm placement by evaluating for chest rise, determining the presence of bilateral breath sounds, assessing the levels of expired carbon choxide, and, if the patient has a perfusing rhythm, Spo_2 levels. After confirming appropriate placement, secure the tube in place and consider the placement of a bite block. If the tube was placed incorrectly and air did not enter the lungs, the tube must be removed and the patient ventilated with an oral airway and a bag-mask device. Indications, contraindications, advantages, and disadvantages of the King Laryngeal Tube Airway are shown in Box 2-11.

BOX 2-11 **King Laryngeal Tube Airway**

Indications
- Unconscious patient
- Patient with an absent gag reflex
- Failure of less invasive airway measures
- Inability to intubate when airway protection is needed

Advantages
- Minimal training and retraining required
- Visualization of the upper airway or use of special equipment not required for insertion
- More compact than the Combitube
- Proximal cuff seals the oropharynx allowing ventilation to take place via the airway openings that lie between the cuffs; distal cuff is designed to seal off the esophagus
- S-shaped design decreases the likelihood of tracheal intubation
- Ability to place suction tube to prevent or relieve gastric distention
- May be less technically difficult to use and determine correct placement than other advanced airways

Contraindications
- Patient with an intact gag reflex
- Patient with known or suspected esophageal disease
- Patient known to have ingested a caustic substance
- Patient with injury to the throat or neck

Disadvantages
- Proximal port may be occluded with secretions
- Soft tissue trauma due to rigidity of tube
- Esophageal or tracheal trauma due to poor insertion technique or use of wrong size device
- Damage to the cuffs by the patient's teeth during insertion

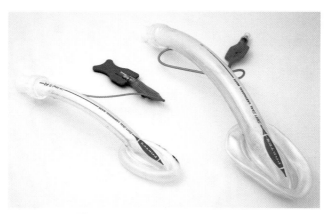

Figure 2-36 Laryngeal mask airways.

The Laryngeal Mask Airway

The LMA may be used as an alternative to a tracheal tube or face mask with either spontaneous or positive pressure ventilation. Healthcare professionals who have been trained to use an LMA can use it as an acceptable alternative to bag-mask ventilation or a tracheal tube for airway management of the patient who is in cardiac arrest.[18]

Because of the relative ease of learning how to use the device, healthcare personnel who work in an emergency setting and are not trained in tracheal intubation can be taught to use the LMA. The LMA may be used as the primary airway, as a channel for a tracheal tube, or as an option for the management of a difficult airway when intubation is unsuccessful.

An LMA consists of a tube that is fused to an elliptical, spoon-shaped mask at a 30-degree angle (Figure 2-36). When inserted, the tube protrudes from the patient's mouth, and it is connected to a ventilation device via a standard connector with a 15-mm inside diameter. The mask resembles a miniature facemask and it has an inflatable rim that is filled with air from a syringe using a pilot valve-balloon system. The tube opens into the middle of the mask by means of three vertical slits that prevent the tip of the epiglottis from falling back and blocking the lumen of the tube.

The LMA is inserted through the mouth and into the pharynx (Figure 2-37). The device is advanced until resistance is felt. The mask is then inflated, and this provides a low-pressure seal around the laryngeal inlet. The inflatable LMA cuff does *not* ensure an airtight seal to protect the lower airway from aspiration.

The posterior aspect of the tube is marked with a longitudinal black line. When the LMA is correctly placed, the black line on the tube should rest in the midline against the patient's upper lip. Confirm placement by evaluating for chest rise, confirming the presence of bilateral breath sounds, assessment of waveform capnography, and, if the patient has a perfusing rhythm, SpO_2 levels. After proper LMA placement has been confirmed, secure the device in place.

Indications, contraindications, advantages, and disadvantages of LMAs are shown in Box 2-12. LMA size recommendations based on weight are shown in Table 2-5.

Tracheal Intubation[1]

Tracheal intubation is an advanced airway procedure in which a tube is placed directly into the trachea. It may be performed for a variety of reasons, including for the delivery of anesthesia, to assist a patient's breathing with positive pressure ventilation, and to protect the patient's airway from aspiration. Intubation requires special training equipment and supplies (Box 2-13).

A laryngoscope is an instrument that consists of a handle and blade that is used for examining the interior of the larynx and for visualizing the glottic opening (i.e., the space between the vocal cords). A standard laryngoscope is made of plastic or stainless steel. The laryngoscope handle contains the batteries for the light source. It attaches to a plastic or stainless steel blade that has a bulb located in the blade's distal tip. The point at which the handle and the blade attach to make electrical contact is called the *fitting*. The bulb on the laryngoscope blade lights up when the blade is attached to the laryngoscope handle and elevated to a right angle (Figure 2-38).

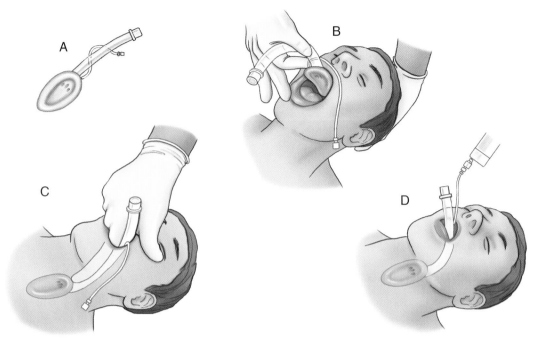

Figure 2-37 A, A laryngeal mask airway (LMA) with the cuff inflated. **B,** LMA placement into the pharynx. **C,** LMA placement using the index finger as a guide. **D,** LMA in place with cuff overlying pharynx.

BOX 2-12   Laryngeal Mask Airway

Indications
- Difficult face mask fit (beards, absence of teeth)
- Patient in whom intubation has been unsuccessful and ventilation is difficult
- Patient in whom airway management is necessary but the healthcare provider is untrained in the technique of visualized orotracheal intubation
- Many elective surgical procedures with relatively short periods of anesthesia

Contraindications
- Healthcare provider untrained in use of laryngeal mask airway
- Contraindicated if a risk of aspiration exists (i.e., patients with full stomachs)

Advantages
- Can be quickly inserted to provide ventilation when bag-mask ventilation is not sufficient and tracheal intubation cannot be readily accomplished
- Tidal volume delivered may be greater than with face mask ventilation
- Less gastric insufflation occurs than with bag-mask ventilation
- Provides ventilation equivalent to the tracheal tube
- Training simpler than with tracheal intubation
- Unaffected by anatomic factors (e.g., beard, absence of teeth)
- No risk of esophageal or bronchial intubation exists
- When compared with tracheal intubation, poses less potential for trauma from direct laryngoscopy and tracheal intubation
- Less coughing, laryngeal spasm, sore throat, and voice changes than with tracheal intubation

Disadvantages
- Does not provide protection against aspiration
- Cannot be used if the mouth cannot be opened more than 0.6 in (1.5 cm)
- May not be effective when respiratory anatomy is abnormal (i.e., abnormal oropharyngeal anatomy or the presence of pathology is likely to result in a poor mask fit)
- May be difficult to provide adequate ventilation if high airway pressures are required

TABLE 2-5	Laryngeal Mask Airway (LMA), Disposable LMA (LMA Unique), and Intubating LMA Size Recommendation Based on Weight		
Weight	**LMA**	**Disposable LMA**	**Intubating LMA**
Less than 5 kg	1	1	—
5-10 kg	1.5	1.5	—
10-20 kg	2	2	—
20-30 kg	2.5	2.5	—
30-50 kg	3	3	3
50-70 kg	4	4	4
70-100 kg	5	5	5
More than 100 kg	6	—	—

Modified from Vrocher D, Hopson LR: Basic airway management and decision-making. In Roberts JR, Hedges JR editors: *Clinical Procedures in Emergency Medicine,* 4th ed, 2004, Philadelphia, Saunders. p. 63.

BOX 2-13	Tracheal Intubation–Equipment and Supplies

- 10-mL syringe for inflation of the tracheal tube cuff (if present)
- Bag-mask device with supplemental oxygen and reservoir
- Bite-block or oral airway
- Commercial tube-holder or tape
- Extra batteries
- Laryngoscope blades
- Laryngoscope handle
- Suction equipment
- Stylet
- Tracheal tubes of various sizes
- Water-soluble lubricant
- Waveform capnography, exhaled CO_2 detector, esophageal detector device

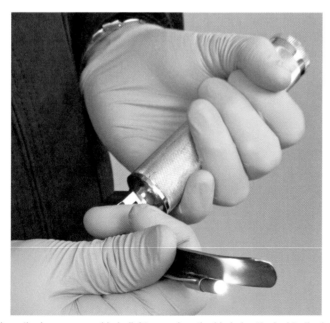

Figure 2-38 The bulb on the laryngoscope blade lights up when the blade is attached to the laryngoscope handle and elevated to a right angle.

Laryngoscope blades are available in a variety of sizes that range from 0 to 4. Size 0 is used for infants and size 4 blade is used for large adults. Select the appropriate blade size with the laryngoscope blade held next to the patient's face. A blade of proper size should reach between the patient's lips and larynx. If you are unsure about the correct size, it is usually best to select a blade that is too long, rather than too short.

There are two types of laryngoscope blades: straight and curved (Figure 2-39). The straight blade is also referred to as the **Miller**, **Wisconsin**, or **Flagg** blade. During tracheal intubation, the tip of the straight blade is positioned under the epiglottis. When the laryngoscope handle is lifted anteriorly, the blade directly lifts the epiglottis out of the way to expose the glottic opening. The curved blade is also called the Macintosh blade. The tip of the curved blade is inserted into the vallecula. When the laryngoscope handle is lifted anteriorly, the blade elevates the tongue and indirectly lifts the epiglottis, thereby allowing for the visualization of the glottic opening.

A tracheal tube is a curved tube that is open at both ends (Figure 2-40). A standard 15-mm connector is located at the proximal end for the attachment of various devices for the delivery of positive pressure ventilation. The distal end of the tube is beveled to facilitate placement between the vocal cords. In addition to the opening on the distal tip of the tube, an additional hole is located near the tube's end; this is called the *Murphy eye*. If the tip of the tube becomes occluded, this feature allows for continued airflow through the tube. Water-soluble lubricant applied to the distal tip of the tracheal tube promotes ease of passage during intubation and decreases the possibility of trauma. A petroleum-based lubricant should never be used because it may damage the tube and cause tracheal inflammation.

> **ACLS Pearl**
>
> A tracheal intubation attempt should not take more than 30 seconds. The 30-second time interval begins when ventilation of the patient ceases, to allow for the insertion of the laryngoscope blade into the patient's mouth, and it ends when the patient is ventilated upon placement of the tracheal tube.

Some tracheal tubes have an inflatable balloon cuff that surrounds the distal tip of the tube. When the distal cuff is inflated, it makes contact with the wall of the trachea as it expands, thereby sealing off the trachea from the remainder of the pharynx and reducing the risk of aspiration. When assembling intubation equipment, ensure that the cuff will hold air because these cuffs are prone to leaks and holes. With a syringe, inflate the cuff with approximately 6 to 10 mL of air after tube placement. The cuff is attached to a one-way valve through a side tube with a pilot balloon that is used to indicate if the cuff is inflated. Be sure to remove the syringe after instilling air into the tube or the pressure exerted from the inflated cuff in the trachea will cause the air to leak out, thus compromising the ability of the cuff to reduce the risk of aspiration. The syringe should remain with the person responsible for the intubation in case of leakage (to inflate more air) or for extubation (if necessary).

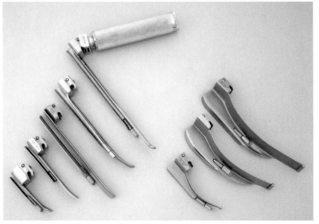

Figure 2-39 Straight and curved laryngoscope blades.

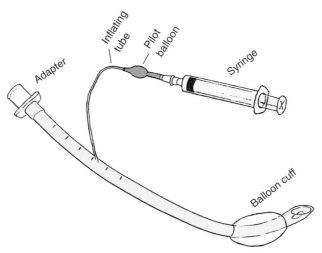

Figure 2-40 Components of the tracheal tube.

Tracheal tubes are measured in millimeters by their internal diameter and their external diameter. They are available in lengths that range from 12 to 32 cm. Internal tube diameters range from 2.5 to 5.5 mm (uncuffed) and from 5 to 10 mm (cuffed) in half-millimeter increments. Imprinted markings are found along the length of the tube that specify its internal diameter as well as centimeters measured from the distal tip of the tube. A radiolucent line is also present in tracheal tubes to allow for the easy detection of tube placement by radiologic studies. In most respects, except for the absence of a cuff and a pilot balloon, the smaller tracheal tubes are essentially the same as the larger ones. However, at the distal tip of the tube is some type of designation that lets you know how far past the vocal cords to pass the tube into the trachea. Depending on the manufacturer, the distal tip may be blackened. When intubating, the tracheal tube is passed until the black portion of the tube has disappeared beyond the vocal cords. In some cases, the tube has a series of solid black lines. Closest to the tip is a single black line, and as you move proximally there is a set of two solid black lines. These lines are a point of reference when advancing the tube so that the initial single line is beyond the vocal cords while the double set remains visible.

The selection of a tracheal tube of the correct size is important. A tube that is too small may provide too little airflow and may lead to the delivery of inadequate tidal volumes. A tube that is too large may cause tracheal edema, vocal cord damage, or both. Select the largest tube size that is appropriate for the patient; larger tubes facilitate the suctioning of secretions and decrease the work of breathing. Common internal diameters of tracheal tubes for adults typically range from 7.5 mm (adult females) to 9 mm (adult males).[43] Because of the size variation in adults, several sizes of tubes should be on hand. At a minimum, have available a tracheal tube that is 0.5 mm smaller and 0.5 mm larger than the estimated tube size.

When the tracheal tube has been properly placed, the centimeter markings on the side of the tube should be observed and recorded. In adults, this value is typically between the 19- and 23-cm mark at the front teeth.

Tracheal tube manufacturers continually develop new types of tubes for use in intubation. Some tubes have ports that allow for medication instillation into the lungs without interrupting ventilation. Others have built-in controls that allow you to manipulate the distal tip of the tube to facilitate passage into the glottic opening.

A stylet is a relatively stiff but flexible metal rod that is covered by plastic for insertion into the tracheal tube. It is used for maintaining the shape of the relatively pliant tracheal tube and for "steering" it into position (Figure 2-41). The appropriately sized stylet is longer than the selected tracheal tube and is only approximately 4 mm in diameter so that after it has been lubricated with a water-soluble lubricant, it easily slides in and out of the length of the tube. The functional shape of the stylet can be described as the approximate shape of a hockey stick, or the letter J.

When a stylet is used, its tip must be recessed approximately 0.5 inch from the end of the tracheal tube to avoid trauma to the airway structures. To prevent the stylet from slipping down into the tube and out of reach, "hook" the manipulation end over the proximal end of the tracheal tube. Stylets are available in a variety of sizes, and they may be used when intubating both pediatric and adult patients.

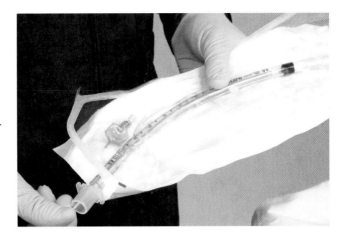

Figure 2-41 Tracheal tube with stylet.

BOX 2-14 **Verifying Tracheal Tube Placement**

Methods that are used to verify the proper placement of a tracheal tube include the following:

- Visualizing the passage of the tracheal tube between the vocal cords
- Auscultating the presence of bilateral breath sounds
- Determining the absence of sounds over the epigastrium during ventilation
- Observing adequate chest rise with each ventilation
- Observing absence of vocal sounds after the placement of the tracheal tube
- Measuring the level of end-tidal carbon dioxide (waveform capnography is preferred)
- Verifying tube placement with the use of an esophageal detector device
- Obtaining a chest radiograph

  Do not rely exclusively on one method or device to detect and monitor for inadvertent esophageal intubation.

After the tracheal tube has been passed through the vocal cords, it is advanced until the proximal end of the cuff lies 0.5 to 1 inch beyond the cords. While firmly holding the tracheal tube, gently withdraw the laryngoscope, and remove the stylet if it was used. Confirm placement by evaluating for chest rise, confirmation of bilateral breath sounds, assessment of waveform capnography, and, if the patient has a perfusing rhythm, Spo_2 levels. Methods used to confirm proper tracheal tube position are listed in Box 2-14.

YOU SHOULD KNOW In cardiac arrest situations, members of the resuscitation team may opt to wait to insert an advanced airway until there is a return of spontaneous circulation. If an advanced airway is not inserted, the patient should be ventilated at a rate of 10 to 12 breaths/min. If the decision is made to insert an advanced airway during the resuscitation effort, ventilation does not require interruption (or even pausing) of chest compressions once the advanced airway is in place. The patient should be ventilated at a rate of 1 breath about every 6 to 8 seconds (about 8 to 10 breaths/min) after an advanced airway is in place.[25] Avoid delivering an excessive number or volume of ventilations.

Esophageal detector devices are used as an aid to help determine if a tracheal tube is in the trachea or the esophagus. There are two types of esophageal detectors: syringes and bulbs (Figure 2-42). These devices operate with the understanding that the esophagus is a collapsible tube and the trachea a rigid one. The syringe device is connected to a tracheal tube with the plunger fully inserted into the barrel of the syringe. If the tube is in the trachea, the plunger can be easily withdrawn from the syringe barrel. If the tracheal tube is in the esophagus, resistance will be felt when the plunger is withdrawn because the walls of the esophagus will collapse when negative pressure is applied to the syringe. The esophageal

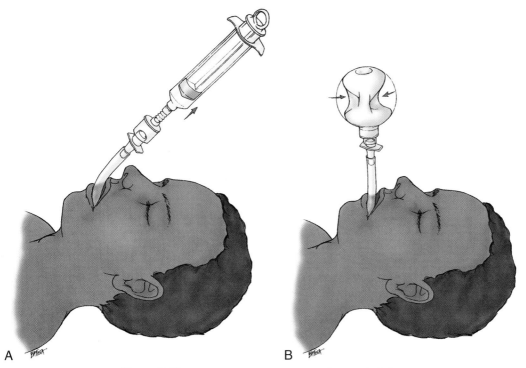

Figure 2-42 Esophageal detector device. **A,** Syringe. **B,** Bulb.

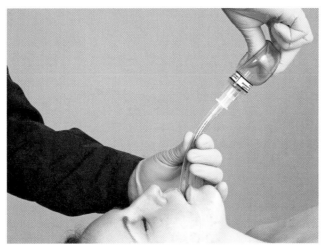

Figure 2-43 An esophageal detector device may be used to assess tracheal tube placement.

detector device should be checked for air leaks before use. If any connections are loose, the leak may allow the syringe to be easily withdrawn, thus mimicking tracheal location of the tube.[26] The bulb device is compressed before it is connected to a tracheal tube. A vacuum is created as the pressure on the bulb is released. If the tube is in the trachea, the bulb will refill easily when pressure is released, indicating proper tube placement. If the tracheal tube is in the esophagus, the bulb will remain collapsed, which indicates improper tube placement. Conditions in which the trachea tends to collapse can result in misleading findings. Examples of these conditions include morbid obesity, late pregnancy, status asthmaticus, and the presence of profuse tracheal secretions.

If an esophageal detector device is used to confirm the placement of the tube, apply the device to the tube before the inflation of the distal cuff (Figure 2-43). Inflating the cuff moves the distal end of the tracheal tube away from the walls of the esophagus. If the tube was inadvertently inserted into the esophagus, this movement will cause the detector bulb to reexpand, which falsely suggests that the tube is in the trachea. If an exhaled CO_2 detector is used to verify tube placement, the lungs will need to be ventilated at least six times before evaluating tracheal tube placement to quickly wash out any retained CO_2.

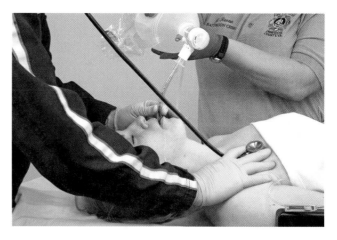

Figure 2-44 Confirm proper placement of the tracheal tube by first auscultating over the epigastrium (should be silent) and then in the midaxillary and anterior chest line on the right and left sides of the patient's chest.

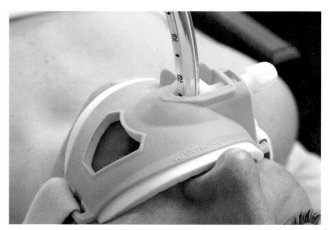

Figure 2-45 After proper tracheal tube position is confirmed, secure it with a commercial tube holder or tape and provide ventilatory support with supplemental oxygen.

While still holding the tracheal tube, inflate the distal cuff with approximately 6 to 10 mL of air; the volume varies with the cuff size. Disconnect the syringe from the inflation valve, attach a ventilation device to the tracheal tube, and ventilate the patient. Confirm the proper placement of the tube by first auscultating over the epigastrium (no sound should be heard) and then in the midaxillary and anterior chest line on the right and left sides of the patient's chest (Figure 2-44). Observe the patient's chest for full movement with ventilation.

If breath sounds are absent bilaterally after intubation and gurgling is heard over the epigastrium, assume esophageal intubation. Deflate the tracheal tube cuff, remove the tube, and preoxygenate before reattempting intubation. If breath sounds are diminished on the left after intubation but present on the right, assume right primary bronchus intubation. Deflate the tracheal tube cuff, pull back the tube slightly, reinflate the cuff, and reevaluate breath sounds. When placement is confirmed, note and record the depth (i.e., centimeter marking) of the tube at the patient's teeth.

After proper tube position the tube confirmed, secure the tube with a commercial tube holder or tape and provide ventilatory support with supplemental oxygen (Figure 2-45). The use of capnography is recommended at this time for the continuous monitoring of tube placement. After securing the tube, recheck and record the tube depth at the patient's teeth.

> **ACLS Pearl**
> An advanced airway that is misplaced or that becomes dislodged can be fatal. Make it a habit to recheck the placement of an advanced airway immediately after insertion, after securing the tube, during intrafacility or interfacility transport, and whenever the patient is moved. Be certain to document the centimeter position of the tube at the patient's teeth/lips. Capnography can be used to immediately alert you to a misplaced or dislodged tube.

Indications, contraindications, advantages, and disadvantages of tracheal intubation are shown in Box 2-15. Possible complications of tracheal intubation are listed in Box 2-16.

BOX 2-15 | Tracheal Intubation

Indications
- Inability of the patient to protect his or her own airway due to the absence of protective reflexes (e.g., coma, respiratory and/or cardiac arrest)
- Inability of the rescuer to ventilate the unresponsive patient with less invasive methods
- Present or impending airway obstruction/respiratory failure (e.g., inhalation injury, severe asthma, exacerbation of chronic obstructive pulmonary disease, severe pulmonary edema, severe flail chest or pulmonary contusion)
- When prolonged ventilatory support is required

Contraindications
- Healthcare provider untrained in tracheal intubation

Advantages
- Keeps the airway open
- Reduces the risk of aspiration
- Ensures delivery of a high concentration of oxygen
- Permits suctioning of the trachea
- Provides a route for administration of some medications
- Ensures delivery of a selected tidal volume to maintain lung inflation

Disadvantages
- Considerable training and experience required; retraining may be needed to ensure competency
- Special equipment needed
- Bypasses physiologic function of upper airway (e.g., warming, filtering, humidifying of inhaled air)
- Requires direct visualization of vocal cords

BOX 2-16 | Tracheal Intubation–Possible Complications

- Arrhythmias
- Aspiration
- Barotrauma
- Bleeding
- Cuff leak
- Esophageal intubation
- Hypoxia due to prolonged or unsuccessful intubation
- Increased intracranial pressure
- Laryngeal or tracheal edema
- Laryngospasm
- Mucosal necrosis
- Occlusion caused by patient biting the tube or secretions
- Right primary bronchus intubation
- Trauma to the lips, teeth, tongue or soft tissues of the oropharynx
- Tube occlusion
- Vocal cord damage

STOP AND REVIEW

True/False

Indicate whether the statement is true or false.

_____ 1. The laryngeal mask airway is available in only one size.

_____ 2. Use of a colorimetric capnometer enables ongoing monitoring to ensure a tracheal tube remains in the trachea.

_____ 3. A greater tidal volume can be delivered with mouth-to-mask ventilation than with a bag-mask device.

_____ 4. Pulse oximetry provides information about the effectiveness of a patient's ventilation.

_____ 5. A bag-mask device can be used for a spontaneously breathing patient as well as a nonbreathing patient.

_____ 6. Use of a supraglottic airway is considered an acceptable alternative to bag-mask ventilation or a tracheal tube for airway management in cardiac arrest, if used by a properly trained healthcare professional.

Multiple Choice

Identify the choice that best completes the statement or answers the question.

_____ 7. Which of the following statements is INCORRECT regarding the nasal airway?
a. The nasal airway may cause a nosebleed if forcefully inserted.
b. Most responsive and semi-responsive patients can tolerate a nasal airway.
c. A nasal airway should be lubricated with a water-soluble lubricant before insertion.
d. The nasal airway is the airway adjunct of choice in patients who have severe craniofacial trauma.

_____ 8. Which of the following statements is correct regarding the use of a Combitube?
a. Esophageal trauma is a possible complication of Combitube use.
b. Direct visualization of the airway is required for insertion of the device.
c. Once the Combitube is positioned, ventilation should begin through the pharyngeal tube.
d. Because it is available in several sizes, the Combitube can be used in patients of all ages, from neonates to adults.

_____ 9. An oral airway:
a. May result in an airway obstruction if improperly inserted
b. Should be lubricated with a petroleum-based lubricant before insertion
c. Is usually well tolerated in the responsive or semi-responsive patient
d. May inadvertently enter the cranial vault if used in a patient with a craniofacial injury

_____ 10. Common internal diameters (I.D.) of tracheal tubes for adults typically range from:
a. 6 to 7.5 mm I.D
b. 7.5 to 9 mm I.D
c. 9 to 10 mm I.D
d. 10 to 10.5 mm I.D

_____ 11.   Tracheal intubation:
a. Is contraindicated in unresponsive patients
b. Eliminates the risk of aspiration of gastric contents
c. Should be preceded by efforts to ventilate by another method
d. When attempted, should be performed in less than 60 seconds

_____ 12.   When using an exhaled carbon dioxide detector to confirm placement of a tracheal tube in a patient with spontaneous circulation, a lack of carbon dioxide on the detector generally means:
a. The tube is correctly placed in the trachea
b. The tube is improperly positioned in the esophagus

Questions 13 and 14 pertain to the following scenario:

You and a coworker arrive to find a 78-year-old woman unresponsive in bed. She is not breathing but does have a pulse.

_____ 13.   You have a pocket face mask on hand that is equipped with an oxygen inlet. After quickly connecting oxygen tubing to the inlet on the mask, you should set the oxygen flow rate at:
a. 1 to 2 L/min
b. 4 to 6 L/min
c. 8 to 10 L/min
d. 10 to 12 L/min

_____ 14.   Which of the following statements is correct regarding mouth-to-mask ventilation for this patient?
a. Take a deep breath before each ventilation and then ventilate at a rate of 6 to 8 breaths/min.
b. Take a deep breath before each ventilation and then ventilate at a rate of 12 to 15 breaths/min.
c. Take a normal breath before each ventilation and ventilate at a rate of 10 to 12 breaths/min.
d. Take a normal breath before each ventilation and ventilate at a rate of 12 to 20 breaths/min.

Completion
Complete each statement.

15. When suctioning, apply intermittent suction while _____ the catheter.

16. A bag-mask used with supplemental oxygen set at a flow rate of 15 L/min with no reservoir will deliver approximately _____% to _____% oxygen to the patient.

Matching
Match each description below with its corresponding answer.

a. Lung _____ refers to the resistance of the patient's lung tissue to ventilation.
b. This device can deliver an oxygen concentration of 22% to 45% at a flow rate of 0.25 to 8 L/min.
c. One of several risk factors for difficult mask ventilation
d. Exhaled carbon dioxide detectors provide information about the effectiveness of _____.
e. A _____ mask is the delivery device of choice when high concentrations of oxygen are needed in the spontaneously breathing patient.
f. With this type of capnometer, the patient's breath causes a chemical reaction on pH-sensitive litmus paper housed in the detector.
g. Oxygen delivery devices such as a nasal cannula and nonrebreather mask are used for _____ breathing patients.

h. The narrowest part of the adult larynx
i. This can be indirectly evaluated by observing the rise and fall of a patient's chest.
j. _____ _____ is a noninvasive method of measuring oxygen saturation of functional hemoglobin.
k. The process of getting oxygen into the body and to its tissues for metabolism.
l. An oxygen flow rate of at least 5 L/min must be used to flush carbon dioxide from this device.
m. A dual-lumen airway
n. The amount of air moved in and out of the respiratory tract in 1 minute
o. An example of a situation in which exhaled carbon dioxide monitoring is recommended

_____ 17. Glottis

_____ 18. Pulse oximetry

_____ 19. Minute volume

_____ 20. Continuous monitoring of tracheal tube position

_____ 21. Colorimetric

_____ 22. Tidal volume

_____ 23. Compliance

_____ 24. Oxygenation

_____ 25. History of snoring

_____ 26. Spontaneously

_____ 27. Simple face mask

_____ 28. Nonrebreather

_____ 29. Ventilation

_____ 30. Nasal cannula

_____ 31. Combitube

Short Answer

32. What type of suction catheter is used to clear secretions from a tracheal tube?

33. How do you determine the correct size nasal airway?

34. Complete the following table.

Device	Approximate Inspired Oxygen Concentration	Liter Flow (Liters/Minute)
Nasal cannula		
Simple face mask		6 to 10
Partial rebreather mask	35% to 60%	6 to 10
Nonrebreather mask		

35. What are the most frequent problems with the use of the bag-mask device?

36. While attempting to insert a nasal airway, you find you are unable to advance the device. How should you proceed?

37. How do you determine the proper size oral airway to use?

REFERENCES

1. Aehlert B: *Paramedic practice today: above and beyond*, St Louis, 2010, Mosby.
2. Brashers VL: Structure and function of the pulmonary system. In McCance KL, Huether SE, editors: *Pathophysiology: the biologic basis for disease in adults and children*, ed 6, St Louis, 2009, Mosby.
3. Douce FH: Pulmonary function testing. In Wilkins RL, Stoller JK, Kacmarek RM, editors: *Egan's fundamentals of respiratory care*, ed 9, St Louis, 2009, Mosby.
4. Huether SE: *Understanding pathophysiology*, ed 4, St Louis, 2007, Mosby.
5. Bell C: Understanding contemporary pulse oximetry, Clinical Window: International Web Journal for Medical Professionals, 2005(19). www.clinicalwindow.liitin.net/dl/Art%2019-1.pdf. Accessed September 11, 2011.
6. Mahlmeister MJ: Sensor selection in pulse oximetry. RT, the Journal for Respiratory Care Practitioners 1998. www.dolphinmedical.com/faqs/respcare-selection-1998.pdf. Accessed April 19, 2010.
7. Schutz SL: Oxygen saturation monitoring by pulse oximetry. In Wiegand DJL-M, Carlson KK, editors: *AACN procedure manual for critical care*, ed 5, Philadelphia, 2005, Saunders.
8. Kleinman ME, Chameides L, Schexnayder SM, et al: Part 14: pediatric advanced life support: 2010 American Heart Association guidelines for cardiopulmonary resuscitation and emergency cardiovascular care, *Circulation* 122(suppl 3):S876–S908, 2010.
9. Poirier MP, Gonzalez Del-Rey JA, McAneney CM, DiGiulio GA: Utility of monitoring capnography, pulse oximetry, and vital signs in the detection of airway mishaps: a hyperoxemic animal model, *Am J Emerg Med* 16:350–352, 1998.
10. Birmingham PK, Cheney FW, Ward RJ: Esophageal intubation: a review of detection techniques, *Anesth Analg* 65:886–891, 1986.
11. Bickler PE, Feiner JR, Severinghaus JW: Effects of skin pigmentation on pulse oximeter accuracy at low saturation, *Anesthesiology* 102(4):715–719, 2005.
12. Feiner JR, Severinghaus JW, Bickler PE: Dark skin decreases the accuracy of pulse oximeters at low oxygen saturation: the effects of oximeter probe type and gender, *Anesth Analg* 105(6 Suppl):S18–S23, 2007.
13. Murphy MF, Krauss B: Monitoring the emergency patient. In Marx JA, editor: *Rosen's emergency medicine*, ed 7, St Louis, 2009, Mosby.
14. Ornato JP, Shipley JB, Racht EM, et al: Multicenter study of a portable, hand-size, colorimetric end-tidal carbon dioxide detection device, *Ann Emerg Med* 21(5):518–523, 1992.
15. Sum Ping ST, Mehta MP, Symreng T: Accuracy of the FEF CO2 detector in the assessment of endotracheal tube placement, *Anesth Analg* 74:415–419, 1992.
16. Ward KR, Yealy DM: End-tidal carbon dioxide monitoring in emergency medicine. Part 2: clinical applications, *Acad Emerg Med* 5(6):637–646, 1998.
17. Cantineau JP, Merckx P, Lambert Y, et al: Effect of epinephrine on end-tidal carbon dioxide pressure during prehospital cardiopulmonary resuscitation, *Am J Emerg Med* 12(3):267–270, 1994.

18. Neumar RW, Otto CW, Link MS, et al: Part 8: adult advanced cardiovascular life support: 2010 American Heart Association guidelines for cardiopulmonary resuscitation and emergency cardiovascular care, *Circulation* 122(Suppl 3):S729–S767, 2010.

19. O'Connor RE, Brady W, Brooks SC, et al: Part 10: acute coronary syndromes: 2010 American Heart Association guidelines for cardiopulmonary resuscitation and emergency cardiovascular care, *Circulation* 122(Suppl 3):S787–S817, 2010.

20. Urden LD: Pulmonary therapeutic management. In *Critical care nursing: diagnosis and management*, ed 6, St Louis, 2009, Mosby.

21. Heuer AJ, Scanlan CL: Medical gas therapy. In Wilkins RL, Stoller JK, Kacmarek RM, editors: *Egan's fundamentals of respiratory care*, ed 9, St Louis, 2009, Mosby.

22. Tiffin NH, Keim MR, Trewen TC: The effects of variations in flow through an insufflating catheter and endotracheal tube and suction catheter size on test lung pressures, *Respir Care* 35:889, 1990.

23. Schade K, Borzotta A, Michaels A: Intracranial malposition of nasopharyngeal airway, *J Trauma* 49:967–968, 2000.

24. Muzzi DA, Losasso TJ, Cucchiara RF: Complication from a nasopharyngeal airway in a patient with a basilar skull fracture, *Anesthesiology* 74:366–368, 1991.

25. Berg RA, Hemphill R, Abella BS, et al: Part 5: adult basic life support: 2010 American Heart Association guidelines for cardiopulmonary resuscitation and emergency cardiovascular care, *Circulation* 122(Suppl 3):S685–S705, 2010.

26. Reardon RF, Mason PE, Clinton JE: Basic airway management and decision-making. In Roberts JR, Hedges JR, editors: *Clinical Procedures in Emergency Medicine*, ed 5, Philadelphia, 2009, Saunders.

27. Rouse M, Frakes M: Airway Management. In *ASTNA patient transport: principles and practice*, 4th ed, St. Louis, 2010, Mosby.

28. Langeron O, Masso E, Huraux C, et al: Prediction of difficult mask ventilation, *Anesthesiology* 92(5):1229–1236, 2000.

29. Birnbaumer DM, Pollack Jr CV: Troubleshooting and managing the difficult airway, *Semin Respir Crit Care Med* 23(1):3–9, 2002.

30. Kheterpal S, Han R, Tremper KK, et al: Incidence and predictors of difficult and impossible mask ventilation, *Anesthesiology* 105(5):885–891, 2006.

31. Rice MJ, Mancuso AA, Gibbs C, et al: Cricoid pressure results in compression of the postcricoid hypopharynx: the esophageal position is irrelevant, *Anesth Analg* 109(5):1546–1552, 2009.

32. Howells TH, Chamney AR, Wraight WJ, Simons RS: The application of cricoid pressure: an assessment and a survey of its practice, *Anaesthesia* 38(5):457–460, 1983.

33. Lawes EG: Cricoid pressure with or without the "cricoid yoke," *Br J Anaesth* 58(12):1376–1379, 1986.

34. Flucker CJ, Hart E, Weisz M, et al: The 50–millilitre syringe as an inexpensive training aid in the application of cricoid pressure, *Eur J Anaesthesiol* 17(7):443–447, 2000.

35. Koziol CA, Cuddeford JD, Moos DD: Assessing the force generated with application of cricoid pressure, *AORN J* 72(6):1018–1028, 1030, 2000.

36. Kopka A, Crawford J: Cricoid pressure: a simple, yet effective biofeedback trainer. *Eur J Anaesthesiol* 21(6):443–447, 2004.

37. Domuracki KJ, Moule CJ, Owen H, et al: Learning on a simulator does transfer to clinical practice, *Resuscitation* 80(3):346–349, 2009.

38. Bhardwaj M, Chhabra B, Kiran S: Evaluation of the effect of cricoid pressure on insertion of laryngeal mask airway, *J Anaesthesiol Clin Pharmacol* 14(3):283–285, 1998.

39. Asai T, Barclay K, Power I, Vaughan RS: Cricoid pressure impedes placement of the laryngeal mask airway and subsequent tracheal intubation through the mask, *Br J Anaesth* 72(1):47–51, 1994.

40. Ansermino JM, Blogg CE: Cricoid pressure may prevent insertion of the laryngeal mask airway, *Br J Anaesth* 69(5):465–467, 1992.

41. Aoyama K, Takenaka I, Sata T, Shigematsu A: Cricoid pressure impedes positioning and ventilation through the laryngeal mask airway, *Can J Anaesth* 43(10):1035–1040, 1996.

42. Brimacombe J, White A, Berry A: Effect of cricoid pressure on ease of insertion of the laryngeal mask airway, *Br J Anaesth* 71(6):800–802, 1993.

43. Simmons KF, Scanlan CL: Airway management. In Wilkins RL, Stoller JK, Kacmarek RM, editors: *Egan's fundamentals of respiratory care*, ed 9, St. Louis, 2009, Mosby.

CHAPTER 3

Rhythms and Management

OBJECTIVES

Upon completion of this chapter, you will be able to:

1. Given a patient situation, describe the electrocardiogram (ECG) characteristics and initial emergency care (including mechanical, pharmacological [including indications, contraindications, doses, and route of administration of applicable medications], and electrical therapy where applicable) for each of the following situations:
   - Too fast rhythms–Narrow-QRS tachycardia, wide-QRS tachycardia, irregular tachycardia
   - Too slow rhythms–Symptomatic bradycardia
   - Cardiac arrest rhythms
2. Identify a patient who is experiencing a cardiac dysrhythmia as asymptomatic, symptomatic but stable, symptomatic but unstable, or pulseless.
3. Describe the role of each member of the resuscitation team.
4. Discuss the "phase response" of code organization.

INTRODUCTION

A prerequisite to participation in most Advanced Cardiac Life Support (ACLS) courses is completion of a basic ECG recognition course. This requirement exists because there simply is not time in an ACLS course to cover detailed information about rhythm recognition. A basic ECG course teaches you how to identify cardiac rhythms. An ACLS course quickly reviews cardiac rhythms, but focuses on teaching how to recognize serious signs and symptoms related to those rhythms and how to treat them.

Normally, the heart beats at a very regular rate and rhythm. If this pattern is interrupted, an abnormal heart rhythm can result. Although *arrhythmia* technically means "absence of rhythm" and *dysrhythmia* means "abnormal heart rhythm," these terms are used interchangeably by healthcare professionals to refer disturbances in cardiac rhythm. To help you understand and recognize cardiac dysrhythmias, this chapter reviews the heart's blood supply and conduction pathways, and ECG lead systems, waveforms, segments, and intervals. Cardiac dysrhythmias, their identifying features, and therapeutic interventions for symptomatic dysrhythmias are also discussed.

SECTION 1

Anatomy Review and Basic Electrophysiology

CORONARY ARTERIES

The right coronary artery (RCA) originates from the right side of the aorta. It travels along the groove between the right atrium and right ventricle (Figure 3-1). Blockage of the RCA can result in inferior wall myocardial infarction (MI), disturbances in atrioventricular (AV) nodal conduction, or both.

The left coronary artery (LCA) originates from the left side of the aorta. The first segment of the LCA is called the left main coronary artery. The left main coronary artery supplies oxygenated blood to its two primary branches: the left anterior descending (LAD), which is also called the *anterior interventricular artery,* and the circumflex artery (Cx). Blockage of the left main coronary artery has been referred to as the *widow maker* because of its association with sudden cardiac arrest when occluded.

The major branches of the LAD are the septal and diagonal arteries. Blockage of the septal branch of the LAD can result in a septal MI. Blockage of the diagonal branch of the LAD can result in an anterior wall MI. Blockage of the LAD can also result in pump failure, intraventricular conduction delays, or both.

> **ACLS Pearl**
>
> A common cause of MI is a blocked coronary artery. When viewing the patient's 12-lead ECG, an understanding of the coronary artery anatomy makes it possible to predict which coronary artery is blocked.

The Cx coronary artery circles around the left side of the heart. Blockage of the Cx artery can result in a lateral wall MI. In some patients, the Cx artery may also supply the inferior portion of the left ventricle. A posterior wall MI may occur because of blockage of the right coronary artery or the Cx. A summary of the coronary arteries is shown in Table 3-1.

BASIC ELECTROPHYSIOLOGY

Myocardial Cell Types

In general, cardiac cells have either a mechanical (contractile) or an electrical (pacemaker) function. **Myocardial cells** (also called **working cells** or **mechanical cells**) contain contractile filaments. When these cells are electrically stimulated, these contractile filaments slide together and cause the myocardial cell to contract. These myocardial cells form the thin muscular layer of the atrial walls and the thicker muscular layer of the ventricular walls (i.e., the myocardium). These cells do not normally generate electrical impulses on their own and they rely on pacemaker cells for this function.

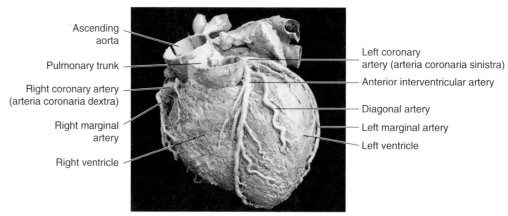

Ascending aorta
Pulmonary trunk
Right coronary artery (arteria coronaria dextra)
Right marginal artery
Right ventricle

Left coronary artery (arteria coronaria sinistra)
Anterior interventricular artery
Diagonal artery
Left marginal artery
Left ventricle

Figure 3-1 Anterior view of the heart with the right and left coronary arteries and some of their branches.

TABLE 3-1	Coronary Arteries		
Coronary Artery and Its Branches	**Portion of Myocardium Supplied**	**Portion of Conduction System Supplied**
Right Posterior descending Right marginal	• Right atrium • Right ventricle • Inferior surface of left ventricle (about 85%)* • Posterior surface of left ventricle (about 85%)*	• SA node (about 60%)* • AV node (85% to 90%)* • Proximal portion of bundle of His • Part of posterior-inferior fascicle of left bundle branch
Left Anterior descending	• Anterior surface of left ventricle • Part of lateral surface of left ventricle • Most of the interventricular septum	• Most of right bundle branch • Anterior-superior fascicle of left bundle branch • Part of posterior-inferior fascicle of left bundle branch
Circumflex	• Left atrium • Part of lateral surface of left ventricle • Inferior surface of left ventricle (about 15%)* • Posterior surface of left ventricle (15%)*	• SA node (about 40%)* • AV node (10% to 15%)*

*Percentage of population.
AV, Atrioventricular; SA, sinoatrial.

Pacemaker cells are specialized cells of the electrical conduction system. Pacemaker cells also may be referred to as **conducting cells** or **automatic cells**. They are responsible for the spontaneous generation and conduction of electrical impulses.

Properties of Cardiac Cells

The heart has pacemaker cells that can generate an electrical impulse without being stimulated by a nerve. The ability of cardiac pacemaker cells to create an electrical impulse without being stimulated by another source is called **automaticity**. The heart's normal pacemaker (the sinoatrial [SA] node) usually prevents other areas of the heart from assuming this function because its cells depolarize more rapidly than other pacemaker cells. Normal concentrations of sodium (Na^+), potassium (K^+), and calcium (Ca^{2+}) are important in maintaining automaticity. Increased blood concentrations of these electrolytes decrease automaticity. Decreased concentrations of K^+ and Ca^{2+} in the blood increase automaticity.

Cardiac muscle is electrically irritable because of an ionic imbalance across the membranes of cells. **Excitability** (irritability) is the ability of cardiac muscle cells to respond to an external stimulus, such as that from a chemical, mechanical, or electrical source. **Conductivity** is the ability of a cardiac cell to receive an electrical impulse and conduct it to an adjoining cardiac cell. All cardiac cells possess this characteristic. The intercalated disks present in the membranes of cardiac cells are responsible for the property of conductivity. They allow an impulse in any part of the myocardium to spread throughout the heart. The speed with which the impulse is conducted can be altered by factors such as sympathetic and parasympathetic stimulation and medications. **Contractility** is the ability of myocardial cells to shorten, thereby causing cardiac muscle contraction, in response to electrical stimulus. The heart normally contracts in response to an impulse that begins in the SA node. The strength of the heart's contraction can be improved with certain medications, such as digitalis, dopamine, and epinephrine.

Cardiac Action Potential

In the normal heart, electrical activity occurs because of ionic changes that occur in the body's cells. Human body fluids contain **electrolytes,** which are elements or compounds that break into charged particles (**ions**) when melted or dissolved in water or another solvent. The main electrolytes that affect the function of the heart are Na⁺, K⁺, Ca²⁺, and chloride (Cl⁻). Electrolytes move about in body fluids and carry a charge, just as electrons moving along a wire conduct a current. The **action potential** of a cardiac cell reflects the rapid sequence of voltage changes that occur across the cell membrane during the electrical cardiac cycle. The configuration of the action potential varies depending on the location, size, and function of the cardiac cell.

Separated electrical charges of opposite polarity (positive vs. negative) have potential energy. The measurement of this potential energy is called **voltage**. Voltage is measured between two points in units of volts or millivolts.

Polarization

In the body, ions spend a lot of time moving back and forth across cell membranes. As a result, a slight difference in the concentrations of charged particles across the membranes of cells is normal. Thus potential energy (voltage) exists because of the imbalance of charged particles. This imbalance makes the cells excitable.

Cell membranes contain pores or channels through which specific electrolytes and other small, water-soluble molecules can cross the cell membrane from the outside to the inside (Figure 3-2). When a cell is at rest, K⁺ leaks out of it. Large molecules such as proteins and phosphates remain inside the cell because they are too big to pass easily through the cell membrane. These large molecules carry a negative charge. This results in more negatively charged ions on the inside of the cell.

When the inside of a cell is more negative than the outside, it is said to be in a **polarized state** (Figure 3-3). The voltage (difference in electrical charges) across the cell membrane is the **membrane potential**. Electrolytes are quickly moved from one side of the cell membrane to the other by

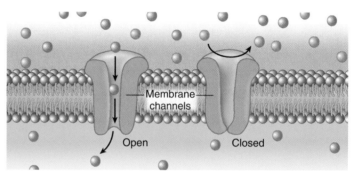

Figure 3-2 Cell membranes contain membrane channels. These channels are pores through which specific ions or other small, water-soluble molecules can cross the cell membrane from outside to inside.

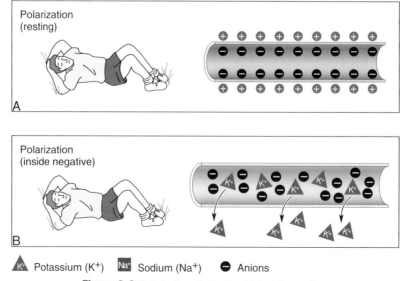

Figure 3-3 Polarization. **A,** Resting. **B,** Inside negative.

means of pumps. These pumps require energy in the form of adenosine triphosphate (ATP) when movement occurs against a concentration gradient. The energy expended by the cells to move electrolytes across the cell membrane creates a flow of current. This flow of current is expressed in volts. Voltage appears on an ECG as spikes or waveforms. Thus an ECG is actually a sophisticated voltmeter.

Depolarization

For a pacemaker cell to "fire" (produce an impulse), a flow of electrolytes across the cell membrane must exist. When a cell is stimulated, the cell membrane changes and becomes **permeable** to Na^+ and K^+. Permeability refers to the ability of a membrane channel to allow passage of electrolytes once it is open. Na^+ rushes into the cell through Na^+ channels. This causes the inside of the cell to become more positive relative to the outside. A spike (waveform) is then recorded on the ECG. The stimulus that alters the electrical charges across the cell membrane may be electrical, mechanical, or chemical.

When opposite charges come together, energy is released. When the movement of electrolytes changes the electrical charge of the inside of the cell from negative to positive, an impulse is generated. The impulse causes channels to open in the next cell membrane and then the next. The movement of charged particles across a cell membrane causing the inside of the cell to become positive is called **depolarization** (Figure 3-4). Depolarization must take place before the heart can mechanically contract and pump blood. Depolarization occurs because of the movement of Na^+ into the cell. Depolarization proceeds from the innermost layer of the heart (endocardium) to the outermost layer (epicardium).

An impulse normally begins in the pacemaker cells found in the SA node of the heart. A chain reaction occurs from cell to cell in the heart's electrical conduction system until all the cells have been stimulated and depolarized. This chain reaction is a wave of depolarization. The chain reaction is made possible because of gap junctions that exist between the cells. Eventually the impulse is spread from the pacemaker cells to the working myocardial cells. The working myocardial cells contract when they are stimulated. When the atria are stimulated, a P wave is recorded on the ECG. Thus the P wave represents atrial depolarization. When the ventricles are stimulated, a QRS complex is recorded on the ECG. Thus the QRS complex represents ventricular depolarization.

> ### ◗ ACLS Pearl
> Depolarization is *not* the same as contraction. Depolarization is an electrical event that is expected to result in contraction, which is a mechanical event. It is possible to see organized electrical activity on the cardiac monitor, even when the assessment of the patient reveals no palpable pulse. This clinical situation is called **pulseless electrical activity (PEA)**.

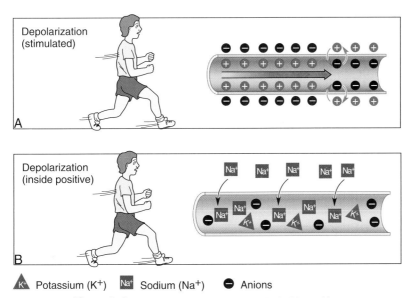

▲ Potassium (K^+)   ■ Sodium (Na^+)   ● Anions

Figure 3-4 Depolarization. **A,** Stimulated. **B,** Inside positive.

Repolarization

After the cell depolarizes, it quickly begins to recover and restore its electrical charges to normal. The movement of charged particles across a cell membrane in which the inside of the cell is restored to its negative charge is called **repolarization**. The cell membrane stops the flow of Na⁺ into the cell and allows K⁺ to leave it. Negatively charged particles are left inside the cell. Thus the cell is returned to its resting state (Figure 3-5). This causes contractile proteins in the working myocardial cells to separate (relax). The cell can be stimulated again if another electrical impulse arrives at the cell membrane. Repolarization proceeds from the epicardium to the endocardium. On the ECG, the ST segment and T wave represent ventricular repolarization.

The action potential of a ventricular myocardial cell consists of five phases labeled 0 to 4. These phases reflect the rapid sequence of voltage changes that occur across the cell membrane during the electrical cardiac cycle. Phases 1, 2, and 3 have been referred to as **electrical systole**. Phase 4 has been referred to as **electrical diastole**. Figure 3-6 shows the action potential of a normal ventricular muscle cell.

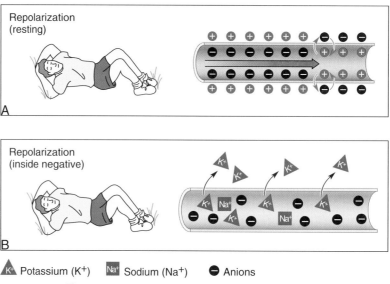

Figure 3-5 Repolarization. **A,** Resting. **B,** Inside negative.

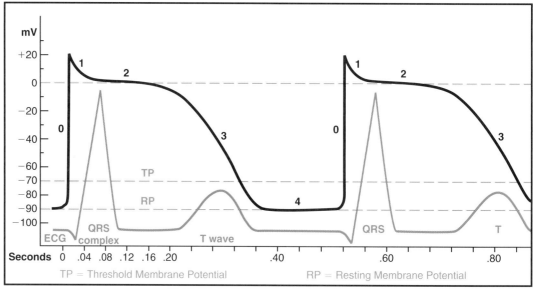

Figure 3-6 Action potential of a ventricular muscle cell.

Keeping It Simple

Polarization = ready state
Depolarization = stimulation
Repolarization = recovery

Refractory Periods

Refractoriness is a term used to describe the period of recovery that cells need after being discharged before they are able to respond to a stimulus. In the heart, the refractory period is longer than the contraction itself.

During the **absolute refractory period**, the cell will not respond to further stimulation within itself. This means that the myocardial working cells cannot contract and the cells of the electrical conduction system cannot conduct an electrical impulse, no matter how strong the internal electrical stimulus. As a result, tetanic (sustained) contractions cannot be provoked in the cardiac muscle. On the ECG, the absolute refractory period corresponds with the onset of the QRS complex to the peak of the T wave.

During the **relative refractory period**, which is also known as the *vulnerable period*, some cardiac cells have repolarized to their threshold potential and thus can be stimulated to respond (i.e., depolarize) to a stronger-than-normal stimulus (Figure 3-7). This period corresponds with the downslope of the T wave on the ECG.

After the relative refractory period is a **supranormal period**. A weaker-than-normal stimulus can cause cardiac cells to depolarize during this period. The supranormal period corresponds with the end of the T wave. Because the cell is more excitable than normal, dysrhythmias can develop during this period.

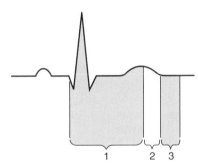

Figure 3-7 Refractory periods. 1, The absolute refractory period; 2, relative refractory period; and 3, the supranormal period.

Conduction System

The specialized electrical (pacemaker) cells in the heart are arranged in a system of pathways called the **conduction system**. In the normal heart, the cells of the conduction system are interconnected. The conduction system makes sure that the chambers of the heart contract in a coordinated fashion. The pacemaker site with the fastest firing rate typically controls the heart.

Sinoatrial Node

The normal heartbeat is the result of an electrical impulse that begins in the SA node. The heart's pacemaker cells have a built-in (intrinsic) rate that becomes slower and slower from the SA node down to the end of the His-Purkinje system. The intrinsic rate of the SA node is 60 to 100 beats/min. The SA node is normally the primary pacemaker because it depolarizes more quickly than other pacemaker sites in the heart (Figure 3-8). Other areas of the heart can assume pacemaker responsibility if:

- The SA node fails to fire (generate an impulse)
- The SA node fires too slowly
- The SA node fails to activate the surrounding atrial myocardium

The SA node is richly supplied by sympathetic and parasympathetic nerve fibers. The fibers of the SA node directly connect with the fibers of the atria. As the impulse leaves the SA node, it is spread from cell to cell in wavelike form across the atrial muscle. As the impulse spreads, it stimulates the

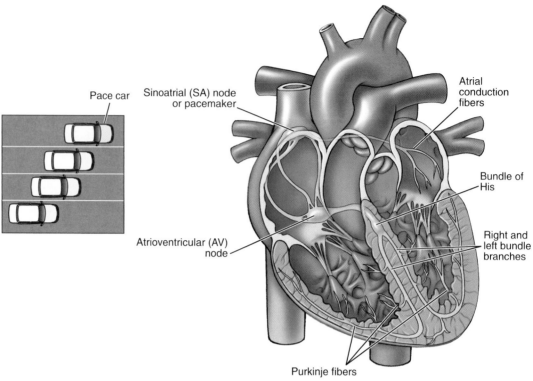

Figure 3-8 The conduction system.

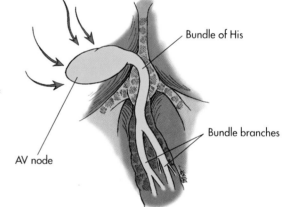

Figure 3-9 The atrioventricular (AV) junction consists of the AV node and the nonbranching portion of the bundle of His.

right atrium, the interatrial septum, and then the left atrium via Bachmann's bundle, which is a small grouping of cells in the left atrium connected by one of four atrial conduction tracts. This results in contraction of the right and left atria at almost the same time.

Conduction through the AV node begins before atrial depolarization is completed. The impulse is spread to the AV node by three internodal pathways that consist of a mixture of working myocardial cells and specialized conducting fibers.

Atrioventricular Junction

The internodal pathways merge gradually with the cells of the AV node. Depolarization and repolarization are slow in the AV node, making this area vulnerable to blocks in conduction (AV blocks). The **AV junction** is made up of the AV node and the nonbranching portion of the bundle of His (Figure 3-9). This area consists of specialized conduction tissue that provides the electrical links between the atria and the ventricles. When the AV junction is bypassed by an abnormal pathway, the abnormal route is called an *accessory pathway*. An accessory pathway is an extra bundle of working myocardial tissue that forms a connection between the atria and the ventricles outside of the normal conduction system.

TABLE 3-2 Normal Pacemaker Sites	
Pacemaker	**Beats/Minute**
Sinoatrial (SA) node (primary pacemaker)	60 to 100
Atrioventricular (AV) junction	40 to 60
Purkinje fibers	20 to 40

Atrioventricular Node

The **AV node** is a group of nerve cells located in the floor of the right atrium immediately behind the tricuspid valve and near the opening of the coronary sinus. The AV node is supplied by both sympathetic and parasympathetic nerve fibers.

As the impulse from the atria enters the AV node, there is a delay in conduction of the impulse to the ventricles. If this delay did not occur, the atria and ventricles would contract at about the same time. The delay in conduction allows the atria to empty blood into the ventricles before the next ventricular contraction begins. This increases the amount of blood in the ventricles, thus increasing stroke volume.

Bundle of His

The **bundle of His** is also called the *common bundle* or *atrioventricular bundle* and is located in the upper portion of the interventricular septum. The AV junction has pacemaker cells that have an intrinsic rate of 40 to 60 beats/min. The bundle of His conducts the electrical impulse to the right and left bundle branches.

Right and Left Bundle Branches

The right bundle branch innervates the right ventricle. The left bundle branch spreads the electrical impulse to the interventricular septum and left ventricle, which is thicker and more muscular than the right ventricle. The left bundle branch divides into three divisions called **fascicles**, which are small bundles of nerve fibers allowing electrical innervation of the larger, more muscular left ventricle.

Purkinje Fibers

The right and left bundle branches divide into smaller and smaller branches and then into a special network of fibers called the **Purkinje fibers**. These fibers spread from the interventricular septum into the papillary muscles. They continue downward to the apex of the heart, making up an elaborate web that penetrates about one third of the way into the ventricular muscle mass. The fibers then become continuous with the muscle cells of the right and left ventricles. The Purkinje fibers have pacemaker cells that have an intrinsic rate of 20 to 40 beats/min (Table 3-2). The electrical impulse spreads rapidly through the right and left bundle branches and the Purkinje fibers to reach the ventricular muscle. The electrical impulse spreads from the endocardium to the myocardium, finally reaching the epicardial surface. The ventricular walls are stimulated to contract in a twisting motion that wrings blood out of the ventricular chambers and forces it into arteries.

THE ELECTROCARDIOGRAM

The ECG records the electrical activity of a large mass of atrial and ventricular cells as specific waveforms and complexes. The electrical activity within the heart can be observed by means of electrodes connected by cables to an ECG machine. Think of the ECG as a voltmeter that records the electrical voltages (potentials) generated by depolarization of the heart's cells. The basic function of the ECG is to detect current flow as measured on the patient's skin.

ECG monitoring may be used for the following purposes:
- To monitor a patient's heart rate
- To evaluate the effects of disease or injury on heart function
- To evaluate pacemaker function
- To evaluate the response to medications (such as antiarrhythmics)
- To obtain a baseline recording before, during, and after a medical procedure
- To evaluate for signs of myocardial ischemia, injury, and infarction

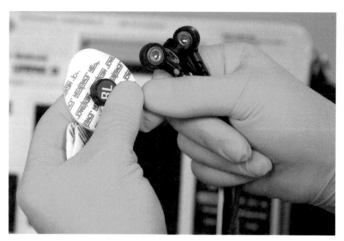

Figure 3-10 Electrodes are applied at specific locations on the patient's chest wall and limbs to view the heart's electrical activity from different angles and planes.

Electrodes

An **electrode** is an adhesive pad containing a conductive substance in the center and that is applied to the patient's skin. Electrodes are applied at specific locations on the patient's chest wall and extremities to view the heart's electrical activity from different angles and planes. The conductive media of the electrode conducts skin surface voltage changes through wires to a cardiac monitor. One end of a monitoring cable, which is also called a **lead wire**, is attached to the electrode and the other end to an ECG machine (Figure 3-10).

Leads

A **lead** is a record (i.e., tracing) of electrical activity between two electrodes. Each lead records the *average* current flow at a specific time in a portion of the heart. Leads allow for the viewing of the heart's electrical activity in two different planes: frontal (coronal) and horizontal (transverse). A 12-lead ECG provides views of the heart in both the frontal and horizontal planes and views the surfaces of the left ventricle from 12 different angles. From this, ischemia, injury, and infarction affecting any area of the heart can be identified.

Frontal Plane Leads

Frontal plane leads view the heart from the front of the body as if it were flat. Directions in the frontal plane are superior, inferior, right, and left (Figure 3-11). Six leads view the heart in the frontal plane. Leads I, II, and III are called *standard limb leads*. Leads aVR, aVL, and aVF are called *augmented limb leads*.

Standard Limb Leads

Leads I, II, and III make up the standard limb leads. If an electrode is placed on the right arm, left arm, and left leg, three leads are formed. The positive electrode is located at the left arm in lead I, while leads II and III both have their positive electrode located at the left leg. The difference in electrical potential between the positive pole and its corresponding negative pole is measured by each lead.

Lead I records the difference in electrical potential between the left arm (+) and right arm (−) electrodes. The positive electrode is placed on the left arm and the negative electrode is placed on the right arm. The third electrode is a ground that minimizes electrical activity from other sources (Figure 3-12A). Lead I views the lateral surface of the left ventricle.

Lead II records the difference in electrical potential between the left leg (+) and right arm (−) electrodes. The positive electrode is placed on the left leg and the negative electrode is placed on the right arm (Figure 3-12B). Lead II views the inferior surface of the left ventricle. This lead is commonly used for cardiac monitoring because positioning of the positive and negative electrodes in this lead most closely resembles the normal pathway of current flow in the heart.

Lead III records the difference in electrical potential between the left leg (+) and left arm (−) electrodes. In lead III the positive electrode is placed on the left leg and the negative electrode is placed

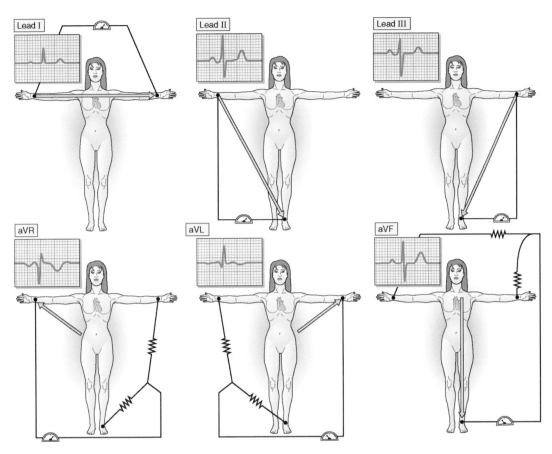

Figure 3-11 Frontal plane leads.

TABLE 3-3	Standard Limb Leads		
Lead	**Positive Electrode**	**Negative Electrode**	**Heart Surface Viewed**
I	Left arm	Right arm	Lateral
II	Left leg	Right arm	Inferior
III	Left leg	Left arm	Inferior

on the left arm (Figure 3-12C). Lead III views the inferior surface of the left ventricle. A summary of the standard limb leads can be found in Table 3-3.

Augmented Limb Leads

Leads aVR, aVL, and aVF are augmented limb leads that record measurements at a specific electrode with respect to a reference electrode. The electrical potential produced by the augmented leads is normally relatively small. The ECG machine augments (i.e., magnifies) the amplitude of the electrical potentials detected at each extremity by about 50% over those recorded at the standard limb leads. The "a" in aVR, aVL, and aVF refers to augmented. The "V" refers to voltage and the last letter refers to the position of the positive electrode. The "R" refers to the right arm, the "L" to left arm, and the "F" to left foot (leg). Therefore, the positive electrode in aVR is located on the right arm, aVL has a positive electrode at the left arm, and aVF has a positive electrode positioned on the left leg (Figure 3-13).

Lead aVR views the heart from the right shoulder (the positive electrode) and views the base of the heart (primarily the atria and the great vessels). This lead does not view any wall of the heart. Lead aVL combines views from the right arm and left leg, with the view being from the left arm and oriented to the lateral wall of the left ventricle. Lead aVF combines views from the right arm and the left arm toward the left leg; it views the inferior surface of the left ventricle from the left leg. A summary of augmented leads can be found in Table 3-4.

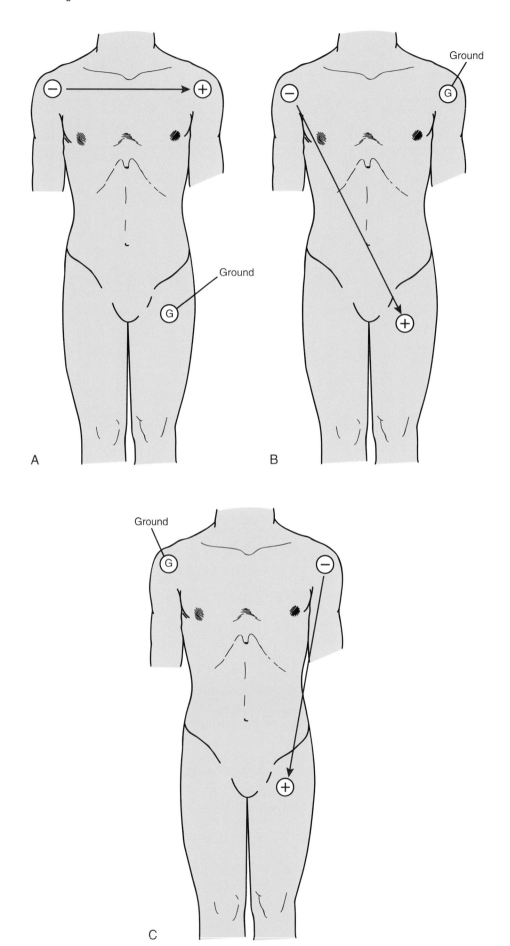

Figure 3-12 Electrode placement on the patient's limbs for **(A)** lead I, **(B)** lead II, and **(C)** lead III.

TABLE 3-4	**Augmented Limb Leads**	
Lead	**Positive Electrode**	**Heart Surface Viewed**
aVR	Right arm	None
aVL	Left arm	Lateral
aVF	Left leg	Inferior

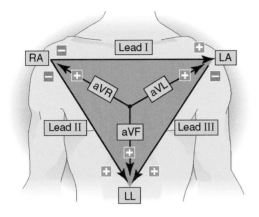

Figure 3-13 View of the standard limb leads and augmented leads.

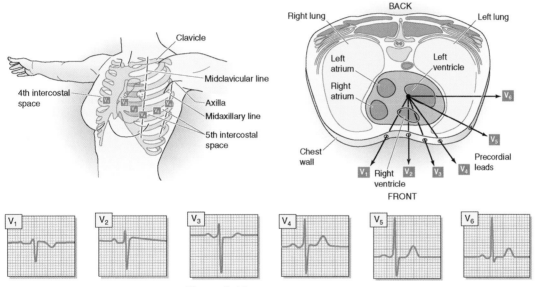

Figure 3-14 Horizontal plane leads.

Horizontal Plane Leads

Horizontal plane leads view the heart as if the body were sliced in half horizontally. Directions in the horizontal plane are anterior, posterior, right, and left. Six chest (precordial or "V") leads view the heart in the horizontal plane (Figure 3-14). This allows a view of the front and left side of the heart.

Chest Leads

The chest leads are identified as V_1, V_2, V_3, V_4, V_5, and V_6. Each electrode placed in a "V" position is a positive electrode. Lead V_1 is recorded with the positive electrode in the fourth intercostal space, just to the right of the sternum. Lead V_2 is recorded with the positive electrode in the fourth intercostal space, just to the left of the sternum. Lead V_3 is recorded with the positive electrode on a line midway between V_2 and V_4. Lead V_4 is recorded with the positive electrode in the left midclavicular line in the fifth intercostal space. To evaluate the right ventricle, lead V_4 may be moved to the same anatomic location but on the right side of the chest. The lead is then called **V_4R** and it is viewed for ECG changes consistent with acute MI. Lead V_5 is recorded with the positive electrode in the left anterior

TABLE 3-5	Chest Leads	
Lead	**Positive Electrode Position**	**Heart Surface Viewed**
V_1	Right side of sternum, fourth intercostal space	Septum
V_2	Left side of sternum, fourth intercostal space	Septum
V_3	Midway between V_2 and V_4	Anterior
V_4	Left midclavicular line, fifth intercostal space	Anterior
V_5	Left anterior axillary line; same level as V_4	Lateral
V_6	Left midaxillary line; same level as V_4	Lateral

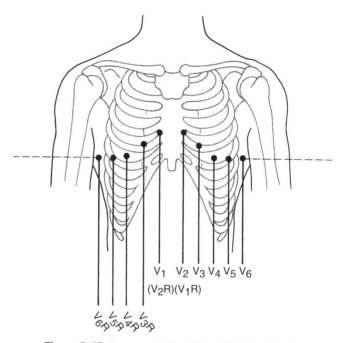

Figure 3-15 Placement of the left and right chest leads.

axillary line at the same level as V_4. Lead V_6 is recorded with the positive electrode in the left midaxillary line at the same level as V_4. A summary of the chest leads can be found in Table 3-5.

Right Chest Leads

Other chest leads that are not part of a standard 12-lead ECG may be used to view specific surfaces of the heart. Right chest leads are used to evaluate the right ventricle (Figure 3-15). The placement of right chest leads is identical to the placement of the standard chest leads except that it is done on the right side of the chest. If time does not permit obtaining all of the right chest leads, the lead of choice is V_4R. A summary of the right chest leads can be found in Table 3-6.

TABLE 3-6	Right Chest Leads and Their Placement
Lead	**Placement**
V_1R	Lead V_2
V_2R	Lead V1
V_3R	Midway between V_2R and V_4R
V_4R	Right midclavicular line, fifth intercostal space
V_5R	Right anterior axillary line; same level as V_4R
V_6R	Right midaxillary line; same level as V_4R

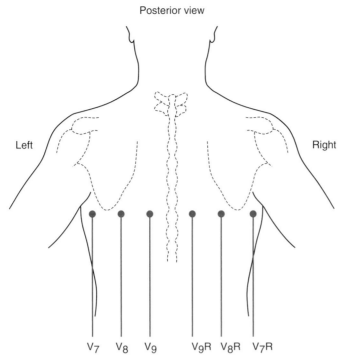

Posterior view

Left

Right

V₇ V₈ V₉   V₉R V₈R V₇R

Figure 3-16 Posterior chest lead placement.

Posterior Chest Leads

On a standard 12-lead ECG, no leads look directly at the posterior surface of the heart. Additional chest leads may be used for this purpose. These leads are placed farther left and toward the back (Figure 3-16). All of the leads are placed on the same horizontal line as V_4 to V_6. Lead V_7 is placed at the posterior axillary line. Lead V_8 is placed at the angle of the scapula (i.e., the posterior scapular line) and lead V_9 is placed over the left border of the spine.

> **ACLS Pearl**
>
> Fifteen- and 18-lead ECGs are being used with increasing frequency to help spot infarctions of the right ventricle and the posterior wall of the left ventricle. The 15-lead ECG uses all of the leads of a standard 12-lead ECG plus leads V_4R, V_8, and V_9. An 18-lead ECG uses all of the leads of the 15-lead ECG plus leads V_5R, V_6R, and V_7. When obtaining a 15- or 18-lead ECG, first obtain a standard 12-lead ECG. Then, move the electrodes (and corresponding wires) to the desired position for the additional leads (such as V_5R, V_6R, and V_7) and run a second ECG. Because the machine will not know that you have repositioned the electrodes, it will be necessary for you to handwrite the electrode position/lead onto the ECG paper to properly indicate the origin of the tracing. The machine's computer-generated interpretation also must be disregarded in the event the cables are moved.

What Each Lead "Sees"[1]

Think of the positive electrode as an eye looking in at the heart. The part of the heart that each lead "sees" is determined by two factors. The first factor is the dominance of the left ventricle on the ECG and the second is the position of the positive electrode on the body. Because the ECG does not directly measure the heart's electrical activity, it does not "see" all of the current flowing through the heart. What the ECG sees from its vantage point on the body's surface is the net result of countless individual currents competing in a tug-of-war. For example, the QRS complex, which represents ventricular depolarization, is not a display of all the electrical activity occurring in the right and left ventricles. It is the net result of a tug-of-war produced by the many individual currents in both the right and left ventricles. Since the left ventricle is much larger than the right, the left overpowers it. What is seen in the QRS complex is the additional electrical activity of the left ventricle, that is, the portion that exceeds the right ventricle. Therefore, in a normally conducted beat, the QRS complex primarily represents the electrical activity occurring in the left ventricle.

The second factor, position of the positive electrode on the body, determines which portion of the left ventricle is seen by each lead. You can commit the view of each lead to memory, or you can easily reason it by remembering where the positive electrode is located. The view of each lead is listed in Table 3-7, while Figure 3-17 demonstrates the portion of the left ventricle that each lead views. Please note that aVR is not included in Table 3-7 or Figure 3-17.

TABLE 3-7	What Each Lead "Sees"
Leads	**Heart Surface Viewed**
II, III, aVF	Inferior
V_1, V_2	Septal
V_3, V_4	Anterior
I, aVL, V_5, V_6	Lateral

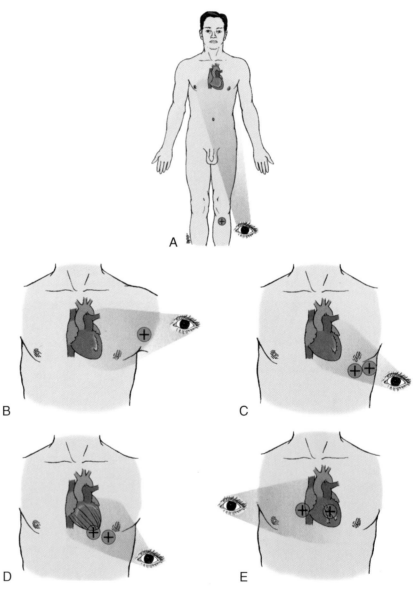

Figure 3-17 The position of the positive electrode on the body determines the portion of the heart "seen" by each lead. **A,** Leads II, III, and aVF each has its positive electrode positioned on the left leg. From the perspective of the left leg, each of them "sees" the inferior wall of the left ventricle. **B,** From their vantage point on the left arm, leads I and aVL "look" in at the lateral wall of the left ventricle. **C,** Leads V_5 and V_6 also "view" the lateral wall because they are positioned on the axillary area of the left chest. **D,** Leads V_3 and V_4 are positioned in the area of the anterior chest. From this perspective, these leads "see" the anterior wall of the left ventricle. **E,** The septal wall is "seen" by leads V_1 and V_2, which are positioned next to the sternum.

Electrocardiogram Paper

ECG paper is graph paper made up of small and large boxes measured in millimeters. The smallest boxes are 1 mm wide and 1 mm high (Figure 3-18). The horizontal axis of the paper corresponds with *time*. Time is used to measure the interval between or duration of specific cardiac events, which is stated in seconds. ECG paper normally records at a constant speed of 25 mm/second. Thus, each horizontal unit (i.e., each 1-mm box) represents 0.04 second (25 mm/sec × 0.04 second = 1 mm). The lines after every five small boxes on the paper are heavier. The heavier lines indicate one large box. Because each large box is the width of five small boxes, a large box represents 0.20 second.

The vertical axis of the graph paper represents the *voltage* or *amplitude* of the ECG waveforms or deflections. Voltage is measured in millivolts (mV). Voltage may appear as a positive or negative value, because voltage is a force with direction as well as amplitude. Amplitude is measured in millimeters (mm). The ECG machine's sensitivity must be calibrated so that a 1-mV electrical signal will produce a deflection that measures exactly 10 mm tall. When properly calibrated, a small box is 1-mm high (0.1 mV), and a large box, which is equal to five small boxes, is 5 mm high (0.5 mV).

Waveforms and Complexes

An ECG waveform is movement away from the baseline (isoelectric line) in either a positive (upward) or negative (downward) direction. Waveforms are named alphabetically, beginning with P, QRS, T, and U (Figure 3-19).

The P wave is the first waveform in the cardiac cycle and represents atrial depolarization and the spread of the electrical impulse throughout the right and left atria. A P wave is normally positive (upright) in standard leads and precedes each QRS complex.

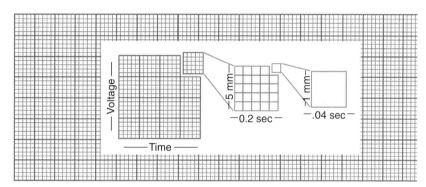

Figure 3-18 Electrocardiogram (ECG) graph paper. The horizontal axis represents time. The vertical axis represents amplitude or voltage.

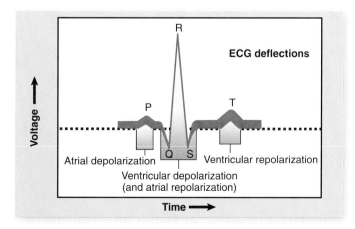

Figure 3-19 Electrocardiogram (ECG) waveforms and complexes.

The QRS complex consists of the Q wave, R wave, and S wave. It represents the spread of the electrical impulse through the ventricles (ventricular depolarization). A QRS complex normally follows each P wave. One or even two of the three waveforms that make up the QRS complex may not always be present.

The QRS complex begins as a downward deflection, the *Q wave*. A Q wave is *always* a negative waveform. It is important to differentiate normal (physiologic) Q waves from pathologic Q waves. With the exception of leads III and aVR, a normal Q wave in the limb leads is less than 0.04 second (one small box) in duration and less than one-third the height of the R wave in that lead. An abnormal (pathologic) Q wave is more than 0.04 second in duration or more than one-third the height of the following R wave in that lead. MI is one possible cause of abnormal Q waves. In the early hours of infarction, an abnormal Q wave may not have developed to its full width or amplitude. Therefore, a single ECG tracing may not identify an abnormal Q wave. In a patient with a suspected MI, be sure to look at Q waves closely. Even if the initial ECG tracings do not show Q waves that are more than 0.04 second in duration or equal to or more than one-third the amplitude of the QRS complex, pathology must be considered if the Q waves become wider or deeper in each subsequent tracing.

In adults, the normal duration of the QRS complex is 0.11 second or less.[2] If the impulse originates in a bundle branch, the duration of the QRS may be only slightly greater than 0.10 second. For example, a QRS duration between 0.10 and 0.12 second in adults is called an *incomplete* bundle branch block (BBB). In adults, a QRS measuring more than or equal to 0.12 second is called a *complete* BBB.

YOU SHOULD KNOW
- If an electrical impulse does not follow the normal ventricular conduction pathway, it will take longer to depolarize the myocardium. This delay in conduction through the ventricle produces a wider QRS complex than normal.
- The width of a QRS complex is most accurately determined when it is viewed and measured in more than one lead. The measurement should be taken from the QRS complex with the longest duration and clearest onset and end.

Ventricular repolarization is represented on the ECG by the T wave. The normal T wave is slightly asymmetric: the peak of the waveform is closer to its end than to the beginning, and the first half has a more gradual slope than the second half. The direction of the T wave is normally the same as the QRS complex that precedes it.

A U wave is a small waveform that, when seen, follows the T wave. The U wave represents repolarization of the Purkinje fibers in the papillary muscle of the ventricular myocardium. Normal U waves are small, round, and less than 1.5 mm in amplitude.

Segments and Intervals

A **segment** is a line between waveforms. It is named by the waveform that precedes or follows it.

The PR segment is the horizontal line between the end of the P wave and the beginning of the QRS complex. It is part of the PR interval and represents activation of the AV node, the bundle of His, the bundle branches, and the Purkinje fibers.

The TP segment is the portion of the ECG tracing between the end of the T wave and the beginning of the following P wave (Figure 3-20). When the heart rate is within normal limits, the TP segment is usually isoelectric. With rapid heart rates, the TP segment is often unrecognizable because the P wave encroaches on the preceding T wave.

The portion of the ECG tracing between the QRS complex and the T wave is the ST segment, which represents the early part of repolarization of the right and left ventricles. The point at which the QRS complex and the ST segment meet is called the *ST junction* or *J-point* (Figure 3-21). Various conditions may cause displacement of the ST segment from the isoelectric line in either a positive or negative direction. Myocardial ischemia, injury, and infarction are among the causes of ST-segment deviation. ST depression in a patient experiencing an acute coronary syndrome suggests the presence of myocardial ischemia and ST elevation suggests myocardial injury. Injured myocardium is tissue that has been cut off from or experienced a severe reduction in its blood and oxygen supply. Injured myocardial tissue is not yet dead and may be salvageable if the blocked vessel can be quickly opened, thereby restoring blood flow and oxygen to the injured area.

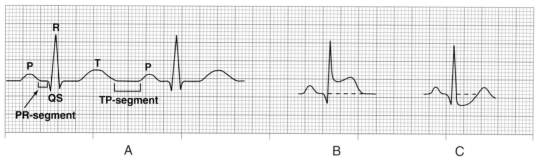

Figure 3-20 Segments. **A,** The TP segment is used as the baseline from which to determine the presence of ST-segment elevation or depression. **B,** ST-segment elevation. **C,** ST-segment depression.

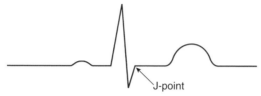

Figure 3-21 The point where the QRS complex and the ST segment meet is called the *ST junction* or *J-point.*

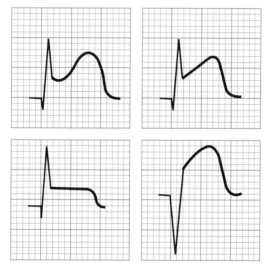

Figure 3-22 Variable shapes of ST-segment elevation seen with acute myocardial infarction.

When looking for ST-segment elevation or depression, we are particularly interested in the *early* portion of the ST segment. First locate the J-point. Next use the TP segment to estimate the position of the isoelectric line and then compare the level of the ST segment with that of the isoelectric line (see Figure 3-20). It may be difficult to clearly determine the J-point in patients with rapid heart rates or hyperkalemia. Some displacement of the ST segment from the isoelectric line is normal and dependent on age, gender, and ECG lead. Possible shapes of ST-segment elevation seen with acute MI are shown in Figure 3-22.

For men 40 years of age and older, the threshold value for abnormal J-point elevation is 2 mm in leads V_2 and V_3 and 1 mm in all other leads. For men younger than 40 years of age, the threshold value for abnormal J-point elevation in leads V_2 and V_3 is 2.5 mm. For women, the threshold value for abnormal J-point elevation is 1.5 mm in leads V_2 and V_3 and greater than 1 mm in all other leads. For men and women, the threshold for abnormal J-point elevation in V_3R and V_4R is 0.5 mm, except for males younger than 30 years of age, for whom 1 mm is more appropriate. For men and women, the threshold value for abnormal J-point elevation in leads V_7 through V_9 is 0.5 mm. For men and women of all ages, ST-segment depression of more than 0.5 mm in leads V_2 and V_3 and of more than 1 mm in all other leads suggests myocardial ischemia.[3,4]

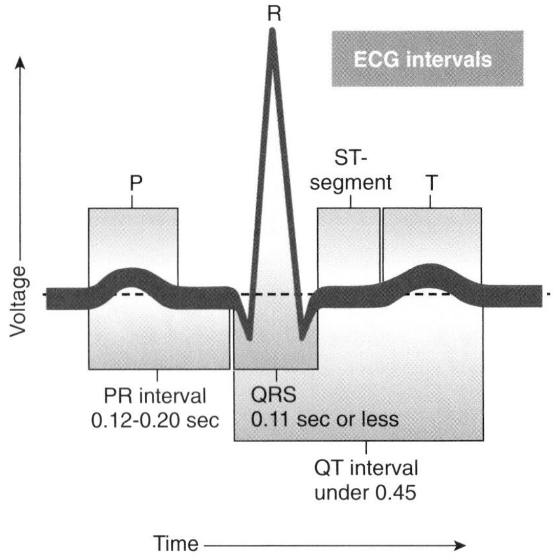

R

ECG intervals

P

ST-segment

T

Voltage

Figure 3-23 Electrocardiogram (ECG) segments and intervals.

PR interval
0.12-0.20 sec

QRS
0.11 sec or less

QT interval
under 0.45

Time

> **ACLS** Pearl
>
> There is some difference of opinion as to where ST-segment deviation should be measured. In general, deviation is measured as the number of millimeters of vertical ST segment displacement from the isoelectric line or from the patient's baseline at a point 0.06 or 0.08 second after the J point. Proper machine calibration is critical when analyzing ST segments. The ST-segment criteria described here apply *only* when the monitor is adjusted to standard calibration.

An **interval** is made up of a waveform and a segment (Figure 3-23). The P wave plus the PR segment equals the PR interval (PRI). The PRI is measured from the point where the P wave leaves the baseline to the beginning of the QRS complex. The term *PQ interval* is preferred by some because it is the period actually measured unless a Q wave is absent. The PRI normally measures 0.12 to 0.20 second in adults. It may be shorter in children and longer in older adults.

The QT interval represents total ventricular activity; this is the time from ventricular depolarization (i.e., activation) to repolarization (i.e., recovery). The QT interval is measured from the beginning of the QRS complex to the end of the T wave. In the absence of a Q wave, the QT interval is measured from the beginning of the R wave to the end of the T wave. The term *QT interval* is used regardless of whether the QRS complex begins with a Q wave or R wave. The duration of the QT interval varies in accordance with age, gender, and heart rate. As the heart rate increases, the QT interval shortens (i.e., decreases). As the heart rate decreases, the QT interval lengthens (i.e., increases). Because of the variability of the QT interval with the heart rate, it can be measured more accurately if it is corrected (i.e., adjusted) for the patient's heart rate. The corrected QT interval is noted as *QTc*. The QT interval is considered short if it is 0.39 second or less or prolonged if it is 0.46 second or longer in women or 0.45 second or longer in men. A number of conditions (e.g., electrolyte disorders) and medications (e.g., amiodarone and sotalol) can prolong the QT interval. A prolonged QT interval indicates a lengthened relative refractory period. A QTc of more than 0.5 second in either gender has been correlated with a higher risk for life-threatening dysrhythmias (e.g., torsades de pointes [TdP]). A prolonged QT interval may be congenital or acquired.

RHYTHM RECOGNITION

Sinus Rhythm

Sinus rhythm is the name given to a normal heart rhythm. Sinus rhythm reflects normal electrical activity; that is, the rhythm starts in the SA node and then heads down the normal conduction pathway through the atria, AV junction, bundle branches, and ventricles. This results in depolarization of the atria and ventricles. The SA node normally produces electrical impulses faster than any other part of the heart's conduction system. As a result, the SA node is normally the heart's primary pacemaker. A person's heart rate varies with age. In adults and adolescents, the SA node normally fires at a regular rate of 60 to 100 beats/min (Table 3-8, Figure 3-24).

TABLE 3-8	Characteristics of Sinus Rhythm
Rate	Within normal limits for age; in adults, 60 to 100 beats/min
Rhythm	Regular
P waves	Uniform in appearance, positive (upright) in lead II, one precedes each QRS complex
PR interval	Within normal limits for age and constant from beat to beat; in adults, 0.12 to 0.20 sec
QRS duration	0.11 sec or less unless an intraventricular conduction delay exists

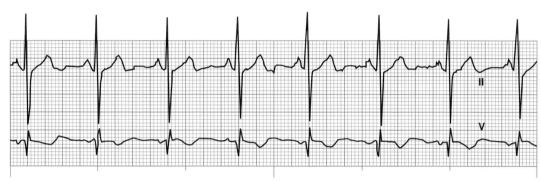

Figure 3-24 Sinus rhythm.

Sinus Arrhythmia

The SA node fires quite regularly most of the time. When it fires irregularly, the resulting rhythm is called a sinus arrhythmia. Sinus arrhythmia that is associated with the phases of breathing and changes in intrathoracic pressure is called *respiratory sinus arrhythmia*. Sinus arrhythmia that is not related to the respiratory cycle is called *nonrespiratory sinus arrhythmia*. A sinus arrhythmia usually occurs at a rate of 60 to 100 beats/min. If sinus arrhythmia is associated with a slower than normal rate, it is called *sinus bradyarrhythmia*. If the rhythm is associated with a faster than normal rate, it is known as *sinus tachyarrhythmia*.

What Causes It?

Respiratory sinus arrhythmia is a normal phenomenon that occurs with changes in intrathoracic pressure. The heart rate increases with inspiration (i.e., R-R intervals shorten) and decreases with expiration (i.e., R-R intervals lengthen). Sinus arrhythmia is most commonly observed in children and adults younger than 30 years of age.

> **ACLS Pearl**
> In respiratory sinus arrhythmia, the changes in rhythm disappear when the patient holds his breath.

Nonrespiratory sinus arrhythmia can be seen in people with normal hearts but is more likely to be found in older individuals and in those with heart disease. It is common after acute inferior wall MI and may be seen with increased intracranial pressure. Nonrespiratory sinus arrhythmia may be the result of the effects of medications (e.g., digitalis, morphine) or carotid sinus pressure.

What Do I Do About It?

Sinus arrhythmia does not usually require treatment unless it is accompanied by a slow heart rate that causes hemodynamic compromise. If hemodynamic compromise is present, intravenous (IV) atropine may be indicated (Table 3-9, Figure 3-25).

TABLE 3-9	Characteristics of Sinus Arrhythmia
Rate	Usually 60 to 100 beats/min, but may be slower or faster
Rhythm	Irregular and phasic with breathing; heart rate increases gradually during inspiration (R-R intervals shorten) and decreases with expiration (R-R intervals lengthen)
P waves	Uniform in appearance; positive (upright) in lead II; one precedes each QRS complex
PR interval	0.12 to 0.20 sec and constant from beat to beat
QRS duration	0.11 sec or less unless an intraventricular conduction delay exists

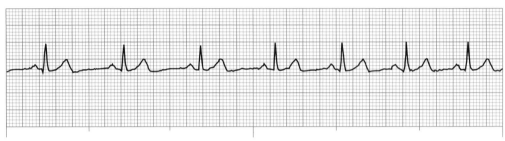

Figure 3-25 Sinus arrhythmia.

SECTION 2

Tachydysrhythmias: Too-Fast Rhythms

[Objectives 1, 2]

Cardiac rhythms can be classified into four main groups: normal, absent/pulseless (cardiac arrest rhythms), slower than normal for age (bradycardia), or faster than normal for age (tachycardia). Some dysrhythmias do not cause serious signs and symptoms, whereas others can be life threatening.

The signs and symptoms experienced by a patient with a tachycardia depend on the following:

- The ventricular rate
- How long the tachycardia lasts
- The patient's general health and the presence of underlying heart disease

The faster the heart rate, the more likely the patient is to have signs and symptoms resulting from the rapid rate.

When a patient presents with signs and symptoms related to a tachycardia, ask yourself these questions:

1. Is the patient stable or unstable?
2. Is the QRS wide or narrow? If it is wide, is it monomorphic or polymorphic?
3. Is the ventricular rhythm regular or irregular?

The answers to these questions will help guide your treatment decisions. Most tachycardias do not cause serious signs and symptoms until the ventricular rate exceeds 150 beats/min unless the patient has impaired ventricular function.[5] Serious signs and symptoms are those that affect vital organ function. Examples of serious signs and symptoms are shown in Box 3-1. If the patient is symptomatic but does not have serious signs and symptoms because of the rapid rate, the patient is considered to be stable. For example, a patient who has symptoms such as lightheadedness or palpitations with stable vital signs is symptomatic, but is not in imminent danger of cardiac arrest. After their ABCs have been assessed, stable patients are given oxygen (if indicated), an IV is started, and drug therapy is begun. Frequent patient reassessment is essential.

If the tachycardia produces serious signs and symptoms (typically with heart rates of 150 beats/min or more), the patient is considered unstable. Unstable patients who have a pulse and serious signs and symptoms due to the tachycardia should receive immediate synchronized cardioversion.

BOX 3-1 | **Signs and Symptoms of Hemodynamic Compromise**

- Acute changes in mental status
- Chest pain
- Cold, clammy skin
- Fall in urine output
- Heart failure
- Low blood pressure
- Pulmonary congestion
- Shortness of breath
- Signs of shock

NARROW-QRS TACHYCARDIAS

Supraventricular arrhythmias begin above the bifurcation of the bundle of His. This means that supraventricular arrhythmias include rhythms that begin in the SA node, atrial tissue, or the AV junction.

Sinus Tachycardia

Normal heart rates vary with age. In adults, the rate associated with sinus tachycardia is usually between 101 and 180 beats/min (Table 3-10, Figure 3-26). Because an infant's or child's heart rate can transiently increase during episodes of crying or pain, or in the presence of a fever, the term *tachycardia* is used to describe a significant and persistent increase in heart rate. In infants, a tachycardia is a heart rate of more than 200 beats/min. In a child older than 5 years of age, a tachycardia is a heart rate of more than 160 beats/min.

What Causes It?

Sinus tachycardia is a normal response to the body's demand for increased cardiac output that results from many conditions (Box 3-2). The patient is often aware of an increase in heart rate. Some patients complain of palpitations, a racing heart, or a feeling of pounding in their chests. Sinus tachycardia is seen in some patients with acute MI, especially in those with an anterior infarction.

ACLS Pearl

The management of patients who present with a tachycardia is often complex. As an ACLS provider, it is important for you to recognize when to consult expert advice regarding rhythm interpretation, medications, or patient management decisions.[5]

TABLE 3-10 | **Characteristics of Sinus Tachycardia**

Rate	101 to 180 beats/min
Rhythm	Regular
P waves	Uniform in appearance; positive (upright) in lead II; one precedes each QRS complex; at very fast rates it may be difficult to distinguish a P wave from a T wave
PR interval	0.12 to 0.20 sec and constant from beat to beat
QRS duration	0.11 sec or less unless an intraventricular conduction delay exists

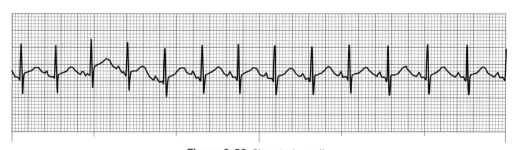

Figure 3-26 Sinus tachycardia.

BOX 3-2 | Causes of Sinus Tachycardia

- Acute myocardial infarction
- Caffeine-containing beverages
- Dehydration, hypovolemia
- Drugs such as cocaine, amphetamines, "ecstasy," cannabis
- Exercise
- Fear and anxiety
- Fever
- Heart failure
- Hyperthyroidism
- Hypoxia
- Infection
- Medications such as epinephrine, atropine, and dopamine
- Nicotine
- Pain
- Pulmonary embolism
- Shock
- Sympathetic stimulation

What Do I Do About It?

In a patient with coronary artery disease, sinus tachycardia can cause problems. The heart's demand for oxygen increases as the heart rate increases. As the heart rate increases, there is less time for the ventricles to fill and less blood for the ventricles to pump out with each contraction. This can lead to decreased cardiac output. Because the coronary arteries fill when the ventricles are at rest, rapid heart rates decrease the time available for coronary artery filling. This decreases the heart's blood supply. Chest discomfort can result if the supplies of blood and oxygen to the heart are inadequate. Sinus tachycardia in a patient who is having an acute MI may be an early warning signal for heart failure, cardiogenic shock, and more serious dysrhythmias.

Treatment for sinus tachycardia is directed at correcting the underlying cause, that is, fluid replacement, relief of pain, removal of offending medications or substances, reducing fever, or anxiety.

ACLS Pearl

Never shock a sinus tachycardia; rather, treat the cause of the tachycardia.

Atrial Tachycardia

The term **supraventricular tachycardia (SVT)** includes three main types of fast rhythms, which are shown in Figure 3-27.
- Atrial tachycardia (AT). During AT, an irritable site in the atria fires automatically at a rapid rate.
- AV nodal reentrant tachycardia (AVNRT). During AVNRT, fast and slow pathways in the AV node form an electrical circuit or loop. The impulse moves in a repeating loop around the AV nodal (junctional) area.
- AV reentrant tachycardia (AVRT). During AVRT, the impulse begins above the ventricles but travels via a pathway other than the AV node and bundle of His.

Keeping It Simple

Some SVTs need the AV node to sustain the rhythm and some do not. For example, AVNRT and AVRT require the AV node as part of the reentry circuit to continue the tachycardia. Other SVTs use the AV node only to conduct the rhythm to the ventricles. For example, atrial tachycardia, atrial flutter, and atrial fibrillation arise from a site (or sites) within the atria; they do not need the AV node to sustain the rhythm.

Atrial tachycardia consists of a series of rapid beats from an irritable site in the atria. This rapid atrial rate overrides the SA node and becomes the pacemaker. Conduction of the atrial impulse to the ventricles is often 1:1, which means that every atrial impulse is conducted through the AV node to the ventricles. This results in a P wave preceding each QRS complex. Although the P waves appear upright, they tend to look different from those seen when the impulse is initiated from the SA node (Table 3-11, Figures 3-28, 3-29).

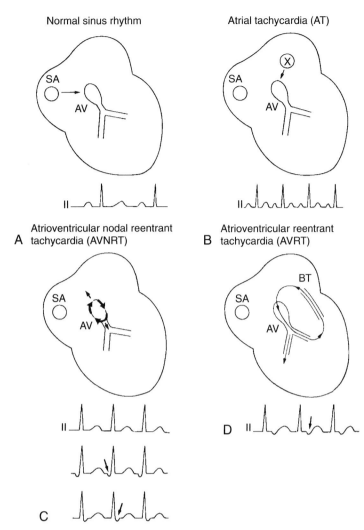

Figure 3-27 Major types of paroxysmal supraventricular tachycardia. **A,** The reference is normal sinus rhythm. **B,** With atrial tachycardia (AT), a focus (X) outside the sinoatrial (SA) node fires off automatically at a rapid rate. **C,** With atrioventricular (AV) nodal reentrant tachycardia (AVNRT), the cardiac stimulus originates as a wave of excitation that spins around the AV nodal (junctional) area. As a result, retrograde P waves may be buried in the QRS or appear immediately before or just after the QRS complex (*arrows*) because of nearly simultaneous activation of the atria and ventricles. **D,** A similar type of reentrant (circus-movement) mechanism may occur with a bypass tract (BT) of the type found in Wolff-Parkinson-White syndrome. This mechanism is referred to as atrioventricular reentrant tachycardia (AVRT). Note the negative P wave (*arrow*) in lead II, somewhat after the QRS complex. (With AVRT, the P wave in lead II may be negative or isoelectric.)

TABLE 3-11	Characteristics of Atrial Tachycardia (AT)
Rate	150 to 250 beats/min
Rhythm	Regular
P waves	One positive P wave precedes each QRS complex in lead II; these P waves differ in shape from sinus P waves; with rapid rates, it may be difficult to distinguish P waves from T waves
PR interval	May be shorter or longer than normal; may be difficult to measure because P waves may be hidden in T waves
QRS duration	0.11 sec or less unless an intraventricular conduction delay exists

ACLS Pearl

It is important to look closely for P waves in all dysrhythmias, but is very important when trying to figure out the origin of a tachycardia. If P waves are not visible in one lead, try looking in another before finalizing your rhythm diagnosis.

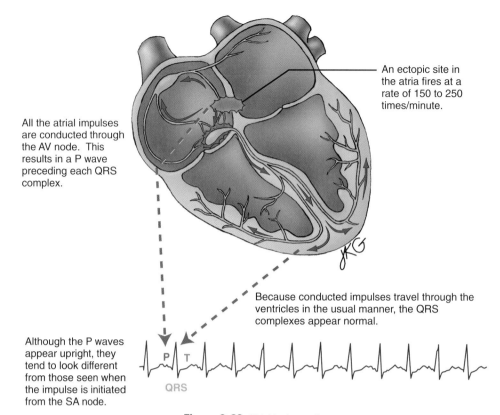

An ectopic site in the atria fires at a rate of 150 to 250 times/minute.

All the atrial impulses are conducted through the AV node. This results in a P wave preceding each QRS complex.

Because conducted impulses travel through the ventricles in the usual manner, the QRS complexes appear normal.

Although the P waves appear upright, they tend to look different from those seen when the impulse is initiated from the SA node.

Figure 3-28 Atrial tachycardia

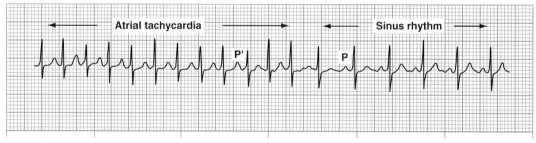

Figure 3-29 Atrial tachycardia is shown that ends spontaneously with the abrupt resumption of sinus rhythm. The P waves of the tachycardia (rate: about 150 beats/min) are superimposed on the preceding T waves.

There is more than one type of atrial tachycardia. Atrial tachycardia that begins in a small area (i.e., focus) within the heart is called *focal atrial tachycardia*. There are several types of focal AT. Focal AT may be due to an automatic, triggered, or reentrant mechanism. A patient with focal AT often presents with paroxysmal AT. The atrial rate is usually between 100 and 250 beats/min; it rarely reaches 300 beats/min.

Automatic AT, which is also called **ectopic AT** is another type of AT in which a small cluster of cells with altered automaticity fire. The impulse is spread from the cluster of cells to the surrounding atrium and then to the ventricles via the AV node. This type of AT often involves a "warm up" period. This means there is a progressive shortening of the P-P interval for the first few beats of the arrhythmia. Automatic AT gradually slows down as it ends, which has been called the "cool down" period. The atrial rate is usually between 100 and 250 beats/min. P waves look different from sinus P waves, but are still related to the QRS complex. Vagal maneuvers do not usually stop the tachycardia, but they may slow the ventricular rate. Multifocal AT is discussed later in this chapter with irregular tachycardias.

Pearl

The term *paroxysmal* is used to describe a rhythm that starts or ends suddenly. Atrial tachycardia that starts or ends suddenly is called *paroxysmal atrial tachycardia (PAT)*. PAT may last for minutes, hours, or days.

What Causes It?

Atrial tachycardia can occur in persons with normal hearts or in patients with organic heart disease. Atrial tachycardia associated with automaticity or reentry is often related to an acute event such as:

- Acute illness with excessive catecholamine release
- Electrolyte imbalance
- Heart disease including coronary artery disease, valvular disease, cardiomyopathies, and congenital heart disease
- Infection
- Stimulant use (e.g., caffeine, albuterol, theophylline, and cocaine)

What Do I Do About It?

When taking the patient's history, try to find out how often the episodes occur, how long they last, and possible triggers. If the patient complains of palpitations, it is important to find out if they are regular or irregular. Palpitations that occur regularly with a sudden onset and end are usually due to AVNRT or AVRT. Irregular palpitations may be due to premature complexes, atrial fibrillation (AFib), or multifocal atrial tachycardia.

If episodes of atrial tachycardia are short, the patient may be asymptomatic. A rhythm that lasts from three beats up to 30 seconds is a nonsustained rhythm. A sustained rhythm is one that lasts more than 30 seconds. If atrial tachycardia is sustained and the patient is symptomatic as a result of the rapid rate, treatment usually includes oxygen (if indicated), IV access, and vagal maneuvers. Although AT will rarely stop with vagal maneuvers, the maneuvers are used to try to stop the rhythm or slow conduction through the AV node. Vagal maneuvers are discussed in the next section of this chapter.

If vagal maneuvers fail, antiarrhythmic medications should be tried. Adenosine is the drug of choice, except for patients with severe asthma (Table 3-12, Figure 3-30). A significant percentage of ATs will terminate with administration of adenosine.[6] If needed, calcium channel blockers (Table 3-13, Figures 3-31 and 3-32) or beta-blockers (Table 3-14, Figure 3-33) may be used to slow the ventricular rate. Synchronized cardioversion seldom stops automatic ATs, but may be successful for ATs due to reentry or triggered automaticity. Synchronized cardioversion should be considered for patients with drug-resistant arrhythmia.[6] Synchronized cardioversion is discussed in Chapter 4.

 YOU SHOULD KNOW Calcium channel blockers inhibit the entry of calcium into vascular smooth muscle cells and myocardial cells, which inhibits both myocardial and vascular smooth muscle contraction. By inhibiting the contractility of vascular smooth muscle and coronary vessels, vascular resistance is reduced, thereby reducing blood pressure.

There are two major categories of calcium channel blockers, the dihydropyridines (including amlodipine and nifedipine) and the nondihydropyridines (including diltiazem and verapamil). The dihydropyridines primarily affect the peripheral vasculature, resulting in peripheral vasodilation, with little or no effect on the SA or AV nodes. The nondihydropyridines decrease heart rate and myocardial contractility, slow conduction through the AV node, and have some peripheral arterial dilatory effects as well. The major adverse effects of calcium channel blockers include hypotension, worsening heart failure, bradycardia, and AV block.

Vagal Maneuvers

Vagal maneuvers are methods used to stimulate baroreceptors located in the internal carotid arteries and the aortic arch. Stimulation of these receptors results in reflex stimulation of the vagus nerve and release of acetylcholine. Acetylcholine slows conduction through the AV node, resulting in a slowing of the heart rate.

TABLE 3-12 **Adenosine**

Adenosine	Mechanism of Action/Effects	Indications	Dosage[5]	Precautions
Trade Name: Adenocard **Class:** Endogenous chemical, antiarrhythmic Figure 3-30	Found naturally in all body cells Rapidly metabolized in the blood vessels Slows sinus rate Slows conduction time through AV node Can interrupt reentry pathways through AV node Half-life is less than 10 sec	Stable narrow-QRS regular tachycardias Unstable narrow-QRS regular tachycardia while preparations are made for synchronized cardioversion Stable, regular, wide-QRS tachycardia If the dysrhythmia is not due to reentry involving the AV node or sinus node (i.e., atrial fibrillation, atrial flutter, atrial or ventricular tachycardias), adenosine will not terminate the dysrhythmia but may produce transient AV block that may clarify the diagnosis	Initial dose = 6 mg rapid IV push over 1 to 3 sec. If no response within 1 to 2 min, give 12 mg rapid IV push. May repeat 12 mg dose once in 1 to 2 min. Follow each dose immediately with a 20-mL normal saline flush and raise the arm for 10 to 20 sec. Due to extremely short half-life, start IV line as proximal to the heart as possible, such as the antecubital fossa.	Constant ECG monitoring is essential. Contraindicated in patients with asthma. Adverse effects (nausea, chest tightness, shortness of breath, headache) common but transient and usually resolve within 1 to 2 min. Discontinue in any patient who develops severe respiratory difficulty. Reduce the dose by one-half in patients on dipyridamole (Persantine), carbamazepine (Tegretol), those with transplanted hearts, or if given via a central IV line. Consider increasing the dose in patients on theophylline, caffeine, or theobromine.

Examples of vagal maneuvers include:

- Coughing.
- Squatting.
- Breath-holding.
- Carotid sinus massage. This procedure is performed with the patient's neck extended. Firm pressure is applied just underneath the angle of the jaw for up to 10 seconds (Figure 3-34). The procedure for performing carotid sinus massage is shown in Skill 3-1. Carotid sinus pressure should be avoided in older adults, in patients who have a history of stroke, in known carotid artery stenosis, or in patients who have a carotid artery bruit on auscultation. Simultaneous, bilateral carotid pressure should *never* be performed.
- Application of a cold stimulus to the face (e.g., a washcloth soaked in iced water, a cold pack, or crushed ice mixed with water in a plastic bag or glove) for up to 10 seconds. This technique is often effective for infants and young children. When using this method, do not obstruct the patient's mouth or nose or apply pressure to the eyes.
- Valsalva maneuver. Instruct the patient to blow through an occluded straw or take a deep breath and bear down, as if having a bowel movement, for up to 10 seconds. This strains the abdominal muscles and increases intrathoracic pressure.
- Gagging. Use a tongue depressor or culturette swab to briefly touch the back of the throat.

TABLE 3-13	**Calcium Channel Blockers**			
Drug	**Mechanism of Action/Effects**	**Indications**	**Dosage[5]**	**Precautions**
diltiazem (Cardizem) **Figure 3-31** verapamil (Calan, Isoptin, Verelan) **Figure 3-32**	Inhibit movement of calcium ions across cell membranes in the heart and vascular smooth muscle, resulting in: • Relaxation of coronary vascular smooth muscle • Dilation of both large and small coronary arteries • Decreased sinoatrial and AV conduction, increased AV node refractoriness • Decreased myocardial oxygen demand • Decreased myocardial contractility Produce antihypertensive effects primarily by relaxation of vascular smooth muscle and a resultant decrease in peripheral vascular resistance	Stable narrow-QRS tachycardia if the rhythm persists despite vagal maneuvers or adenosine or the tachycardia is recurrent To control the ventricular rate in patients with atrial fibrillation or atrial flutter	Diltiazem: Initial dose 0.25 mg/kg IV bolus over 2 min. If needed, follow in 15 min with 0.35 mg/kg over 2 min. Subsequent IV bolus doses should be individualized for each patient. Verapamil: 2.5- to 5-mg slow IV push over 2 minutes (give over 3 to 4 min in older adults or when BP is within the lower range of normal). May repeat with 5 to 10 mg in 15 to 30 min (if no response and BP remains normal or elevated). Maximum total dose 20 to 30 mg.	Can worsen hypotension and should not be given to patients with a systolic BP of less than 90 mm Hg. Use with caution in patients with mild to moderate hypotension. Monitor BP, heart rate, and ECG closely. Avoid in patients with heart failure and atrial fibrillation or atrial flutter associated with known pre-excitation (e.g., Wolff-Parkinson-White [WPW]) syndrome. Avoid in patients with wide-QRS tachycardia (may precipitate ventricular fibrillation). IV calcium channel blockers and IV beta-blockers should not be given together or in close proximity (within a few hours)—may cause severe hypotension.

Atrioventricular Nodal Reentrant Tachycardia

AVNRT is the most common type of SVT. It is caused by reentry in the area of the AV node. In the normal AV node, there is only one pathway through which an electrical impulse is conducted from the SA node to the ventricles. Patients with AVNRT have two conduction pathways within the AV node that conduct impulses at different speeds and recover at different rates. The fast pathway conducts impulses rapidly but has a long refractory period (slow recovery time). The slow pathway conducts impulses slowly but has a short refractory period (fast recovery time). Under the right conditions, the fast and slow pathways can form an electrical circuit or loop (Figure 3-35). As one side of the loop is recovering, the other is firing.

AVNRT is usually caused by a premature atrial complex (PAC) that is spread by the electrical circuit. This allows the impulse to spin around in a circle indefinitely and to reenter the normal electrical pathway with each pass around the circuit. The result is a very rapid and regular rhythm that ranges from 150 to 250 beats/min (Table 3-15, Figure 3-36).

TABLE 3-14	**Beta-blockers**		
Drug	**Mechanism of Action/Effects**	**Indications**	**Precautions**
atenolol (Tenormin); esmolol (Brevibloc); labetalol (Normodyne, Trandate); metoprolol (Lopressor); propranolol (Inderal)	Slow sinus rate Depress AV conduction Reduce blood pressure Decrease myocardial oxygen consumption	Stable narrow-QRS tachycardias if the rhythm persists despite vagal maneuvers or adenosine or the tachycardia is recurrent For ventricular rate control in atrial fibrillation and atrial flutter if no signs of heart failure Specific forms of polymorphic ventricular tachycardia	In general, patients with reactive airway disease should not receive beta-blockers. Some beta-blockers should be used with caution in patients with impaired renal or liver function. Adverse effects include hypotension, bradycardia, and precipitation of heart failure. Avoid in patients with decompensated heart failure and pre-excited atrial fibrillation or atrial flutter.

Figure 3-33

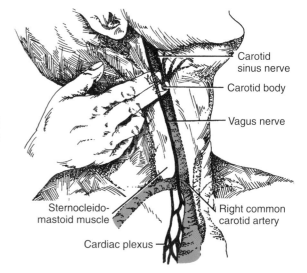

Figure 3-34 Carotid sinus massage. The carotid sinus (carotid body) is located at the bifurcation of the carotid artery at the angle of the jaw.

Carotid sinus nerve
Carotid body
Vagus nerve
Sternocleido-mastoid muscle
Right common carotid artery
Cardiac plexus

SKILL 3-1 Carotid Sinus Massage

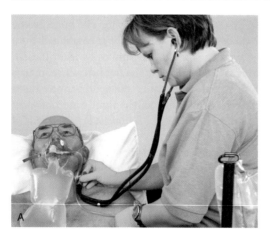

Step 1 Before performing this procedure, take appropriate standard precautions. Make sure that suction, a defibrillator, and emergency medications are available and that you have a physician's order to perform the procedure. Place the patient on oxygen (if indicated), assess the patient's vital signs, establish IV access, and apply ECG electrodes. Explain the procedure to the patient. Gently palpate each carotid artery separately to assess pulse quality. If the pulses are markedly unequal, consult a physician before performing the procedure. Check for carotid bruits by listening to each carotid artery with a stethoscope. A bruit is a blowing or rushing sound created by the turbulence within the vessel. If a bruit is heard, do not perform this procedure.

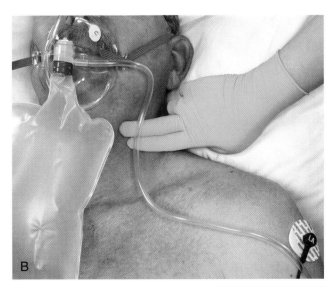

Step 2 If no bruit is heard and no contraindications are present, turn the patient's head to one side. Press "Print" or "Record" on the cardiac monitor to run a continuous ECG strip during the procedure. With two fingers, locate the carotid pulse just underneath the angle of the jaw. With firm pressure, press the carotid artery toward the cervical vertebrae but do not apply so much pressure as to occlude the vessel. Begin an up-and-down motion and perform this for no longer than 10 seconds. Never massage both carotid arteries at the same time. Visually monitor the patient and ECG throughout the procedure. Note the onset and end of the vagal maneuver on the rhythm strip.

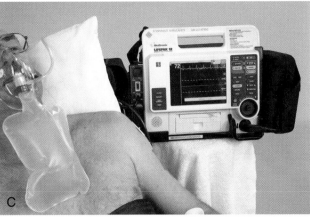

Step 3 After the procedure, reassess the patient's vital signs and the ECG rhythm.

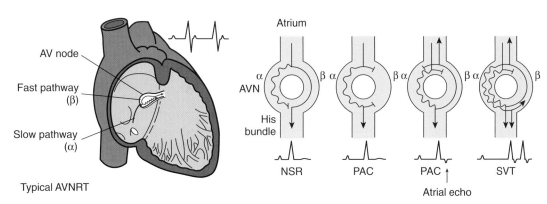

Figure 3-35 Schematic for supraventricular tachycardia (SVT) due to AV nodal reentry (AVNRT). AV, AV node; NSR, normal sinus rhythm; PAC, premature atrial complex.

TABLE 3-15	Characteristics of Atrioventricular Nodal Reentrant Tachycardia (AVNRT)
Rate	150 to 250 beats/min; typically 180 to 200 beats/min in adults
Rhythm	Ventricular rhythm is usually very regular
P waves	P waves are often hidden in the QRS complex; if the ventricles are stimulated first and then the atria, a negative (inverted) P wave will appear after the QRS in leads II, III, and aVF; when the atria are depolarized after the ventricles, the P wave typically distorts the end of the QRS complex
PR interval	P waves are not seen before the QRS complex; therefore, the PR interval is not measurable
QRS duration	0.11 sec or less unless an intraventricular conduction delay exists

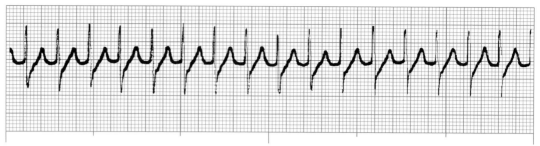

Figure 3-36 Atrioventricular (AV) nodal reentrant tachycardia (AVNRT).

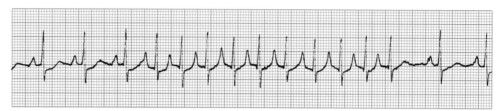

Figure 3-37 Paroxysmal supraventricular tachycardia (PSVT).

What Causes It?

AVNRT can occur at any age. Whether a person is born with a tendency to have AVNRT or whether it develops later in life for an unknown reason has not been clearly determined. AVNRT is common in young, healthy persons with no structural heart disease. It occurs more often in women than in men. AVNRT also occurs in persons with chronic obstructive pulmonary disease (COPD), coronary artery disease, valvular heart disease, heart failure, and digitalis toxicity. AVNRT can cause angina or MI in patients with coronary artery disease.

What Do I Do About It?

Treatment depends on the severity of the patient's signs and symptoms. Signs and symptoms that may be associated with rapid ventricular rates include:

- Chest pain or pressure
- Dyspnea
- Heart failure
- Lightheadedness
- Nausea
- Neck vein pulsations

- Nervousness, anxiety
- Palpitations (common)
- Signs of shock
- Syncope or near-syncope
- Weakness

If the patient is stable but symptomatic (and symptoms are the result of rapid heart rate), treatment usually includes oxygen (if indicated), IV access, and vagal maneuvers. If vagal maneuvers are contraindicated or do not slow the rate or cause conversion of the tachycardia to a sinus rhythm, the first antiarrhythmic given is adenosine. If the patient is unstable, treatment should include oxygen, IV access, and sedation (if the patient is awake and time permits), followed by synchronized cardioversion.

A regular, narrow-QRS tachycardia that starts or ends suddenly is called **paroxysmal supraventricular tachycardia (PSVT)** (Figure 3-37). (PSVT is discussed here since most supraventricular tachycardias are the result of AVNRT). P waves are seldom seen because they are hidden in T waves of preceding beats. The QRS is narrow unless there is a problem with conduction of the impulse through the ventricles, as in a BBB.

> **ACLS Pearl**
>
> ST-segment changes (usually depression) are common in patients with SVTs. In most patients, these ST-segment changes are thought to be the result of repolarization changes. However, in older adults and those with a high likelihood of ischemic heart disease, ST-segment changes may represent ECG changes consistent with an acute coronary syndrome. The patient should be watched closely. Appropriate laboratory tests and a 12-lead ECG should be obtained to rule out infarction as needed.

Atrioventricular Reentrant Tachycardia

AVRT is the second most common type of SVT. Remember that the AV node is normally the only electrical connection between the atria and ventricles. The term **pre-excitation** is used to describe rhythms that originate from above the ventricles but in which the impulse travels via a pathway other than the AV node and bundle of His. Thus the supraventricular impulse excites the ventricles earlier than would be expected if the impulse traveled by way of the normal conduction system. Patients with pre-excitation syndromes, such as Wolff-Parkinson-White (WPW) syndrome and Lown-Ganong-Levine (LGL) syndrome, are prone to AVRT.

What Causes It?

During fetal development, strands of myocardial tissue form connections between the atria and ventricles, outside the normal conduction system. These strands normally become nonfunctional shortly after birth; however, in patients with pre-excitation syndrome, these connections persist as congenital malformations of working myocardial tissue. Because these connections bypass part or all of the normal conduction system, they are called **accessory pathways.** The term **bypass tract** is used when one end of an accessory pathway is attached to normal conductive tissue. This pathway may connect the right atrial and ventricular walls, the left atrial and ventricular walls, or the atrial and ventricular septa on either the right or the left side.

There are three major forms of pre-excitation syndrome, each differentiated by its accessory pathways or bypass tracts[7] (Figure 3-38).

- In **Wolff-Parkinson-White** (WPW) **syndrome**, the accessory pathway is called the Kent bundle. This bundle connects the atria directly to the ventricles, completely bypassing the normal conduction system. WPW syndrome is the most common pre-excitation syndrome. It is more common in men than women and 60% to 70% of people with WPW syndrome have no associated heart disease. WPW syndrome is one of the most common causes of tachydysrhythmias in infants and children. Although the accessory pathway in WPW syndrome is believed to be congenital in origin, symptoms associated with pre-excitation often do not appear until young adulthood.
- In **Lown-Ganong-Levine** (LGL) **syndrome**, the accessory pathway is called the *James bundle.* This bundle connects the atria directly to the lower portion of the AV node, thus partially bypassing the AV node. In LGL syndrome, one end of the James bundle is attached to normal conductive tissue. This congenital pathway may be called a *bypass tract.*
- Another unnamed pre-excitation syndrome involves the Mahaim fibers. These fibers do not bypass the AV node but originate below the AV node and insert into the ventricular wall, bypassing part or all of the ventricular conduction system.

Delta waves are produced with accessory pathways that insert directly into ventricular muscle. A **delta wave** is the initial slurred deflection at the beginning of the QRS complex. It results from initial activation of the QRS by conduction over the accessory pathway (Figure 3-39). Characteristics of WPW syndrome appear in Table 3-16. Examples of AV nodal rhythm disturbances are shown in Figure 3-40.

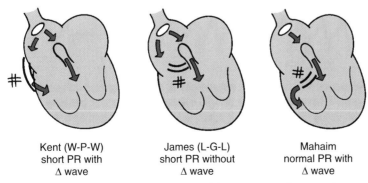

Kent (W-P-W)	James (L-G-L)	Mahaim
short PR with	short PR without	normal PR with
Δ wave	Δ wave	Δ wave

Figure 3-38 The three major forms of pre-excitation. Location of the accessory pathways and corresponding electrocardiogram (ECG) characteristics.

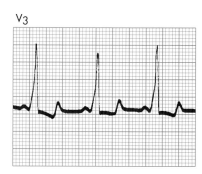

Figure 3-39 Lead V₃. Typical Wolff-Parkinson-White (WPW) syndrome pattern showing the short PR interval, delta wave, wide QRS complex, and secondary ST and T wave changes.

TABLE 3-16	**Characteristics of Wolff-Parkinson-White (WPW) Syndrome**
Rate	Usually 60 to 100 beats/min, if the underlying rhythm is sinus in origin
Rhythm	Regular, unless associated with atrial fibrillation
P waves	Upright in lead II unless WPW is associated with atrial fibrillation
PR interval	If P waves are observed, 0.12 sec or less because the impulse travels very quickly across the accessory pathway, bypassing the normal delay in the AV node
QRS duration	Usually more than 0.12 sec; slurred upstroke of the QRS complex (delta wave) may be seen in one or more leads

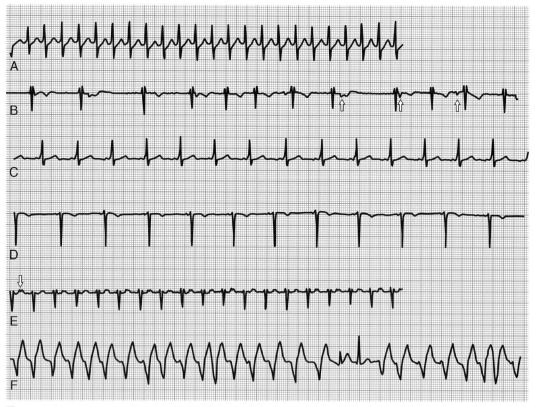

Figure 3-40 Atrioventricular (AV) nodal rhythm disturbances. **A,** AV nodal reentrant tachycardia (AVNRT) at a rate of 185 beats/min. The retrograde P waves are hidden in the QRS complexes. **B,** Automatic junctional tachycardia. Note the presence of AV dissociation during tachycardia. The P waves (*arrows*) are dissociated form the QRS complexes. **C,** Normal sinus rhythm in a patient with Wolff-Parkinson-White (WPW) syndrome. Note the short PR interval (less than 0.12 sec), the slurring of the initial portion of the QRS (delta wave), and the wide QRS complex. **D,** Normal sinus rhythm in a patient with Lown-Ganong-Levine (LGL) pattern. Note the short PR interval without the presence of a delta wave or wide QRS complex. **E,** Orthodromic AV reentrant tachycardia at a rate of 146 beats/min in a patient with WPW syndrome. The retrograde P waves are clearly seen altering the normal T wave contour (*arrow*). **F,** Atrial fibrillation in a patient with WPW syndrome. Note the rapid and irregular ventricular response with widening of the QRS secondary to pre-excitation.

Keeping It Simple

Recognizing Wolff-Parkinson-White Syndrome
- Short PR interval
- Delta wave
- Widening of the QRS

What Do I Do About It?

Persons with WPW syndrome are syndrome predisposed to tachydysrhythmias and most commonly to AFib, atrial flutter, or PSVT. This is because the accessory pathway bypasses the protective blocking mechanism provided by the AV node and provides a mechanism for reentry. Common signs and symptoms associated with WPW syndrome and a rapid ventricular rate include palpitations, light-headedness, shortness of breath, anxiety, weakness, dizziness, chest discomfort, and signs of shock.

If the patient is symptomatic because of the rapid ventricular rate, treatment will depend on how unstable the patient is, the width of the QRS complex (i.e., wide or narrow), and the regularity of the ventricular rhythm. Consultation with a cardiologist is recommended when caring for a patient with AVRT. Do not give drugs that slow or block conduction through the AV node (e.g., adenosine, digoxin, diltiazem, verapamil) because they may speed up conduction through the accessory pathway, resulting in a further *increase* in heart rate. If the patient is unstable, preparations should be made for synchronized cardioversion.

Junctional Tachycardia

Junctional tachycardia is an ectopic rhythm that begins in the pacemaker cells found in the bundle of His. When three or more sequential premature junctional complexes (PJCs) occur at a rate of more than 100 beats/min, a junctional tachycardia exists. Nonparoxysmal (i.e., gradual onset) junctional tachycardia usually starts as an accelerated junctional rhythm but the heart rate gradually increases to more than 100 beats/min. The usual ventricular rate for nonparoxysmal junctional tachycardia is 101 to 140 beats/min. Paroxysmal junctional tachycardia, which is also known as **focal** or **automatic junctional tachycardia**, is an uncommon dysrhythmia that starts and ends suddenly and is often precipitated by a PJC. The ventricular rate for paroxysmal junctional tachycardia is generally faster, at a rate of 140 beats/min or more.

If the AV junction paces the heart, the electrical impulse must travel in a backward (retrograde) direction to activate the atria. If a P wave is seen, it will be upside down in leads II, III, and aVF because the impulse is traveling away from the positive electrode (Table 3-17, Figure 3-41).

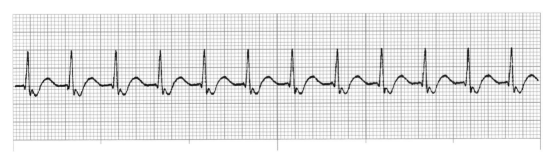

Figure 3-41 Junctional tachycardia.

TABLE 3-17	**Characteristics of Junctional Tachycardia**
Rate	101 to 180 beats/min
Rhythm	Very regular
P waves	May occur before, during, or after the QRS; if visible, the P wave is inverted in leads II, III, and aVF
PR interval	If a P wave occurs before the QRS, the PR interval will usually be 0.12 sec or less; if no P wave occurs before the QRS, there will be no PR interval
QRS duration	0.11 sec or less unless an intraventricular conduction delay exists

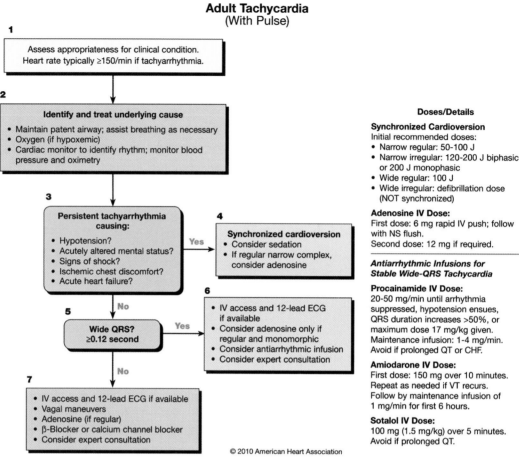

Figure 3-42 The American Heart Association ACLS tachycardia algorithm. CHF, congestive heart failure; NS, normal saline; VT, ventricular tachycardia.

What Causes It?

Junctional tachycardia may occur because of an acute coronary syndrome, heart failure, theophylline administration, or digitalis toxicity (common cause).

What Do I Do About It?

With sustained ventricular rates of 150 beats/min or more, the patient may complain of a "racing heart" and severe anxiety. Because of the fast ventricular rate, the ventricles may be unable to fill completely, resulting in decreased cardiac output. Junctional tachycardia associated with an acute coronary syndrome may:

- Cause heart failure, hypotension, or cardiogenic shock
- Extend the size of an MI
- Increase myocardial ischemia
- Increase the frequency and severity of chest pain
- Predispose the patient to ventricular dysrhythmias

Treatment depends on the severity of the patient's signs and symptoms, and expert consultation is advised. The ACLS tachycardia algorithm appears in Figure 3-42.

WIDE-QRS TACHYCARDIAS

A wide-QRS tachycardia has a QRS duration of 0.12 second or more. Most wide-complex tachycardias are ventricular tachycardia (VT). Some wide-complex tachycardias are actually SVT with BBB or aberrant conduction. Still others are ventricular paced rhythms or a tachycardia with AV conduction

TABLE 3-18	Procainamide			
Procainamide	Mechanism of Action/Effects	Indications	Dosage[5]	Precautions
Trade Name: Pronestyl, Procan SR **Class:** Class IA antiarrhythmic	Prolongs the effective refractory period and action potential duration in the atria, ventricles, and His-Purkinje system Suppresses ectopy in atrial and ventricular tissue Prolongs the PR and QT intervals Exerts a peripheral vasodilatory effect	To control the ventricular rate in the patient with pre-excited atrial fibrillation Stable monomorphic ventricular tachycardia	20 to 50 mg/min IV infusion or 100 mg every 5 min until one of the following occurs: Dysrhythmia resolves Hypotension ensues QRS prolongs by more than 50% of original width Total dose of 17 mg/kg administered Maintenance infusion 1 to 4 mg/min	During administration, carefully monitor the patient's ECG and blood pressure. If the blood pressure falls 15 mm Hg or more, temporarily discontinue administration. Watch the ECG closely for increasing PR and QT intervals, prolonging of the QRS complex, heart block, and/or onset of TdP. Reduce maintenance infusion rate in liver dysfunction, renal failure. Avoid in patients with QT prolongation or heart failure.

associated with or mediated by an accessory pathway (i.e., pre-excited tachycardia). It is best to seek expert consultation when treating a patient who has a wide-complex tachycardia.

If the patient is stable, the QRS is wide, the rhythm is regular, and the QRS complexes are of similar shape (i.e., monomorphic), but you are unsure of the origin of the rhythm, adenosine is the first drug that should be given. With few exceptions, adenosine will generally have no effect if the rhythm is VT. If the wide-QRS rhythm is actually SVT with aberrancy, adenosine administration will usually result in transient slowing or conversion to a sinus rhythm. For pharmacologic termination of a stable wide-QRS tachycardia that is most likely VT, procainamide (Table 3-18), amiodarone (Table 3-19, Figure 3-43), or sotalol (Table 3-20) may be used. These medications are considered first-line antiarrhythmics for monomorphic VT and have complex mechanisms of action. They are used for both atrial and ventricular dysrhythmias. Although lidocaine is a ventricular antiarrhythmic, it is considered a second-line antiarrhythmic for the management of monomorphic VT because it is reportedly less effective for the termination of VT than the first-line agents. Lidocaine is discussed later in this chapter. If the decision is made to administer procainamide, amiodarone, or sotalol, it is recommended that expert consultation be sought before another drug is administered.[5] If the diagnosis of SVT cannot be proved or cannot be made easily, then the patient should be treated as if VT were present.

ACLS Pearl

If the patient presents with serious signs and symptoms caused by the tachycardia, a specific diagnosis of the origin of the tachycardia is irrelevant; the patient requires *immediate* electrical therapy (synchronized cardioversion) (see Chapter 4).

Intraventricular Conduction Defects

A delay or block can occur in any part of the intraventricular conduction system. If a delay or block occurs in one of the bundle branches, the ventricles will not depolarize at the same time (Figure 3-44). The impulse travels first down the unblocked branch and stimulates that ventricle. Because of the

TABLE 3-19 **Amiodarone**

Amiodarone	Mechanism of Action/Effects	Indications	Dosage[5]	Precautions
Trade Name: Cordarone **Class:** Class III antiarrhythmic Figure 3-43	Directly depresses the automaticity of the SA and AV nodes Slows conduction through the AV node and in the accessory pathway of patients with Wolff-Parkinson-White syndrome Inhibits alpha- and beta-adrenergic receptors Possesses both vagolytic and calcium-channel blocking properties Coronary and peripheral vasodilator Mild decrease in myocardial contractility however, cardiac output may actually increase due to decreased afterload	Pulseless VT/VF (after CPR, defibrillation, and a vasopressor) Stable narrow-QRS tachycardias if the rhythm persists despite vagal maneuvers or adenosine or the tachycardia is recurrent To control ventricular rate in atrial fibrillation To control ventricular rate in pre-excited atrial dysrhythmias with conduction over an accessory pathway Stable monomorphic VT Polymorphic VT with normal QT interval	Pulseless VT/VF Initial bolus of 300-mg IV/IO bolus. Can be followed by one dose of 150 mg. If return of spontaneous circulation, consider continuous IV infusion (1 mg/min infusion for 6 hours and then a 0.5 mg/min maintenance infusion over 18 hours). Maximum daily dose 2.2 g IV per 24 hours. Other indications: Loading dose–150 mg IV over 10 min. May repeat every 10 min if needed. After conversion, follow with a 1 mg/min infusion for 6 hours and then a 0.5 mg/min maintenance infusion over 18 hours. Maximum cumulative dose 2.2 g IV per 24 hours.	Hypotension, bradycardia, and AV block are adverse effects of amiodarone administration. Slow the infusion rate or discontinue if seen. Prolongs the PR, QRS, and QT intervals, and has an additive effect with other medications that prolong the QT interval (e.g., procainamide, phenothiazines, some tricyclic antidepressants, thiazide diuretics, sotalol). Although prolongation of the QRS duration and QT interval may be beneficial in some patients, it may also increase the risk for TdP.

TABLE 3-20 **Sotalol**

Sotalol	Mechanism of Action/Effects	Indications	Dosage[5]	Precautions
Trade Name: Betapace **Class:** Class III antiarrhythmic	Slows heart rate Decreases AV nodal conduction Increases AV nodal refractoriness Prolongs the effective refractory period of atrial muscle, ventricular muscle, and AV accessory pathways (where present) in both anterograde and retrograde directions Negative inotrope	Stable monomorphic VT Note: Sotalol is not a first-line antiarrhythmic	1.5 mg/kg IV is the dose used in clinical studies U.S. packaging label recommends that any dose should be infused slowly over 5 hours	Monitor heart rate and blood pressure carefully. Monitor for bradycardia, hypotension, and new dysrhythmias. Use with caution in patients with bronchospastic disease. Avoid in patients with long QT interval and uncontrolled heart failure.

block, the impulse must then travel from cell to cell through the myocardium (rather than through the normal conduction pathway) to stimulate the other ventricle. This means of conduction is slower than normal and the QRS complex appears widened on the ECG. The ventricle with the blocked bundle branch is the last to be depolarized.

Essentially two conditions must exist for the suspicion of BBB. First, the QRS complex must have an abnormal duration (0.12 second or more in width if a complete BBB), and second, the QRS complex must arise as the result of supraventricular activity (this excludes ventricular beats and paced ventricular complexes). If these two conditions are met, delayed ventricular conduction is assumed to be present, and BBB is the most common cause of this abnormal conduction.[8]

A QRS complex measuring 0.10 to 0.12 second is called an *incomplete* right or left BBB. A QRS measuring more than 0.12 second is called a *complete* right or left BBB. If the QRS is wide but there is no BBB pattern, the terms *wide QRS* or *intraventricular conduction delay* are used to describe the QRS.

To determine right versus left BBB, take the following steps:
- Look at lead V_1.
- Move from the J-point back into the QRS complex and determine if the terminal portion (i.e., last 0.04 second) of the QRS complex is a positive (i.e., upright) or negative (i.e., downward) deflection (Figures 3-45 and 3-46).
- If the two criteria for BBB are met and the terminal portion of the QRS is positive, a right BBB is most likely present. If the terminal portion of the QRS is negative, a left BBB is most likely present.

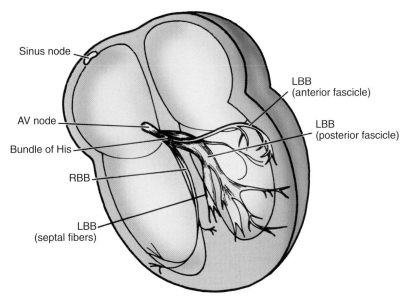

Figure 3-44 Cardiac conduction system. AV, atrioventricular; LBB, left bundle branch; RBB, right bundle branch.

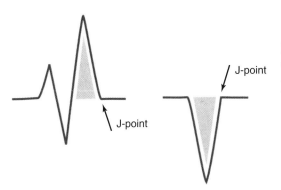

Figure 3-45 Move from the J-point back into the QRS complex and determine if the terminal portion (i.e., last 0.04 second) of the QRS complex is a positive or negative deflection. If the two criteria for bundle branch block (BBB) are met and the terminal portion of the QRS is positive, a right BBB is most likely present. If the terminal portion of the QRS is negative, a left BBB is most likely present.

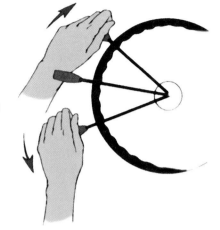

Figure 3-46 Differentiating right versus left BBB. Use the "turn signal theory"—right is up, left is down—to remember the difference.

Accelerated Idioventricular Rhythm

An **accelerated idioventricular rhythm** (AIVR) exists when three or more ventricular beats occur in a row at a rate of 41 to 100 beats/min (Table 3-21, Figure 3-47). Although this heart rate is not considered a tachycardia, AIVR is discussed here because some cardiologists consider the upper end of the rate range to be about 120 beats/min.

AIVR is usually considered a benign escape rhythm that appears when the sinus rate slows and disappears when the sinus rate speeds up. Episodes of AIVR usually last a few seconds to a minute.

What Causes It?

AIVR occurs most often in the setting of acute MI, most often during the first 12 hours. It is particularly common after successful reperfusion therapy. AIVR has been observed in patients with:
- Acute myocarditis
- Cocaine toxicity
- Digitalis toxicity
- Dilated cardiomyopathy
- Hypertensive heart disease
- Subarachnoid hemorrhage

What Do I Do About It?

AIVR generally requires no treatment because the rhythm is protective and often transient, spontaneously resolving on its own. However possible dizziness, lightheadedness, or other signs of hemodynamic compromise may occur because of the loss of atrial kick.

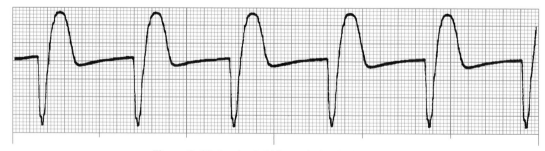

Figure 3-47 Accelerated idioventricular rhythm (AIVR).

TABLE 3-21	**Characteristics of Accelerated Idioventricular Rhythm (AIVR)**
Rate	41 to 100 (41 to 120 per some cardiologists) beats/min
Rhythm	Essentially regular
P waves	Usually absent or, with retrograde conduction to the atria, may appear after the QRS (usually upright in the ST segment or T wave)
PR interval	None
QRS duration	Greater than 0.12 sec; T wave usually in opposite direction of the QRS complex

Ventricular Tachycardia

VT exists when three or more premature ventricular complexes (PVCs) occur in immediate succession at a rate greater than 100 beats/min. VT may occur as a short run lasting less than 30 seconds (i.e., nonsustained) (Figure 3-48), but more commonly persists for more than 30 seconds (i.e., sustained). VT may occur with or without pulses and the patient may be stable or unstable with this rhythm.

VT, like PVCs, may originate from an ectopic focus in either ventricle. When the QRS complexes of VT are of the same shape and amplitude, the rhythm is called *monomorphic VT* (Table 3-22, Figure 3-49). When the QRS complexes of VT vary in shape and amplitude from beat to beat, the rhythm is called *polymorphic VT*. In polymorphic VT, the QRS complexes appear to twist from upright to negative or negative to upright and back. Polymorphic VT is discussed later in this chapter with irregular tachycardias.

> **ACLS Pearl**
>
> A rapid, wide-QRS rhythm associated with pulselessness, shock, or heart failure should be presumed to be ventricular tachycardia until proven otherwise.

What Causes It?

Sustained monomorphic VT is often associated with underlying heart disease, particularly myocardial ischemia. It rarely occurs in patients without underlying heart disease. Common causes of VT include:

- Acid-base imbalance
- Acute coronary syndromes
- Cardiomyopathy
- Cocaine abuse
- Digitalis toxicity
- Electrolyte imbalance (e.g., hypokalemia, hyperkalemia, hypomagnesemia)
- Mitral valve prolapse
- Trauma (e.g., myocardial contusion, invasive cardiac procedures)
- Tricyclic antidepressant overdose
- Valvular heart disease

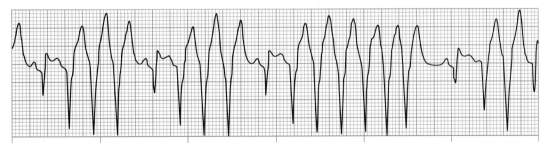

Figure 3-48 Nonsustained ventricular tachycardia.

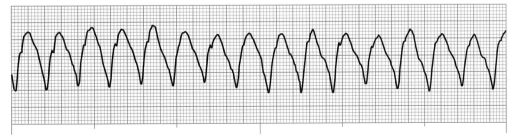

Figure 3-49 Sustained ventricular tachycardia (VT). When the QRS complexes of VT are of the same shape and amplitude, the rhythm is called monomorphic VT.

TABLE 3-22	**Characteristics of Monomorphic Ventricular Tachycardia**
Rate	101 to 250 beats/min
Rhythm	Essentially regular
P waves	Usually not seen; if present, they have no set relationship to the QRS complexes, appearing between them at a rate different from that of the VT
PR interval	None
QRS duration	0.12 sec or more; often difficult to differentiate between the QRS and T wave

What Do I Do About It?

Signs and symptoms associated with VT vary. VT may occur with or without pulses. The patient who has sustained monomorphic VT may be stable for long periods. However, when the ventricular rate is very fast, or when myocardial ischemia is present, monomorphic VT can degenerate to polymorphic VT or ventricular fibrillation. Syncope or near-syncope may occur because of an abrupt onset of VT. The patient's only warning symptom may be a brief period of lightheadedness.

> **YOU SHOULD KNOW** Sustained VT does not always produce signs of hemodynamic instability.

Treatment is based on the patient's signs and symptoms and the type of VT. If the rhythm is monomorphic VT (and the patient's symptoms are caused by the tachycardia):

- Cardiopulmonary resuscitation (CPR) and defibrillation are used to treat the *pulseless* patient with VT.
- Stable but symptomatic patients are treated with oxygen (if indicated), IV access, and ventricular antiarrhythmics (e.g., procainamide, amiodarone, sotalol) to suppress the rhythm. Procainamide should be avoided if the patient has a prolonged QT interval or signs of heart failure. Sotalol should also be avoided if the patient has a prolonged QT interval.
- Unstable patients (usually a sustained heart rate of 150 beats/min or more) are treated with oxygen, IV access, and sedation (if awake and time permits) followed by synchronized cardioversion.

In all cases, an aggressive search must be made for the cause of the VT.

> **ACLS Pearl**
>
> A supraventricular tachycardia with an intraventricular conduction delay may be difficult to distinguish from VT. Keep in mind that VT is considered a potentially life-threatening dysrhythmia. If you are unsure whether a regular, wide-QRS tachycardia is VT or SVT with an intraventricular conduction delay, treat the rhythm as VT until proven otherwise. Obtaining a 12-lead ECG may help differentiate VT from SVT, but do not delay treatment if the patient is unstable.

IRREGULAR TACHYCARDIAS

The severity of signs and symptoms associated with an irregular tachycardia varies depending on the ventricular rate, how long the rhythm has been present, and the patient's cardiovascular status. The patient may be asymptomatic and not require treatment or may experience serious signs and symptoms. It is best to seek expert consultation when treating a patient who has an irregular tachycardia.

Multifocal Atrial Tachycardia

Wandering atrial pacemaker is a rhythm in which the size, shape, and direction of the P waves vary, sometimes from beat to beat. The difference in the look of the P waves is a result of the gradual shifting of the dominant pacemaker between the SA node, the atria, and the AV junction. When a wandering atrial pacemaker is associated with a ventricular rate greater than 100 beats/min, the rhythm is called *multifocal atrial tachycardia* (MAT) (Table 3-23, Figure 3-50). MAT is also called *chaotic atrial tachycardia*.

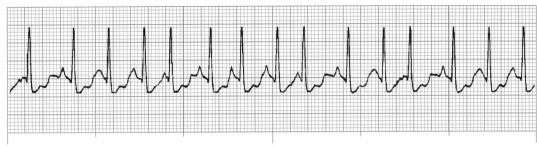

Figure 3-50 Multifocal atrial tachycardia (MAT).

TABLE 3-23	Characteristics of Multifocal Atrial Tachycardia (MAT)
Rate	Ventricular rate is greater than 100 beats/min
Rhythm	May be irregular as the pacemaker site shifts from the SA node to ectopic atrial locations and the AV junction
P waves	Size, shape, and direction may change from beat to beat; at least three different P wave configurations (seen in the same lead) are required for a diagnosis of wandering atrial pacemaker or multifocal atrial tachycardia
PR interval	Variable
QRS duration	0.11 sec or less unless an intraventricular conduction delay exists

What Causes It?

In MAT, multiple ectopic sites stimulate the atria. MAT is most often seen in the following disease states:

- Acute coronary syndromes
- Digoxin toxicity
- Electrolyte imbalances
- Hypoxia
- Rheumatic heart disease
- Severe chronic obstructive pulmonary disease (COPD)
- Theophylline toxicity

What Do I Do About It?

The treatment of MAT is directed at the underlying cause. If you know the rhythm is MAT and the patient is symptomatic, it is best to consult a cardiologist before starting treatment. If the patient is stable and symptomatic but you are uncertain that the rhythm is MAT, you can try a vagal maneuver (as long as there are no contraindications). If vagal maneuvers are contraindicated or ineffective, you can try IV adenosine. Remember that MAT is the result of random and chaotic firing of multiple sites in the atria. MAT does not involve reentry through the AV node. Therefore, it is unlikely that vagal maneuvers or giving adenosine will terminate the rhythm. However, they may momentarily slow the rate enough so that you can look at the P waves and determine the specific type of tachycardia. By determining the type of tachycardia, treatment specific to that rhythm can be given.

Atrial Flutter and Atrial Fibrillation

Atrial flutter is an ectopic atrial rhythm in which an irritable site fires regularly at a very rapid rate. Because of this extremely rapid stimulation, waveforms are produced that resemble the teeth of a saw, or a picket fence; these are called *flutter waves* (Table 3-24). Flutter waves are best observed in leads II, III, aVF, and V_1. If each impulse were sent to the ventricles, the ventricular rate would equal 300 beats/min or more. The healthy AV node protects the ventricles from these extremely fast atrial rates.

Atrial flutter with an atrial rate of 300 beats/min and a ventricular rate of 150 beats/min results in 2:1 conduction; 100 beats/min is 3:1 conduction; 75 beats/min is 4:1 conduction; 50 beats/min is 6:1 conduction, and so on. Although conduction ratios in atrial flutter are often even (i.e., 2:1, 4:1, 6:1), variable conduction can also occur, producing an irregular ventricular rhythm.

AFib occurs because of altered automaticity in one or several rapidly firing sites in the atria or reentry involving one or more circuits in the atria (Table 3-25, Figure 3-51). These rapid impulses

TABLE 3-24	Characteristics of Atrial Flutter
Rate	With type I atrial flutter, the atrial rate ranges from 250 to 350 beats/min; with type II atrial flutter, the atrial rate ranges from 350 to 450 beats/min; the ventricular rate varies and is determined by AV blockade; the ventricular rate will usually not exceed 180 beats/min due to the intrinsic conduction rate of the AV junction
Rhythm	Atrial regular; ventricular regular or irregular depending on AV conduction and blockade
P waves	No identifiable P waves; saw-toothed "flutter" waves are present
PR interval	Not measurable
QRS duration	Usually 0.11 sec or less but may be widened if flutter waves are buried in the QRS complex or an intraventricular conduction delay exists

TABLE 3-25	Characteristics of Atrial Fibrillation
Rate	Atrial rate usually 400 to 600 beats/min; ventricular rate variable
Rhythm	Ventricular rhythm usually irregularly irregular
P waves	No identifiable P waves; fibrillatory waves present; erratic, wavy baseline
PR interval	Not measurable
QRS duration	Usually 0.11 sec or less but may be widened if an intraventricular conduction delay exists

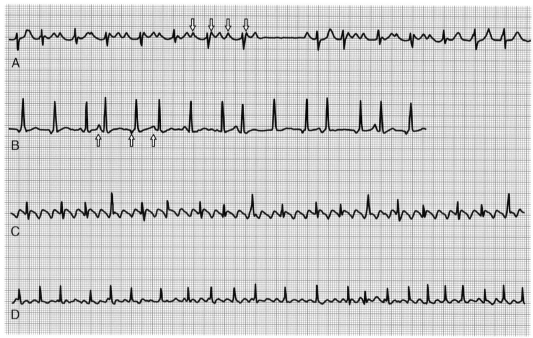

Figure 3-51 Atrial tachydysrhythmias. **A,** Atrial tachycardia (AT) with 2:1 and variable atrioventricular (AV) conduction. Note the presence of more P waves (*arrows*) than QRS complexes. **B,** Multifocal AT demonstrating an irregularly irregular rhythm at a rate of approximately 110 beats/min, with at least three different P wave morphologies (*arrows*) and without a dominant underlying rhythm. **C,** Atrial flutter. Flutter waves are seen as the discrete undulations of the baseline (saw-tooth pattern). The conduction rate is variable. **D,** Atrial fibrillation. The rhythm is irregularly irregular without evidence of organized atrial electrical activity.

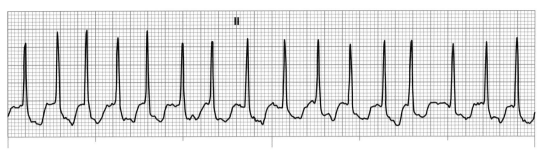

Figure 3-52 Atrial fibrillation with a rapid ventricular response (RVR).

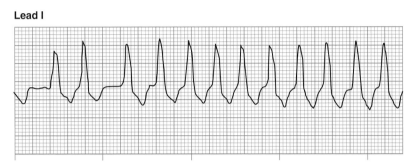

Figure 3-53 Atrial fibrillation with a rapid ventricular response and left bundle branch block (BBB).

cause the muscles of the atria to quiver (fibrillate). This results in ineffectual atrial contraction, decreased stroke volume, a subsequent decrease in cardiac output, and loss of atrial kick.

Atrial flutter or AFib that has a ventricular rate of more than 100 beats/min is described as *uncontrolled*. The ventricular rate is considered rapid when it is 150 beats/min or more (Figures 3-52, 3-53). New-onset atrial flutter or AFib is often associated with a rapid ventricular rate. Atrial flutter or AFib with a rapid ventricular response is commonly called *Aflutter with RVR* or *AFib with RVR*". Atrial flutter or AFib that has a ventricular rate of less than 100 beats/min, is described as controlled. A controlled ventricular rate may be the result of a healthy AV node protecting the ventricles from very fast atrial impulses or of drugs used to control (block) conduction through the AV node, decreasing the number of impulses reaching the ventricles.

What Causes It?
Atrial flutter is usually caused by a reentry circuit in which an impulse circles around a large area of tissue, such as the entire right atrium. It is usually a paroxysmal rhythm that is precipitated by a premature atrial complex. It may last for seconds to hours and occasionally 24 hours or more. Chronic atrial flutter is unusual. This is because the rhythm usually converts to sinus rhythm or AFib, either on its own or with treatment. AFib can occur in patients with or without detectable heart disease or related symptoms.

What Do I Do About It?
When atrial flutter is present with 2:1 conduction, it may be difficult to tell the difference between atrial flutter and sinus tachycardia, atrial tachycardia, AVNRT, AVRT, or SVT. Vagal maneuvers may help identify the rhythm by temporarily slowing AV conduction and revealing the underlying flutter waves (Figure 3-54).

Treatment decisions are based on the ventricular rate, the duration of the rhythm, the patient's general health, and how he or she is tolerating the rhythm. Patients who experience AFib are at increased risk of having a stroke. Because the atria do not contract effectively and expel all of the blood within them, blood may pool within them and form clots. A stroke can result if a clot moves from the

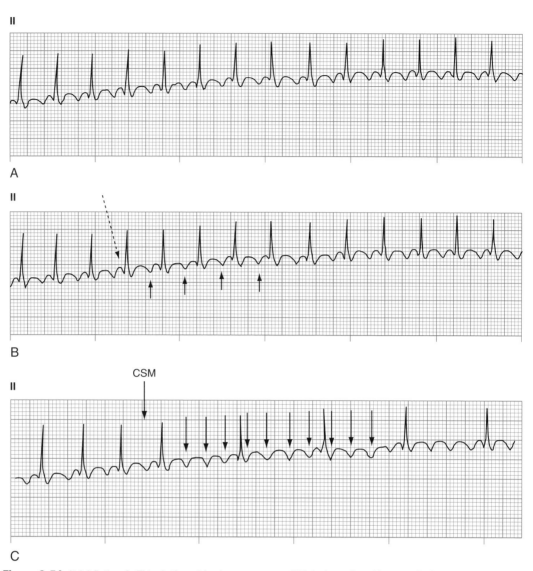

Figure 3-54 Atrial flutter. **A,** This rhythm strip shows a narrow-QRS tachycardia with a ventricular rate just under 150 beats/min. **B,** The same rhythm shown in A with *arrows* added indicating possible atrial activity. **C,** When carotid sinus massage (CSM) is performed, the rate of conduction through the AV node slows, revealing atrial flutter.

atria and lodges in an artery in the brain. If the rhythm has been present for 48 hours or longer, anticoagulation is recommended before attempting to convert the rhythm with medications, synchronized cardioversion, or catheter ablation. A widely accepted practice is to begin anticoagulation 2 to 3 weeks before and continue therapy for about 4 weeks after conversion. If atrial flutter or AFib is associated with a rapid ventricular rate, treatment may be directed toward controlling the ventricular rate or converting the rhythm to a sinus rhythm. "Electric or pharmacologic cardioversion (conversion to normal sinus rhythm) should *not be attempted* in these patients unless the patient is unstable."[5] It is best to obtain a 12-lead ECG and seek expert consultation when treating the symptomatic patient with atrial flutter or AFib.

Synchronized cardioversion should be considered for any patient with atrial flutter or AFib who has serious signs and symptoms because of the rapid ventricular rate (e.g., hypotension, signs of shock, heart failure). If synchronized cardioversion is performed, atrial flutter may be successfully converted to a sinus rhythm using low energy levels. Because the rhythm is more disorganized, AFib generally requires higher energy levels (see Chapter 4).

TABLE 3-26	**Characteristics of Polymorphic Ventricular Tachycardia (PVT)**
Rate	150 to 300 beats/min, typically 200 to 250 beats/min
Rhythm	May be regular or irregular
P waves	None
PR interval	None
QRS duration	0.12 sec or more; there is a gradual alteration in amplitude and direction of the QRS complexes; a typical cycle consists of 5 to 20 QRS complexes

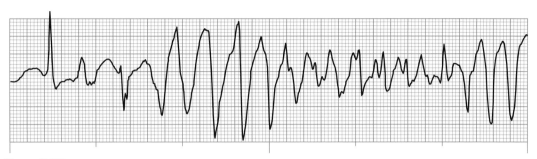

Figure 3-55 When the QRS complexes of ventricular tachycardia (VT) vary in shape and amplitude, the rhythm is termed polymorphic VT.

Polymorphic Ventricular Tachycardia

In polymorphic ventricular tachycardia (PMVT), the QRS complexes appear to twist from upright to negative or negative to upright and back (Table 3-26, Figure 3-55).

What Causes It?

Several types of PMVT and their possible causes have been identified as follows:

- Polymorphic VT that occurs in the presence of a long QT interval (typically 0.45 second or more and often 0.50 second or more) is called *torsades de pointes*. A long QT interval may be congenital, acquired (typically precipitated by antiarrhythmic drug use or hypokalemia, which are typically associated with bradycardia), or idiopathic (neither familial nor with an identifiable acquired cause).
- Polymorphic VT can occur in the presence of an abnormally short QT interval (typically less than 0.32 second). This type of polymorphic VT is called *short QT-PMVT*.
- Polymorphic VT that occurs in the presence of a normal QT interval is simply referred to as *polymorphic VT* or *normal QT-PMVT*.
- Polymorphic VT that is triggered by stress or exercise and occurs in the absence of QT prolongation or structural heart disease is called *catecholaminergic PMVT*.
- Polymorphic VT that is associated with an ECG pattern consisting of right bundle branch-like conduction and ST elevation in the right chest leads without evidence of QT prolongation or structural heart disease is called *Brugada syndrome*.
- Polymorphic VT that is caused by acute myocardial ischemia or infarction and occurs in the absence of QT prolongation is called *ischemic PMVT*.
- Polymorphic VT without QT prolongation that cannot be attributed to one of the above mechanisms is called *idiopathic normal QT PMVT*.

What Do I Do About It?

Symptoms are usually related to the decreased cardiac output that occurs because of the fast ventricular rate. Signs of shock are often present. The patient may experience a syncopal episode or seizures. The rhythm may occasionally terminate spontaneously and recur after several seconds or minutes, or it may deteriorate to ventricular fibrillation. The patient with sustained PMVT is rarely hemodynamically stable.

It is best to seek expert consultation when treating the patient with PMVT because of the diverse mechanisms of PMVT, for which there may or may not be clues as to its specific cause at the time of the patient's presentation. Treatment options vary and can be contradictory. For example, a medication

TABLE 3-27	Magnesium Sulfate			
Magnesium Sulfate	**Mechanism of Action/Effects**	**Indications**	**Dosage[5]**	**Precautions**
Trade Name: Magnesium sulfate **Class:** Antiarrhythmic, electrolyte 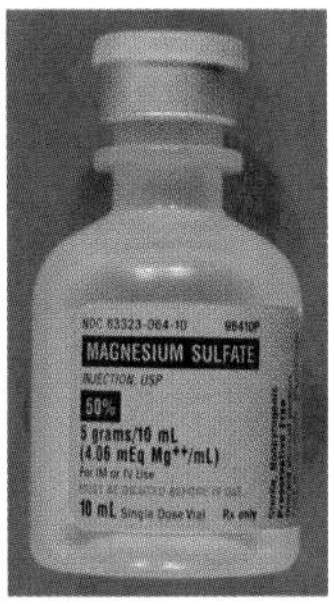 Figure 3-56	Essential for activity of many enzyme systems Plays an important role with regard to neurochemical transmission and muscular excitability	Polymorphic VT with prolonged QT interval	If pulseless, give 1 to 2 g IV diluted in 10 mL D$_5$W. If pulse present, give 1 to 2 g IV diluted in 50 to 100 mL D$_5$W over 15 min.	Use with caution in patients receiving digitalis, patients with impaired renal function, and patients with preexisting heart blocks. Calcium is the antidote for magnesium toxicity.

that may be appropriate for the treatment of TdP may be contraindicated when treating another form of PMVT. In general, if the patient is symptomatic as a result of the tachycardia, treat ischemia (if it is present), correct electrolyte abnormalities, and discontinue any medications that the patient may be taking that prolong the QT interval. If the patient is stable, the use of IV amiodarone (if the QT interval is normal), magnesium (Table 3-27, Figure 3-56), or beta-blockers may be effective, depending on the cause of the PMVT. If the patient is unstable or has no pulse, proceed with defibrillation as for VF (see Chapter 4).

> **ACLS Pearl**
> Because amiodarone, procainamide, and sotalol are antiarrhythmics that can cause prolongation of the QT interval, they are not used for dysrhythmias such as polymorphic VT associated with a long QT interval (TdP).

SECTION 3

Bradydysrhythmias: Too-Slow Rhythms

[Objectives 1, 2]

Cardiac output = Stroke volume × Heart rate. Therefore, a decrease in either stroke volume or heart rate may result in a decrease in cardiac output. An **absolute bradycardia** is a heart rate of less than 60 beats/min. When a patient has a **relative bradycardia**, his or her heart rate may be more than 60 beats/min. This may occur when a hypotensive patient needs a tachycardia (as in hypovolemia) but is unable to increase his or her heart rate as a result of SA node disease, beta-blockers, or other medications. A patient with an unusually slow heart rate may complain of weakness or dizziness and fainting (syncope) can occur. Decreasing cardiac output will eventually produce hemodynamic compromise.

> **ACLS Pearl**
> Many patients tolerate a heart rate of 50 to 60 beats/min but become symptomatic when the rate drops below 50.

TABLE 3-28 **Atropine**

Atropine Sulfate	Mechanism of Action/Effects	Indications	Dosage[5]	Precautions
Trade Name: Atropine **Class:** Vagolytic, parasympatholytic, antimuscarinic, muscarinic antagonist, anticholinergic, parasympathetic antagonist, parasympathetic blocker	Increases heart rate Increases conduction velocity Relaxes bronchial smooth muscle Decreases body secretions Dilates pupils	First-line drug for symptomatic bradycardia	0.5 mg IV every 3 to 5 min to a total dose of 3 mg	Do not push slowly or in smaller than recommended doses May result in tachycardia, palpitations, and ventricular ectopy Use with caution in acute coronary syndromes; excessive increases in heart rate may further worsen ischemia or increase size of infarction. Atropine may paradoxically cause high-degree AV block in patients after cardiac transplantation[9,10]

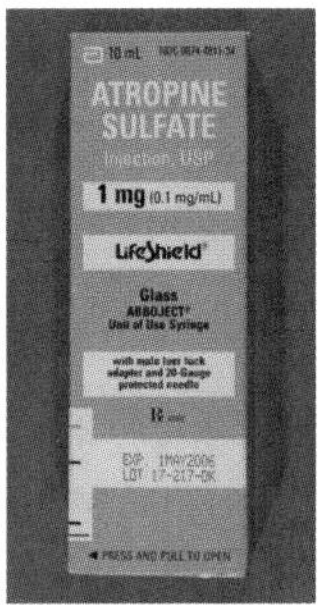

Figure 3-57

BOX 3-3 **Symptomatic Bradycardia—Serious Signs and Symptoms**

- Acute altered mental status
- Dizziness
- Fatigue
- Heart failure
- Low blood pressure
- Ongoing chest discomfort
- Pulmonary congestion
- Signs of shock
- Weakness

If a patient presents with a bradycardia, assess how the patient is tolerating the rhythm. If the patient has no symptoms, no treatment is necessary but he or she should be observed closely. Examples of serious signs and symptoms are shown in Box 3-3. The initial treatment of any patient with a symptomatic bradycardia should focus on support of airway and breathing. Assess the patient's oxygen saturation and determine if signs of increased work of breathing are present (e.g., retractions, tachypnea, or paradoxic abdominal breathing). Give supplemental oxygen if oxygenation is inadequate and assist ventilation if breathing is inadequate. Although atropine (Table 3-28, Figure 3-57) is recommended as the first-line drug for symptomatic bradycardia,[5] it is important to recognize that some bradycardias are unlikely to respond to atropine (e.g., complete AV blocks, wide-QRS AV blocks). Other interventions that may be used in the treatment of symptomatic bradycardia include epinephrine, dopamine, or isoproterenol IV infusions (discussed later in this chapter), or transcutaneous pacing (see Chapter 4).

SINUS BRADYCARDIA

If the SA node fires at a rate slower than normal for the patient's age, the rhythm is called sinus bradycardia. The rhythm starts in the SA node and then heads down the normal pathway of conduction through the atria, AV junction, bundle branches, and Purkinje fibers. This results in atrial and

TABLE 3-29	Characteristics of Sinus Bradycardia
Rate	Less than 60 beats/min
Rhythm	Regular
P waves	Uniform in appearance, positive (upright) in lead II, one precedes each QRS complex
PR interval	0.12 to 0.20 sec and constant from beat to beat
QRS duration	0.11 sec or less unless an intraventricular conduction delay exists

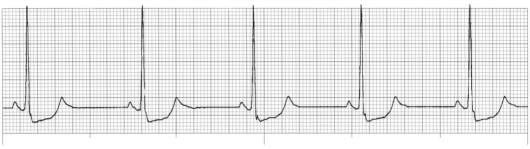

Figure 3-58 Sinus bradycardia with ST-segment depression.

ventricular depolarization. In adults and adolescents, a sinus bradycardia is a heart rate of less than 60 beats/min (Table 3-29, Figure 3-58).

What Causes It?

Sinus bradycardia occurs in adults during sleep and in well-conditioned athletes. It is also present in up to 35% of people younger than 25 years of age while at rest. Sinus bradycardia is common in some MIs. Stimulation of the vagus nerve can also result in slowing of the heart rate. For example, coughing, vomiting, straining to have a bowel movement or sudden exposure of the face to cold water can result in slowing of the heart rate. Carotid sinus pressure can also slow the heart rate. In people who have a sensitive carotid sinus, slowing of the heart rate can occur when a tight collar is worn or with the impact of the stream of water on the neck while in the shower. Other causes of sinus bradycardia are shown in Box 3-4.

BOX 3-4	Causes of Sinus Bradycardia

- Disease of the SA node
- Hyperkalemia
- Hypothermia
- Hypothyroidism
- Hypokalemia
- Hypoxia
- Increased intracranial pressure
- Inferior myocardial infarction
- Medications such as calcium channel blockers, digitalis, beta-blockers, amiodarone, and sotalol
- Obstructive sleep apnea
- Post heart transplantation
- Posterior myocardial infarction
- Vagal stimulation

What Do I Do About It?

Assess how the patient tolerates the rhythm at rest and with activity. If the patient has no symptoms, no treatment is necessary. If the patient is symptomatic because of the slow rate, initial treatment generally includes supplemental oxygen (if indicated), starting an IV, and giving IV atropine.

YOU SHOULD KNOW In the setting of an MI, sinus bradycardia is often temporary. A slow heart rate can be beneficial in the patient who has had an MI (and no symptoms are caused by the slow rate). This is because the heart's demand for oxygen is less when the heart rate is slow.

JUNCTIONAL ESCAPE RHYTHM

Remember that the SA node is normally the heart's pacemaker. The AV junction may assume responsibility for pacing the heart if:
- The SA node fails to discharge (such as sinus arrest)
- An impulse from the SA node is generated but blocked as it exits the SA node (such as SA block)
- The rate of discharge of the SA node is slower than that of the AV junction (such as a sinus bradycardia or the slower phase of a sinus arrhythmia)
- An impulse from the SA node is generated and is conducted through the atria but is not conducted to the ventricles (such as an AV block)

The intrinsic rate of the AV junction is 40 to 60 beats/min. Because a junctional rhythm starts from above the ventricles, the QRS complex is usually narrow and its rhythm is very regular (Table 3-30, Figure 3-59). If the AV junction paces the heart at a rate slower than 40 beats/min, the resulting rhythm is called a *junctional bradycardia*. This may seem confusing because the AV junction's normal pacing rate (40 to 60 beats/min) *is* bradycardic; however, the term junctional bradycardia refers to a rate slower than normal for the AV junction.

TABLE 3-30	Characteristics of Junctional Escape Rhythm
Rate	40 to 60 beats/min
Rhythm	Very regular
P waves	May occur before, during, or after the QRS; if visible, the P wave is inverted in leads II, III, and aVF
PR interval	If a P wave occurs before the QRS, the PR interval will usually be 0.12 sec or less; if no P wave occurs before the QRS, there will be no PR interval
QRS duration	0.11 sec or less unless an intraventricular conduction delay exists

What Causes It?

Causes of a junctional rhythm include the following:
- Acute coronary syndromes (particularly inferior wall MI)
- Effects of medications including digitalis, quinidine, beta-blockers, and calcium channel blockers
- Hypoxia
- Immediate period after cardiac surgery
- Increased parasympathetic tone
- Rheumatic heart disease
- SA node disease
- Valvular disease

What Do I Do About It?

The patient may be asymptomatic with a junctional escape rhythm or may experience signs and symptoms that may be associated with the slow heart rate and decreased cardiac output. Treatment depends on the cause of the dysrhythmia and the patient's presenting signs and symptoms. If the dysrhythmia

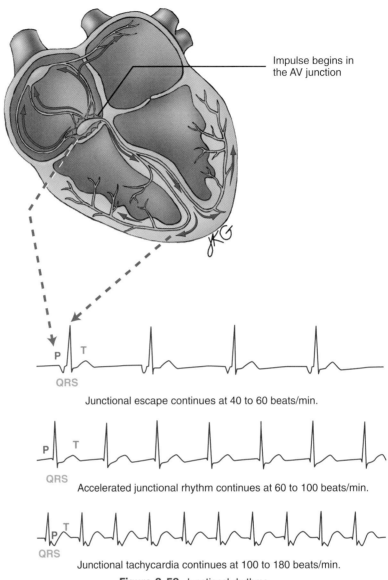

Impulse begins in the AV junction

Junctional escape continues at 40 to 60 beats/min.

Accelerated junctional rhythm continues at 60 to 100 beats/min.

Junctional tachycardia continues at 100 to 180 beats/min.

Figure 3-59 Junctional rhythms.

is caused by digitalis toxicity, this medication should be withheld and administration of a digoxin immune Fab (such as Digibind may be considered). If the patient's signs and symptoms are related to the slow heart rate, atropine should be considered. Other interventions that may be used for the treatment of symptomatic bradycardia include epinephrine (Table 3-31, Figure 3-60), dopamine (Table 3-32, Figure 3-61), or isoproterenol (Table 3-33) IV infusions, or transcutaneous pacing.

> **YOU SHOULD KNOW**
>
> **Important Terms to Commit to Memory**
> Agonist—A drug or substance that produces a predictable response (stimulates action)
> Antagonist—An agent that exerts an action opposite to another (blocks action)
> Chronotrope—A substance that affects the heart rate; positive chronotrope = ↑ heart rate, negative chronotrope = ↓ heart rate
> Dromotrope—A substance that affects AV conduction velocity; positive dromotrope = ↑ AV conduction velocity, negative dromotrope = ↓ AV conduction velocity
> Inotrope—A substance that affects myocardial contractility; positive inotrope = ↑ force of contraction, negative inotrope = ↓ force of contraction

TABLE 3-31   Epinephrine

Epinephrine	Mechanism of Action/Effects	Indications	Dosage[5]	Precautions
Trade Name: Adrenalin **Class:** Natural catecholamine; sympathomimetic; adrenergic agonist Figure 3-60	Stimulates alpha, beta$_1$, and beta$_2$ receptors • Alpha-agonist— constricts arterioles in skin, mucosa, kidneys, and viscera → increased systemic vascular resistance • Beta$_1$ agonist— increases force of contraction (+ inotropic effect), increases heart rate (+ chronotropic effect) → increased myocardial workload and oxygen requirements • Beta$_2$ agonist— relaxes bronchial smooth muscle, dilates vessels in skeletal muscle; dilates cerebral, pulmonary, coronary, and hepatic vessels	Symptomatic bradycardia Hypotension Cardiac arrest–VF, pulseless VT, asystole, pulseless electrical activity	Symptomatic bradycardia or hypotension: • Continuous infusion at 2 to 10 mcg/min Cardiac arrest: • IV/IO: 1 mg (10-mL) of 1:10,000 solution IV push, follow with 20-mL fluid flush. May repeat 1-mg dose every 3 to 5 min • Tracheal: 2 to 2.5 mg diluted in 5 to 10 mL of sterile water or normal saline Post–cardiac arrest care: • Continuous IV infusion of 0.1 to 0.5 mcg/kg/ min (in 70-kg adult, 7 to 35 mcg/ min)	Increases myocardial oxygen demand; may cause postresuscitation myocardial dysfunction and ventricular dysrhythmias.[11] Avoid mixing with sodium bicarbonate. Administer an epinephrine infusion via an infusion pump. Check IV site frequently for evidence of tissue sloughing. Should not be administered in the same IV line as alkaline solutions– inactivates epinephrine. Epinephrine is available in different concentrations and in different medication containers. Read the label carefully before giving epinephrine to ensure you are giving the right dose and using the right concentration of the drug.

ACLS Pearl

Sympathetic (adrenergic) receptors are located in different organs and have different physiologic actions when stimulated. There are five main types of sympathetic receptors: alpha$_1$, alpha$_2$, beta$_1$, beta$_2$, and dopamine (also called dopaminergic).

- Alpha$_1$ receptors are found in the eyes, blood vessels, bladder, and male reproductive organs. Stimulation of alpha$_1$ receptor sites results in constriction.
- Alpha$_2$ receptor sites are found in parts of the digestive system and on presynaptic nerve terminals in the peripheral nervous system. Stimulation results in decreased secretions, decreased peristalsis, and suppression of norepinephrine release.
- Beta receptor sites are divided into beta$_1$ and beta$_2$. Beta$_1$ receptors are found in the heart and kidneys. Stimulation of beta$_1$ receptor sites in the heart results in increased heart rate and increased contractility. Stimulation of beta$_1$ receptor sites in the kidneys results in the release of renin into the blood. Renin promotes the production of angiotensin, a powerful vasoconstrictor. Beta$_2$ receptor sites are found in the arterioles of the heart, lungs, and skeletal muscle. Stimulation of beta$_2$ receptor sites in the smooth muscle of the bronchi results in dilation.
- Dopamine receptors are found in the renal, mesenteric, and visceral blood vessels. Stimulation results in dilation.

TABLE 3-32	Dopamine			
Dopamine	**Mechanism of Action/ Effects**	**Indications**	**Dosage[5]**	**Precautions**
Trade Name: Intropin, Dopastat **Class:** Direct- and indirect-acting sympathomimetic; cardiac stimulant and vasopressor, natural catecholamine **Figure 3-61**	Naturally occurring immediate precursor of norepinephrine in the body Effects of dopamine are dose-related (there is some "overlap" of effects). • Low dose (dopaminergic effects)—dilates renal, mesenteric, and visceral vascular beds • Medium dose (beta effects; "cardiac dose")—improves myocardial contractility, increases SA rate, enhances impulse conduction in the heart • High dose (alpha effects; "pressor dose")—stimulates alpha$_1$ and alpha$_2$ receptors, BP and systemic vascular resistance increase	Temporizing measure in the management of symptomatic bradycardia that has not responded to atropine, or for which atropine is inappropriate, while awaiting availability of a pacemaker Hypotension that occurs after return of spontaneous circulation Hemodynamically significant hypotension in the absence of hypovolemia	Give as a continuous IV infusion of 2 to 10 mcg/kg/min; increase infusion rate according to blood pressure and other clinical responses	Correct hypovolemia before beginning dopamine therapy for the treatment of hypotension and shock. Administer via an infusion pump. Extravasation into surrounding tissue may cause necrosis and sloughing. Gradually taper drug before discontinuing the infusion. Monitor blood pressure, ECG, and drip rate closely.

TABLE 3-33	Isoproterenol			
Isoproterenol	**Mechanism of Action/Effects**	**Indications**	**Dosage[5]**	**Precautions**
Trade Name: Isuprel **Class:** Sympathomimetic, beta-adrenergic receptor agonist, antiarrhythmic	Produces pronounced stimulation of both beta$_1$ and beta$_2$ receptors of the heart, bronchi, skeletal muscle vasculature, and the GI tract Increases heart rate Produces vasodilation Onset of action is immediate	Temporizing measure in the management of symptomatic bradycardia that has not responded to atropine, or for which atropine is inappropriate, while awaiting availability of a pacemaker	Give as a continuous IV infusion of 2 to 10 mcg/min Titrate infusion rate according to heart rate and rhythm response	Administer via an infusion pump. Monitor blood pressure, ECG, and drip rate closely because it may cause hypotension and tachycardia

> ⚙ **ACLS** Pearl
>
> It is important to recognize the similarities and differences among dopamine, epinephrine, and isoproterenol administration when treating a symptomatic bradycardia. Although these drugs are given by continuous IV infusion, their dosing differs. Because the correct infusion rate for dopamine depends on the patient's weight, its dose range is 5 to 10 *mcg/kg/min*. An isoproterenol infusion is *not* based on the patient's weight and is infused at 2 to 10 *mcg/min*. In symptomatic bradycardia, an epinephrine infusion is infused at a dose range of 2 to 10 *mcg/min*; however, during post–cardiac arrest care, epinephrine is infused at a rate of 0.1 to 0.5 *mcg/kg/min*. In all cases, the infusion is titrated to the desired clinical response.

VENTRICULAR ESCAPE RHYTHM

A ventricular escape or idioventricular rhythm (IVR) exists when three or more ventricular beats occur in a row at a rate of 20 to 40 beats/min (Table 3-34, Figure 3-62).

TABLE 3-34	Characteristics of Ventricular Escape (Idioventricular) Rhythm
Rate	20 to 40 beats/min
Rhythm	Essentially regular
P waves	Usually absent or, with retrograde conduction to the atria, may appear after the QRS (usually upright in the ST segment or T wave)
PR interval	None
QRS duration	0.12 sec or greater, T wave frequently in opposite direction of the QRS complex

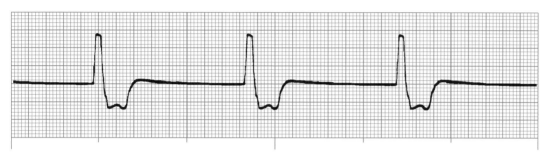

Figure 3-62 Ventricular escape rhythm.

What Causes It?

A ventricular escape rhythm may occur when:
- The SA node and the AV junction fail to initiate an electrical impulse
- The rate of discharge of the SA node or AV junction becomes less than the intrinsic rate of the ventricles
- Impulses generated by a supraventricular pacemaker site are blocked

A ventricular escape rhythm may also occur because of MI, digitalis toxicity, or metabolic imbalances.

What Do I Do About It?

Because the ventricular rate associated with a ventricular escape rhythm is very slow (i.e., 20 to 40 beats/min) with a loss of atrial kick, the patient may experience serious signs and symptoms as a result of decreased cardiac output. If the patient has a pulse and is symptomatic because of the slow rate, atropine may be attempted but is unlikely to be effective. Transcutaneous pacing or a dopamine, epinephrine, or isoproterenol IV infusion may be tried if atropine is ineffective. Medications such as lidocaine should be avoided in the management of this rhythm because lidocaine may abolish ventricular activity, possibly causing asystole in a patient with a ventricular escape rhythm. If the patient is not breathing and has no pulse despite the appearance of organized electrical activity on the cardiac monitor, pulseless electrical activity (PEA) exists. The management of PEA is discussed later in this chapter.

ATRIOVENTRICULAR BLOCKS

AV blocks are divided into three main types: first-, second-, and third-degree (i.e., complete) AV block (Figure 3-63). The clinical significance of an AV block depends on:
- The degree (severity) of the block
- The rate of the escape pacemaker (junctional vs. ventricular)
- The patient's response to that ventricular rate

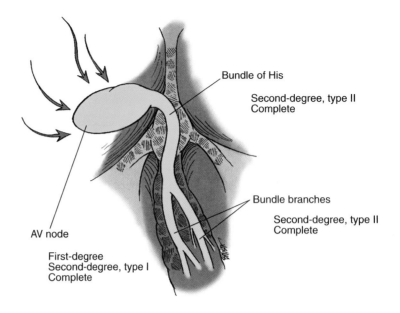

Figure 3-63 Locations of atrioventricular (AV) block.

First-Degree Atrioventricular Block

First-degree AV block is not a dysrhythmia itself; it is a condition that describes the consistent prolonged PR interval seen on the ECG rhythm strip. In first-degree AV block, impulses from the SA node to the ventricles are *delayed* (not blocked) (Figure 3-64). First-degree AV block usually occurs at the AV node (Table 3-35, Figure 3-65).

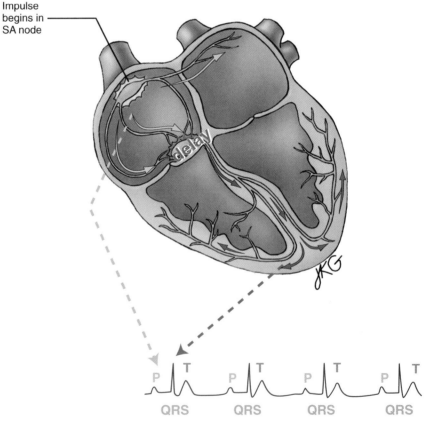

Figure 3-64 First-degree atrioventricular (AV) block.

TABLE 3-35 Characteristics of First-Degree AV Block

Rate	Usually within normal range, but depends on underlying rhythm
Rhythm	Regular
P waves	Normal in size and shape; one positive (upright) P wave before each QRS in leads II, III, and aVF
PR interval	Prolonged (more than 0.20 sec) but constant
QRS duration	0.11 sec or less unless an intraventricular conduction delay exists

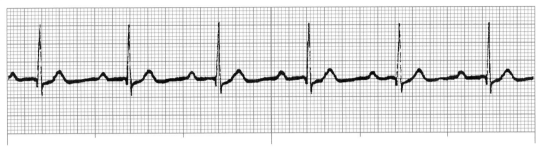

Figure 3-65 Sinus rhythm at 60 beats/min with a first-degree atrioventricular (AV) block.

What Causes It?

First-degree AV block may be a normal finding in individuals with no history of cardiac disease, especially in athletes. In some people, mild prolongation of the PR interval may be a normal variant, especially with sinus bradycardia during rest or sleep. First-degree AV block may also occur because of:

- Acute myocardial infarction
- Hyperkalemia
- Increased vagal tone
- Ischemia or injury to the AV node or junction
- Medications
- Rheumatic heart disease

What Do I Do About It?

The patient with a first-degree AV block is often asymptomatic; however, marked first-degree AV block can lead to symptoms even in the absence of higher degrees of AV block.[12] First-degree AV block that occurs with acute MI should be monitored closely. If first-degree AV block accompanies a symptomatic bradycardia, treat the bradycardia.

Keeping It Simple
A Quick Look at P Waves and AV Blocks

AV Block	P Wave Conduction
First-degree	All P waves conducted but delayed
Second-degree	Some P waves conducted, others blocked
Third-degree	No P waves conducted

Second-Degree Atrioventricular Block

With second-degree AV blocks, there is an *intermittent* disturbance in conduction of impulses between the atria and ventricles. The site of block in second-degree AV block type I is typically at the AV node. The site of block in second-degree AV block type II is the bundle of His or, more commonly, the bundle branches.

Second-Degree Atrioventricular Block, Type I (Wenckebach, Mobitz Type I)

Second-degree AV block type I is also known as *Mobitz type I* or *Wenckebach*. The Wenckebach pattern is the progressive lengthening of the PR interval followed by a P wave with no QRS complex (Figure 3-66). The conduction delay in second-degree AV block type I usually occurs at the level of the AV node (Table 3-36, Figure 3-67).

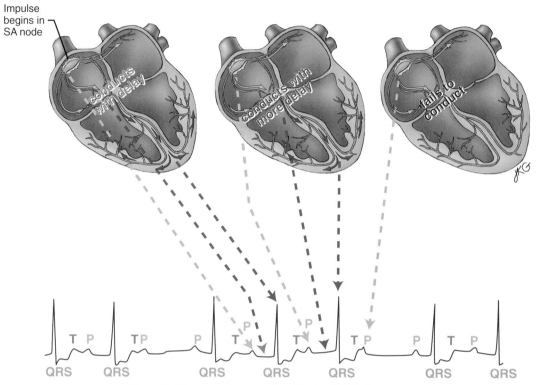

Figure 3-66 Second-degree atrioventricular (AV) block, type I.

TABLE 3-36	Characteristics of Second-Degree AV Block Type I
Rate	Atrial rate is greater than the ventricular rate
Rhythm	Atrial regular (P's plot through on time), ventricular irregular
P waves	Normal in size and shape; some P waves are not followed by a QRS complex (i.e., more P's than QRSs)
PR interval	Lengthens with each cycle (although this may be very slight), until a P wave appears without a QRS complex. (The PRI *after* the nonconducted beat is shorter than the interval preceding the nonconducted beat)
QRS duration	Usually 0.11 sec or less but is periodically dropped

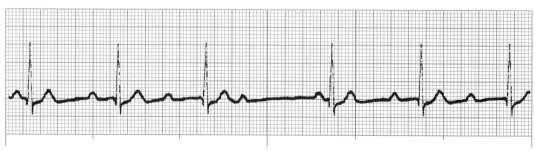

Figure 3-67 Second-degree atrioventricular (AV) block, type I.

What Causes It?

Second-degree AV block type I is usually caused by a conduction delay within the AV node. Remember that the right coronary artery supplies the AV node in 90% of the population. Thus right coronary artery occlusions are associated with AV block occurring in the AV node. If the right coronary artery is blocked, ischemia may develop in the AV node. As a result of this ischemia, there can be a disturbance in the balance between the parasympathetic and sympathetic divisions of the autonomic nervous system, resulting in an increase in parasympathetic tone. Once parasympathetic tone increases, conduction through the AV node is slowed. This slowing may manifest itself as a prolonged PR interval or as dropped beats. An increase in parasympathetic tone is the cause of most AV blocks complicating right coronary artery occlusions (e.g., inferior wall infarctions and right ventricular infarction).

What Do I Do About It?

The patient with this type of AV block is usually asymptomatic because the ventricular rate often remains nearly normal and cardiac output is not significantly affected. If the patient is symptomatic and the rhythm is a result of medications, these substances should be withheld. If the heart rate is slow and serious signs and symptoms occur because of the slow rate, atropine is the drug of choice. When it is associated with an acute inferior wall MI, this dysrhythmia is usually transient and resolves within 48 to 72 hours as the effects of parasympathetic stimulation disappear. When this rhythm occurs in conjunction with acute MI, the patient should be observed for increasing AV block.

Second-Degree Atrioventricular Block, Type II (Mobitz Type II)

Second-degree AV block type II is also called *Mobitz Type II* AV block. The conduction delay in second-degree AV block type II occurs below the AV node, either at the bundle of His or, more commonly, at the level of the bundle branches (Figure 3-68). This type of block (Table 3-37,

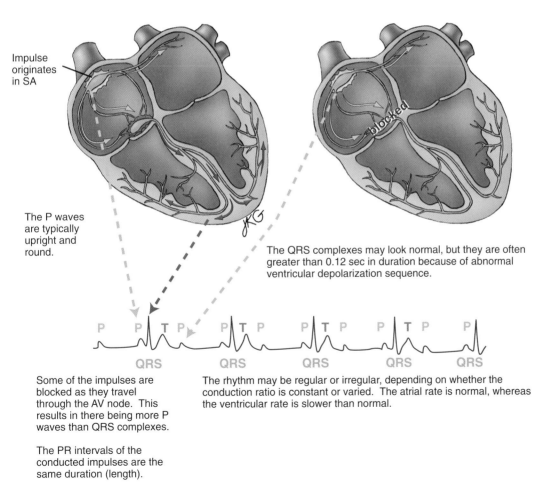

Impulse originates in SA

The P waves are typically upright and round.

The QRS complexes may look normal, but they are often greater than 0.12 sec in duration because of abnormal ventricular depolarization sequence.

Some of the impulses are blocked as they travel through the AV node. This results in there being more P waves than QRS complexes.

The PR intervals of the conducted impulses are the same duration (length).

The rhythm may be regular or irregular, depending on whether the conduction ratio is constant or varied. The atrial rate is normal, whereas the ventricular rate is slower than normal.

Figure 3-68 Second-degree atrioventricular (AV) block, type II.

TABLE 3-37	Characteristics of Second-Degree AV Block, Type II
Rate	Atrial rate is greater than the ventricular rate; ventricular rate often slow
Rhythm	Atrial regular (Ps plot through on time), ventricular irregular
P waves	Normal in size and shape; some P waves are not followed by a QRS complex (i.e., more Ps than QRSs).
PR interval	Within normal limits or slightly prolonged but *constant* for the conducted beats; there may be some shortening of the PR interval that follows a nonconducted P wave
QRS duration	Usually 0.11 sec or greater; periodically absent after P waves

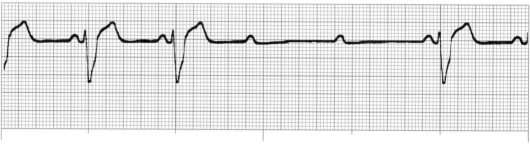

Figure 3-69 Second-degree atrioventricular (AV) block, type II.

Figure 3-69) is more serious than second-degree AV block type I and can progress to third-degree AV block.

What Causes It?

The bundle branches receive their primary blood supply from the left coronary artery. Thus disease of the left coronary artery or an anterior MI is usually associated with blocks that occur within the bundle branches. Second-degree AV block type II may also occur because of acute myocarditis or other types of organic heart disease.

What Do I Do About It?

The patient's response to this rhythm is usually related to the ventricular rate. If the ventricular rate is within normal limits, the patient may be asymptomatic. More commonly, the ventricular rate is significantly slowed and serious signs and symptoms result because of the slow rate and decreased cardiac output.

Second-degree AV block type II may progress to third-degree AV block without warning. In this situation, atropine administration will usually not improve the block but rather will increase the rate of discharge of the SA node. This may trigger a situation in which even fewer impulses are conducted through to the ventricles and the ventricular rate is further slowed. Transcutaneous pacing or a dopamine, epinephrine, or isoproterenol IV infusion may be tried if atropine is ineffective. Second-degree AV block type II usually is an indication for a permanent pacemaker.

Second-Degree Atrioventricular Block, 2:1 Conduction (2:1 Atrioventricular Block)

In 2:1 AV block, two P waves occur for every one QRS complex (2:1 conduction). Since there are no two PQRST cycles in a row from which to compare PR intervals, the decision as to what to term the rhythm is based on the width of the QRS complex (Table 3-38). A 2:1 AV block associated with a narrow QRS complex (i.e., 0.11 second or less) usually represents a form of second-degree AV block, type I (Figure 3-70). A 2:1 AV block associated with a wide QRS complex (i.e., greater than 0.11 sec) and is usually associated with a delay in conduction below the bundle of His; thus, it is usually a type II block (Figure 3-71). The causes are those of type I or type II block previously described. A comparison of the types of second-degree AV blocks is shown in Figure 3-72.

TABLE 3-38	**Characteristics of Second-Degree AV Block 2 : 1 Conduction (2 : 1 AV Block)**
Rate	Atrial rate twice the ventricular rate
Rhythm	Atrial regular (Ps plot through), ventricular regular
P waves	Normal in size and shape; every other P wave is followed by a QRS complex (i.e., more Ps than QRSs)
PR interval	Constant
QRS duration	Within normal limits if the block occurs above the bundle of His (probably type I); wide if the block occurs below the bundle of His (probably type II); absent after every other P wave

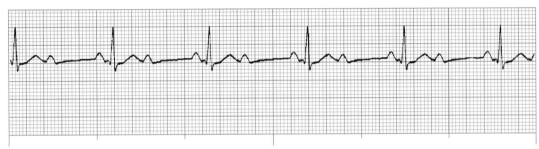

Figure 3-70 Second-degree atrioventricular (AV) block, 2:1 conduction, probably type I.

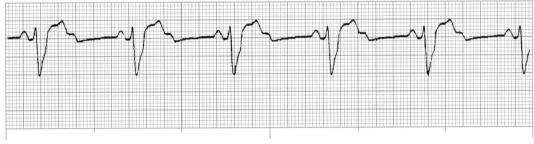

Figure 3-71 Second-degree atrioventricular (AV) block, 2:1 conduction, probably type II.

Third-Degree Atrioventricular Block

In third-degree AV block, there is a *complete* block in conduction of impulses between the atria and ventricles. The site of block in a third-degree AV block may be the AV node or, more commonly, the bundle of His or bundle branches (Table 3-39, Figure 3-73). A secondary pacemaker (either junctional or ventricular) stimulates the ventricles; therefore, the QRS may be narrow or wide, depending on the location of the escape pacemaker and the condition of the intraventricular conduction system.

What Causes It?

Third-degree AV block associated with an inferior MI is thought to be the result of a block above the bundle of His. It often occurs after progression from first-degree AV block or second-degree AV block type I. The resulting rhythm is usually stable because the escape pacemaker is usually junctional (i.e., narrow QRS complexes) with a ventricular rate of more than 40 beats/min (Figure 3-74).

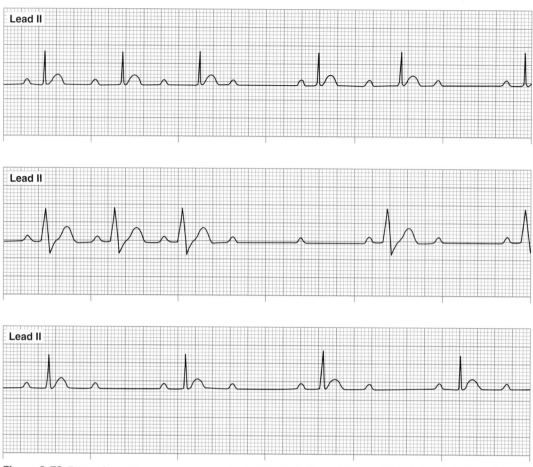

Figure 3-72 Types of second-degree atrioventricular (AV) block. **A,** Second-degree AV block type I. **B,** Second-degree AV block type II. **C,** 2:1 AV block.

TABLE 3-39	Characteristics of Third-Degree AV Block
Rate	Atrial rate greater than (and independent of) the ventricular rate; the ventricular rate is determined by the origin of the escape rhythm
Rhythm	Atrial regular (Ps plot through), ventricular regular; no relationship between the atrial and ventricular rhythms
P waves	Normal in size and shape
PR interval	None: the atria and the ventricles beat independently of each other, thus there is no true PR interval
QRS duration	Narrow or wide, depending on the location of the escape pacemaker and the condition of the intraventricular conduction system (narrow = junctional pacemaker, wide = ventricular pacemaker).

Third-degree AV block associated with an anterior MI is usually preceded by second-degree AV block type II or an intraventricular conduction delay (i.e., right or left BBB). The resulting rhythm is usually unstable because the escape pacemaker is usually ventricular (i.e., wide QRS complexes) with a ventricular rate of less than 40 beats/min (Figure 3-75).

What Do I Do About It?

The patient's signs and symptoms will depend on the origin of the escape pacemaker (i.e., junctional vs. ventricular) and the patient's response to a slower ventricular rate. If the patient is symptomatic as a result of the slow rate, atropine may be tried (but is unlikely to be effective). Other interventions that may be used include epinephrine, dopamine, or isoproterenol IV infusions, or transcutaneous pacing. The ACLS bradycardia algorithm is shown in Figure 3-76.

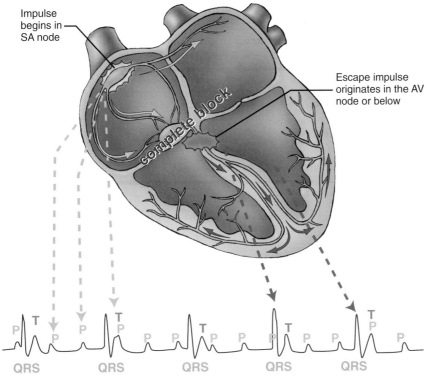

Impulse begins in SA node

Escape impulse originates in the AV node or below

complete block

Figure 3-73 Third-degree atrioventricular (AV) block.

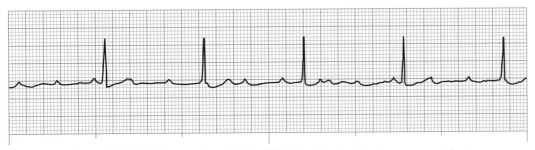

Figure 3-74 Third-degree atrioventricular (AV) block with a junctional escape pacemaker.

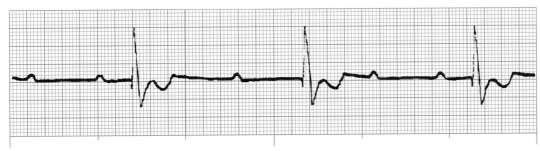

Figure 3-75 Third-degree atrioventricular (AV) block with a ventricular escape pacemaker.

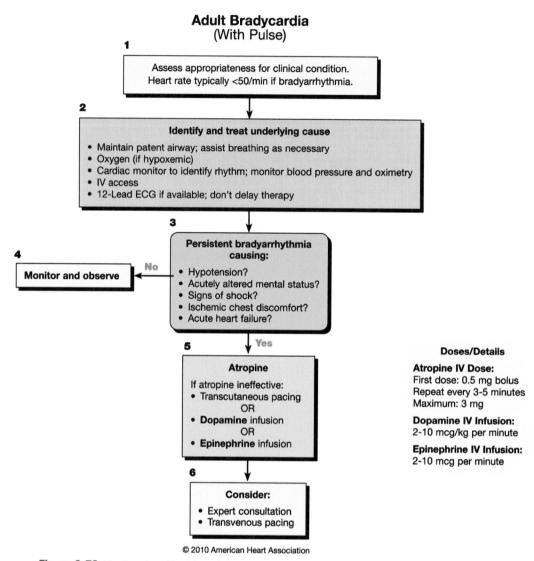

Figure 3-76 The American Heart Association Advanced Cardiac Life Support (ACLS) bradycardia algorithm.

SECTION 4

Cardiac Arrest Rhythms

[Objectives 1, 2]

The initial rhythm recorded by emergency personnel is generally considered the electrical mechanism of a cardiac arrest.[13] This information is important because it affects patient outcome. Patients who are in sustained VT at the time of initial contact have the best outcome, whereas those who present with a bradyarrhythmia or asystole at initial contact have the worst prognosis. If the initial rhythm recorded is VF, the patient's outcome is intermediate between the outcomes associated with sustained VT and bradyarrhythmia and asystole.[13]

VENTRICULAR TACHYCARDIA

Monomorphic VT and polymorphic VT have already been discussed. If either of these rhythms presents without a pulse, the rhythm is treated as ventricular fibrillation (VF).

VENTRICULAR FIBRILLATION

VF is a chaotic rhythm that begins in the ventricles. In VF, there is no organized depolarization of the ventricles (Table 3-40, Figures 3-77 and 3-78). The ventricular muscle quivers. As a result, there is no effective myocardial contraction and no pulse.

What Causes It?

Factors that increase the susceptibility of the myocardium to fibrillate include:
- Acute coronary syndromes
- Antiarrhythmics and other medications
- Dysrhythmias
- Electrolyte imbalance
- Environmental factors (e.g., electrocution)
- Heart failure
- Hypertrophy
- Increased sympathetic nervous system activity
- Vagal stimulation

What Do I Do About It?

Because no drugs used for the treatment of cardiac arrest have been shown to improve survival to hospital discharge, the priorities of care in cardiac arrest due to pulseless VT or VF are high-quality CPR and defibrillation (see Chapter 4).[5] Medications used in pulseless VT/VF include epinephrine, vasopressin, amiodarone, and lidocaine (if amiodarone is unavailable).

TABLE 3-40	Characteristics of Ventricular Fibrillation (VF)
Rate	Cannot be determined because there are no discernible waves or complexes to measure
Rhythm	Rapid and chaotic with no pattern or regularity
P waves	Not discernible
PR interval	Not discernible
QRS duration	Not discernible

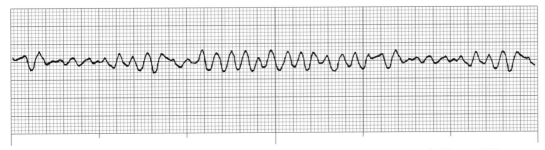

Figure 3-77 Ventricular fibrillation (VF) with waves that are 3 mm high or more is called "coarse" VF.

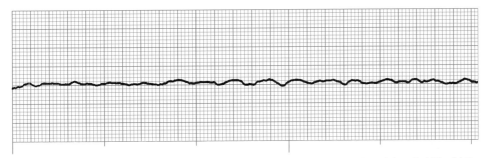

Figure 3-78 Ventricular fibrillation (VF) with low amplitude waves (less than 3 mm) is called "fine" VF.

Epinephrine and vasopressin are vasopressors. Epinephrine has many beneficial actions including bronchodilation, increased heart rate, and increased force of contraction. However, epinephrine is given in cardiac arrest primarily for its vasoconstricting (alpha-adrenergic) properties. Vasoconstriction helps increase coronary and cerebral perfusion pressures.[11] Epinephrine can also have adverse effects including increased myocardial oxygen consumption and necrosis, postresuscitation myocardial dysfunction and ventricular dysrhythmias.[11]

> **ACLS Pearl**
>
> During circulatory collapse or cardiac arrest, the preferred vascular access site is the largest, most accessible vein that does not require the interruption of resuscitation efforts. If no IV is in place before the arrest, establish IV access using a peripheral vein–preferably the antecubital or external jugular vein. During cardiac arrest, give IV drugs rapidly by bolus injection. Follow each drug with a 20-mL bolus of IV fluid and raise the extremity for 10 to 20 seconds to aid delivery of the drug(s) to the central circulation. If peripheral IV access is unsuccessful during cardiac arrest, consider an intraosseous (IO) infusion before considering placement of a central line. To improve flow rates during an IO infusion, the use of a pressure bag or infusion pump may be necessary.

Epinephrine should be given IV or IO in cardiac arrest. Because the effects of epinephrine do not last long, epinephrine should be repeated every 3 to 5 minutes as long as the patient is in cardiac arrest. Although it can be given tracheally, some studies suggest that tracheal epinephrine can produce a transient *decrease* in blood pressure.[14-16] This effect is presumed to be due to beta$_2$-adrenergic receptor stimulation. This can cause hypotension and *lower* coronary perfusion pressure, which may lessen the probability for a return of spontaneous circulation.

> **YOU SHOULD KNOW** Studies have shown that naloxone, atropine, vasopressin, epinephrine, and lidocaine are medications that are absorbed via the trachea. The tracheal route of drug administration is not preferred because multiple studies have shown that giving resuscitation drugs tracheally results in lower blood concentrations than the same dose given IV. The recommended dose of some medications that can be given via the tracheal route is generally 2 to 2.5 times the IV dose, although the optimal tracheal dose of most drugs is unknown.

Vasopressin causes constriction of peripheral, coronary, and renal vessels (Table 3-41, Figure 3-79). When used, 40 units are given once in place of the first or second dose of epinephrine in cardiac arrest. "To date no placebo-controlled trials have shown that administration of any vasopressor agent at any

TABLE 3-41 **Vasopressin**

Vasopressin	Mechanism of Action/Effects	Indications	Dosage[5]	Precautions
Trade Name: Pitressin **Class:** Pituitary hormone, antidiuretic	Causes constriction of peripheral, cerebral, pulmonary, and coronary vessels	Cardiac arrest	One-time dose of 40 units IV/IO push may be used in place of first or second dose of epinephrine in cardiac arrest. Tracheal: 2 to 2.5 times IV/IO dose	Can increase peripheral vascular resistance and provoke cardiac ischemia and angina pectoris. Nausea and vomiting. Tremors. Tissue necrosis if extravasation occurs.

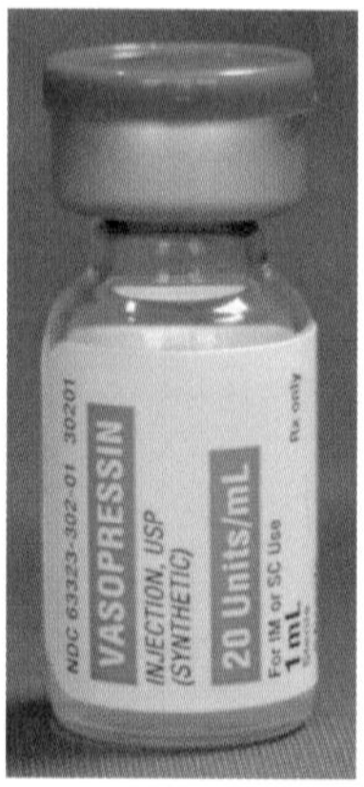

Figure 3-79

TABLE 3-42 Lidocaine

Lidocaine	Mechanism of Action/Effects	Indications	Dosage[5]	Precautions
Trade Name: Xylocaine **Class:** Class 1B antiarrhythmic	Decreases conduction in ischemic cardiac tissue without adversely affecting normal conduction	Stable monomorphic VT Pulseless VT/VF that persists after defibrillation and vasopressor administration (if amiodarone is not available)	Initial dose: 1 to 1.5 mg/kg IV/IO bolus. Consider repeat dose (0.5 to 0.75 mg/kg) in 5 to 10 min. Cumulative IV/IO bolus dose should not exceed 3 mg/kg Maintenance infusion: 1 to 4 mg/min. Tracheal dose: 2 to 3 mg/kg (2 to 2.5 times IV dose)	Only bolus therapy is used in cardiac arrest. Lidocaine may be *lethal* for a patient with bradycardia with a ventricular escape rhythm.

stage during management of VF, pulseless VT, PEA, or asystole increases the rate of neurologically intact survival to hospital discharge."[5]

If pulseless VT/VF continues despite CPR, defibrillation, and administration of a vasopressor, administer an antiarrhythmic. Amiodarone is an antiarrhythmic that blocks sodium channels, inhibits sympathetic stimulation, and blocks potassium channels as well as calcium channels. Amiodarone is the first antiarrhythmic given during cardiac arrest because it reportedly has been demonstrated to improve the rate of return of spontaneous circulation (ROSC) and hospital admission in adults with refractory VF/pulseless VT.[5] Lidocaine may be considered if amiodarone is not available (Table 3-42). If polymorphic VT associated with a long QT interval is present (TdP), magnesium may be considered.[5]

ASYSTOLE (CARDIAC STANDSTILL)

Asystole, which is also called *ventricular asystole*, is a total absence of ventricular electrical activity (Table 3-43, Figure 3-80). There is no ventricular rate or rhythm, no pulse, and no cardiac output. Some atrial electrical activity may be evident. If atrial electrical activity is present, the rhythm is called *"P wave" asystole* or *ventricular standstill* (Figure 3-81). *Bradyasystole* refers to a cardiac rhythm that has a ventricular rate of less than 60 beats/min in adults, periods of absent heart rhythm (i.e., asystole), or both. Bradyasystolic states are clinical situations during which bradyasystole is the dominant heart rhythm.[17]

TABLE 3-43 Characteristics of Asystole

Rate	Ventricular not discernible but atrial activity may be observed (i.e., "P wave" asystole)
Rhythm	Ventricular not discernible, atrial may be discernible
P waves	Usually not discernible
PR interval	Not measurable
QRS duration	Absent

What Causes It?

Use the memory aids "PATCH-4-MD" and "The 5 H's and 5 T's" to recall possible treatable causes of cardiac arrest (see Chapter 1). In addition, ventricular asystole may occur temporarily following termination of a tachycardia with medications, defibrillation, or synchronized cardioversion (Figure 3-82).

What Do I Do About It?

When asystole is observed on a cardiac monitor, confirm that the patient is unresponsive and has no pulse, and then begin CPR. Additional care includes establishing vascular access, considering the possible causes of the arrest, administering epinephrine, and possibly inserting an advanced airway.

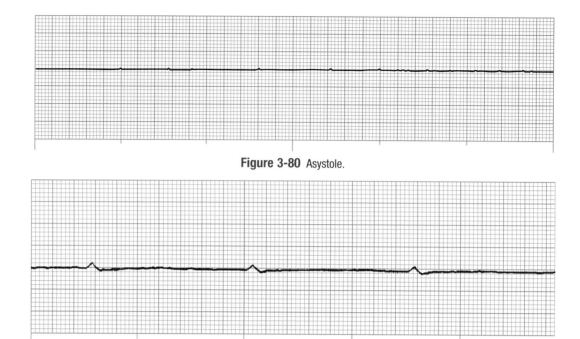

Figure 3-80 Asystole.

Figure 3-81 "P wave" asystole.

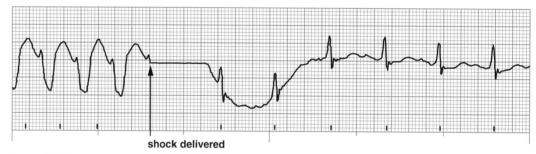

shock delivered

Figure 3-82 This rhythm strip is from a 62-year-old man complaining of palpitations. The patient's initial rhythm was monomorphic ventricular tachycardia. A synchronized shock was delivered, resulting in a sinus rhythm with a prolonged PR interval.

PULSELESS ELECTRICAL ACTIVITY (PEA)

PEA is a clinical situation, not a specific dysrhythmia. PEA exists when organized electrical activity (other than VT) is observed on the cardiac monitor, but the patient is unresponsive and not breathing, and a pulse cannot be felt (Figure 3-83). PEA was formerly called *electromechanical dissociation*. The term was changed from EMD to PEA because research using ultrasonography and indwelling pressure catheters revealed that the electrical activity seen in some of these situations is indeed associated with mechanical contractions; however, the contractions are simply too weak to produce a palpable pulse or measurable blood pressure.

What Causes It?

Use the memory aids "PATCH-4-MD" and "The 5 Hs and 5 Ts" to recall possible treatable causes of cardiac arrest.

What Do I Do About It?

PEA has a poor prognosis unless the underlying cause can be rapidly identified and appropriately managed. Treatment includes high-quality CPR, establishing vascular access, the administration of epinephrine, and an aggressive search for possible causes of the situation and the possible insertion of an advanced airway. The ACLS cardiac arrest and post–cardiac arrest algorithms are shown in Figure 3-84.

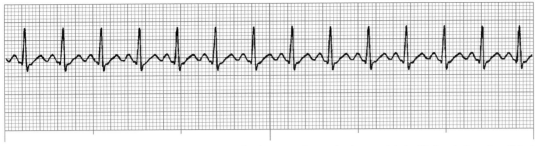

Figure 3-83 The rhythm shown is a sinus tachycardia; however, if no pulse is associated with the rhythm, the clinical situation is termed pulseless electrical activity (PEA).

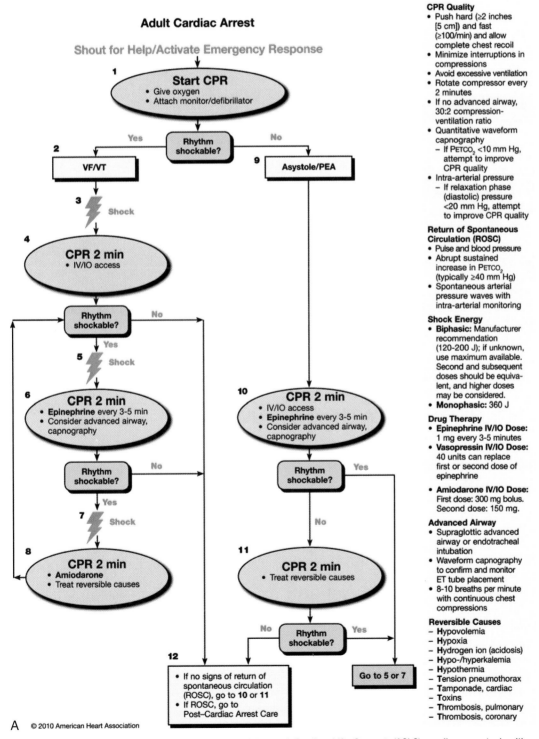

Figure 3-84 A, The American Heart Association Advanced Cardiac Life Support (ACLS) cardiac arrest algorithm.

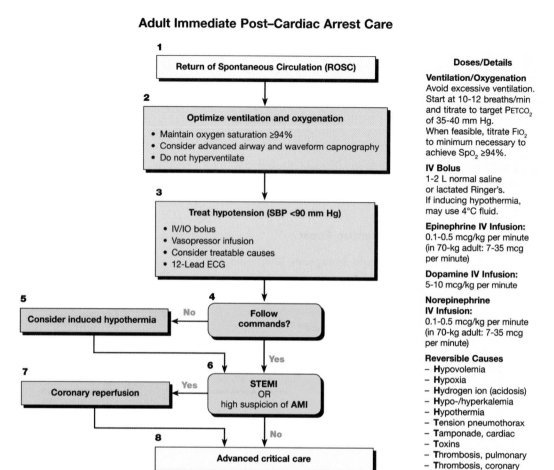

Figure 3-84, con't B, The American Heart Association post–cardiac arrest algorithm. AMI, acute myocardial infarction; CPR, cardiopulmonary resuscitation; ECG, electrocardiogram; ET, endotracheal; IO, intraosseous; PEA, pulseless electrical activity; SBP, systolic blood pressure; STEMI, ST-elevation myocardial infarction.

THE RESUSCITATION TEAM

As a healthcare professional, it is important to know what to do if you encounter a patient who is in cardiac arrest. If you are off duty and encounter an unresponsive patient, activate the emergency medical services (EMS) system by calling 9-1-1.

In the prehospital setting, Emergency Medical Technicians (EMTs) and paramedics often work in teams of two to four. The number varies depending on the environment in which the EMT or paramedic works. For example, a fire department crew that responds to an EMS call may be staffed with two EMTs and two paramedics on the vehicle. Although staffing may differ, the ambulance that arrives on the scene is typically staffed with two EMTs or an EMT and a paramedic.

Healthcare facilities have policies and procedures in place for activating the resuscitation team. Just as it is important to know how to use a piece of equipment before using it in an emergency, you must know your facility's procedure for activating the team. Members of the resuscitation team often carry pagers that are activated by the facility operator. For example, team activation procedures may include pressing a "Code button" at the patient's bedside, calling a specific phone extension, or use a "quick dial button" located on telephones within the facility. When the operator is reached, the type of emergency and its location are stated. Once the operator is notified of the emergency, members of the team are usually activated via pagers and/or an overhead page.

How the team is activated may vary depending on the location and nature of the emergency. For example, a Code/Emergency Response Team is typically called for patients who are not in cardiac arrest but need emergency medical care as well as for patients who have experienced a respiratory or cardiac arrest. This team generally responds within the healthcare facility. Members of the team typically include a critical care or emergency department nurse (depending on the location of the emergency within the facility), a nurse anesthetist or anesthesiologist, a respiratory therapist, a pharmacist or pharmacy technician, an administrative supervisor, a nurse from the patient care area in which the emergency occurs, a chaplain, and at least one physician.

If the facility is a hospital, the Code Team may not be the same team to respond to an emergency that occurs within 250 yards of the hospital's main buildings. A response to an emergency within 250 yards of the facility usually involves an Emergency Response Team from the hospital's emergency department (called an EMTALA Response Team in some facilities) and may also involve an EMS response. Because the emergency is located outside of the main hospital, activation of this team may require procedures different from those used for an in-hospital emergency.

As you can see, it is important to know, learn, and practice your facility's code procedure. It is also important to learn what is expected of you as a member of the resuscitation team.

Goals of the Resuscitation Team

During a resuscitation effort, an interdisciplinary group of healthcare professionals work together to provide coordinated and comprehensive patient care. Teamwork helps to ensure that the patient's many needs are met throughout the resuscitation effort.

Regardless of where a cardiac arrest occurs, the goals of the resuscitation team are to restore spontaneous breathing and circulation and to preserve vital organ function.

Configuration of the Resuscitation Team

[Objective 3]

Every resuscitation effort must have someone who assumes responsibility for overseeing the actions of the resuscitation team. If more than one person attempts to make decisions regarding the patient's care, confusion reigns and chaos will most likely result. The person in charge of the resuscitation effort is typically called the code director or team leader. The team leader directs the members of the team and oversees the resuscitation effort, making sure each team member performs his or her tasks safely and correctly.

In the hospital setting, the team leader is usually an intensivist or emergency department physician who is experienced in cardiac arrest management. Some small hospitals permit a nurse who is trained in ACLS to direct the resuscitation team's activities in a cardiac arrest. Nurses may use standing physician orders to guide decision making during the resuscitation effort; however, in most institutions ACLS is considered the standard of care in a cardiac arrest situation and, in the absence of a physician, emergency care may be initiated by appropriately trained nurses with no physician order per that institution's policy. In the prehospital setting, resuscitation efforts are usually led by a paramedic who operates under standing physician orders, local protocols, or both.

Ideally, the team leader should be in a position to "stand back" to view and direct the resuscitation effort instead of performing specific tasks. However, the size of a resuscitation team and the skills of each team member vary. Some tasks can be performed by personnel with basic life support training, while others require advanced training.

A resuscitation effort requires coordination of four critical tasks:
1. Chest compressions
2. Airway management
3. ECG monitoring and defibrillation
4. Vascular access and drug administration

If the code team consists of five individuals, each of these critical tasks is assigned to a team member and the team leader oversees their actions (Figure 3-85). If the roles of each member of the code team have not been preassigned, the team leader must quickly assign these tasks as the team members are assembled.

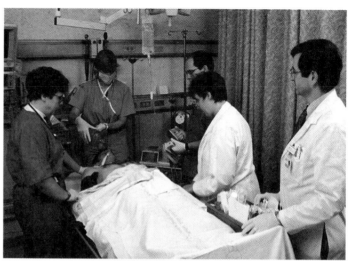

Figure 3-85 The team leader assigns the four critical resuscitation tasks: chest compressions and airway management, electrocardiogram (ECG) monitoring and defibrillation, and vascular access and drug administration.

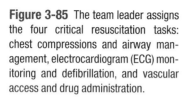
ACLS Pearl

Knowledge of the algorithms is essential to successful completion of an ACLS course. During an ACLS course, your knowledge of the ACLS algorithms is evaluated in simulated situations and on the course post-test. The simulations (also called "cases") are evaluated by an ACLS instructor. The cardiac arrest algorithms are evaluated in the Cardiac Arrest Management (also called the Mega Code) station. In this station, you work in teams of four or five persons. Each person takes a turn as the team leader and as individual resuscitation team members, performing each of the critical tasks of resuscitation. The team leader is evaluated on his or her knowledge of the ACLS algorithms, ability to manage the resuscitation team, and his or her decisions regarding patient management. Although the team leader is responsible for directing the overall actions of the team, a resuscitation effort requires *teamwork*. Each member of the team must know his or her responsibilities and be able to anticipate the team leader's instructions. This is true in real life, as well as in simulated situations.

Team Leader Responsibilities

The team leader has many responsibilities during the resuscitation effort. The team leader:

- Assesses the patient.
- Orders emergency care according to protocols.
- Considers reasons for the cardiac arrest and possible reversible causes.
- Supervises team members (and ensures that each member of the team performs his or her tasks safely and correctly).
- Evaluates the adequacy of chest compressions (including hand position, depth of cardiac compressions, proper rate, and ratio of compressions to ventilations).
- Ensures that the patient receives appropriate oxygen therapy throughout the resuscitation effort.
- Evaluates the adequacy of ventilation (by assessing bilateral and symmetrical chest expansion with each ventilation).
- Ensures that defibrillation, when indicated, is performed safely and correctly.
- Ensures the correct choice and placement of vascular access.
- Confirms proper positioning of an advanced airway (if used).
- Ensures correct drug, dose, and route of administration (also ensures that the medications given are appropriate for the clinical situation or dysrhythmia and that IV bolus medications are followed with a 20-mL fluid flush and the brief elevation of the affected extremity.
- Ensures the safety of all team members, (especially when procedures such as defibrillation are performed).
- Problem-solves (including re-evaluating possible causes of the arrest and recognizing malfunctioning equipment and misplaced or displaced tubes or lines).
- Decides when to terminate resuscitation efforts (in consultation with team members).

Team Member Responsibilities

Nurses who respond to a cardiac arrest must be familiar with the layout of the crash cart and the location of all items contained therein. Recognizing that institutional preferences may vary, the typical contents of a crash cart are shown in Table 3-44. In the prehospital setting, paramedics must be familiar with the location of all medications in their drug box and the resuscitation-related equipment in their emergency bags and vehicles, if applicable.

Airway Management Team Member

The ACLS team member responsible for airway management should know how to do the following:

- Perform the head tilt–chin lift maneuver and the jaw thrust without head tilt maneuver.
- Correctly size and insert an oral airway and a nasal airway.
- Correctly apply and understand the indications, contraindications, advantages, disadvantages, complications, liter flow ranges, and concentrations of delivered oxygen for oxygen delivery devices, including the nasal cannula, simple face mask, pocket mask, nonrebreathing mask, and bag-mask device.
- Suction the upper airway by selecting an appropriate suction device and catheter and by using correct technique.
- Know the indications, contraindications, advantages, disadvantages, complications, equipment, and techniques for insertion of an advanced airway, if this is within his or her scope of practice.
- Know how to confirm placement of an advanced airway.
- Know how to use waveform capnography, an exhaled carbon dioxide detector, and an esophageal detector device.
- Know how to properly secure an advanced airway.

> **ACLS** Pearl
>
> In the hospital, an anesthesiologist or nurse anesthetist typically assumes responsibility for the patient's oxygenation and ventilation and is aided by a respiratory therapist who assists with suctioning, equipment set up, and manual ventilation of the patient. In some institutions, the respiratory therapist performs tracheal intubation.

CPR Team Member

The ACLS or basic life support (BLS) team member responsible for CPR must be able to properly perform CPR and provide chest compressions of adequate rate, force, and depth in the correct location.

Electrocardiography/Defibrillation Team Member

The ACLS team member responsible for ECG monitoring and defibrillation should know:

- How to operate an AED and a manual defibrillator.
- The difference between defibrillation and synchronized cardioversion, as well as the indications for and potential complications of these procedures.
- The proper placement of hand-held defibrillator paddles and combination adhesive pads.
- The safety precautions that must be considered when performing electrical therapy.
- The indications for and possible complications of transcutaneous pacing.
- How to problem-solve with regard to equipment failure.

Vascular Access and Medications Team Member

The ACLS team member responsible for vascular access and medication administration must be familiar with the location of the emergency medications, IV fluids, and related supplies that may be used during a resuscitation effort. In addition, this team member should know:

- The site(s) of first choice for vascular access if no IV catheter is in place at the time of cardiac arrest.
- The procedure for performing IO access in an adult.
- The importance of following each medication given during a cardiac arrest with a 20-mL IV fluid bolus and brief (i.e., 10 to 20 second) elevation of the affected extremity.
- The routes of administration and appropriate dosages for IV, IO, and tracheal resuscitation medications.

TABLE 3-44	Contents of a Typical Crash Cart	
Usual Location	Item	Related Supplies
Top of cart	Monitor-defibrillator with transcutaneous pacing capability Sharps container ACLS algorithms, drug calculation charts Cardiac arrest record and crash cart inventory checklist with clipboard Airway equipment box (alternatively, a drawer may be used for airway supplies) Medication box (alternatively, a drawer may be used for emergency medications)	ECG lead wires, electrodes, conductive gel or adhesive pads
Side of cart	Portable suction machine, oxygen tubing, bag-mask device with oxygen reservoir	Suction canister and tubing, portable oxygen tank with regulator
Back of cart	Cardiac board	
First and second drawers	Emergency medications	Adenosine, amiodarone, atropine sulfate, calcium chloride, dexamethasone, 50% dextrose, diphenhydramine, dobutamine, dopamine (premixed bags), epinephrine 1:10,000, etomidate, flumazenil, furosemide, glucagon, lidocaine, magnesium sulfate, methylprednisolone, naloxone, nitroglycerin (IV), nitroprusside, norepinephrine, sodium bicarbonate, vasopressin, verapamil
Third drawer	Airway equipment	Oral and nasal airways, laryngoscope handle, straight and curved laryngoscope blades, batteries, Magill forceps, stylets, assortment of tracheal tubes, esophageal detector device, tracheal tube securing device, tape, $EtCO_2$ detector, rigid and soft suction catheters, nasal cannula, face masks, tongue blades, oxygen wrench, suction tubing, water-soluble lubricant, tracheostomy tubes (assorted sizes)
Fourth drawer	IV and blood draw supplies	Assorted IV catheters, syringes of various sizes, IV tubing, blood collection tubes, tourniquets, tape, injectable saline, sterile water, alcohol swabs, heparinized aspirators, sutures, gauze pads, needles and needleless adaptors, IV fluids (normal saline, Ringer's lactate solution, 5% dextrose in water), IV start kits, IV tubing, 3-way stopcocks
Fifth drawer	Miscellaneous supplies	Nasogastric tubes, chest tubes, blood pressure cuffs, pacemaker magnet, extra ECG recording paper, sterile and nonsterile gloves, arm boards, restraints, petroleum gauze
Sixth drawer	Procedure kits	Kits for intraosseous and central venous catheter insertion, cutdown tray, arterial blood gas kit, chest tube tray, tracheostomy kit

Support Roles

Support roles in a resuscitation effort include:
- Management of supplies
- Assistance with procedures
- Documentation of the resuscitation effort
- Liaison functions
- Crowd control
- Pastoral care, social workers, or other nursing staff for family support

---

ACLS Pearl

ACLS algorithms are general guidelines for the management of specific dysrhythmias and clinical conditions. A change in the rhythm or a change in the pulse changes the algorithm. Continually reassess the patient–conditions change.

Code Organization–"Phase Response"

Phase I–Anticipation

[Objective 4]

During the anticipation phase of a resuscitation effort, rescuers either respond to the scene of a possible cardiac arrest or await the patient's arrival from outside of the hospital. Important steps to take at this time include the following:
- Analyzing initial information such as patient age, weight (this allows rescuers to anticipate weight-based drug dosages), estimated time of arrest, circumstances surrounding the arrest, and presence of a do-not-attempt-resuscitation (DNAR) order
- Assembling the resuscitation team
- Identifying the team leader
- Assigning critical resuscitation tasks
- Preparing advanced life support equipment and positioning the code cart for easy access to defibrillator pads or paddles, oxygen, suction equipment, medications and supplies, as well as for viewing the ECG monitor
- Positioning the team leader and resuscitation team members to begin or continue resuscitation efforts

Phase II–Entry

During the entry phase, the team leader identifies himself or herself and begins to obtain information as the resuscitation effort begins or continues.

In the field, care should begin where the patient is found unless EMS personnel do not have enough space in which to resuscitate the patient or conditions exist that may be hazardous to them or the patient. Check for signs of obvious death such as lividity, rigor mortis, hemisection, decapitation, or decomposition. If obvious signs of death are present, do not begin CPR. If there are no signs of obvious death and the patient is unresponsive, not breathing, and has no central pulse, make sure the patient is on a firm surface while a team member quickly checks for documentation or other evidence of a DNAR order. If a properly completed DNAR form exists, do not begin CPR. If a DNAR order exists but its validity is questionable, place the patient on a cardiac monitor and consult with a physician immediately for directions regarding how to proceed. Follow your local protocol for what should be done on the scene in these situations while waiting to talk with medical direction. If no DNAR order exists and there are no signs of obvious death, begin resuscitation.

In the hospital, the team leader ensures that a code board is placed under the patient. Most hospital beds have a "code" feature that quickly places the bed flat and deflates cushioning devices at the same time. If the patient is being transferred from another bed, the team leader makes sure that the transfer occurs in a safe and orderly manner from the stretcher or gurney to the resuscitation bed.

The team leader:

- Instructs team members to obtain baseline physical examination information and communicate this information to the team leader.
- Provides a concise history of the event and care given to the team leader who is accepting the patient, when applicable. For example, a first responder relays information to arriving paramedics. Paramedics relay information to the emergency department nurse or physician.
- Considers baseline laboratory values and other relevant data if necessary.
- Evaluates the information at hand and acts on that information.

ACLS Pearl

Although not always available, information related to the arrest should be sought including:
- When and where did the arrest occur?
- Was the arrest witnessed?
- Was CPR performed? If yes, how long was the patient down before CPR was started?
- What was the patient's initial cardiac rhythm? If VF or pulseless VT, when was the first shock delivered?
- Are there any special circumstances to consider such as hypothermia, trauma, drug overdose, DNAR orders?
- What treatment has been given?
- What information is available regarding the patient's past medical history?

Phase III–Resuscitation

During this phase, the team leader directs the resuscitation team through the various resuscitation protocols. As the team leader, it is essential that your manner, attitude, words, and skills be professional throughout the resuscitation effort. It is likely that anyone who has been involved in, or simply observed, a resuscitation effort can recall at least one chaotic event where the team leader shouted at everyone and the team members became flustered, not knowing what to anticipate next. It is best to speak in a calm and confident tone to the members of your team. Generally, speaking in a normal, composed tone has a calming effect on those present. Be open to and actively seek suggestions from team members.

Ask your team members to tell you when there is any change in the status of the patient's pulse, oxygenation, or ventilation. Also ask that they tell you when procedures are completed and drugs are given. For example, if you instructed a team member to establish an IV or give a drug, he or she should respond by saying something like, "IV started, left antecubital vein" or "1 mg 1:10,000 epinephrine given IV" when the task is completed. Team members should be instructed to ask you for clarification if your instructions are unclear.

Remember that during a cardiac arrest, your two most important priorities are CPR and, if a shockable rhythm is present, defibrillation (see Chapter 4). Vascular access, giving drugs, and inserting an advanced airway are of secondary importance. The rhythm present on the cardiac monitor will guide the sequence of procedures that need to be done next. For example, if the patient is in cardiac arrest and the cardiac monitor shows no electrical activity, asystole is present. If the monitor shows an organized rhythm despite no central pulse when you assess the patient, PEA is present. Defibrillation is not indicated for asystole or PEA. If the monitor shows VF or VT, defibrillation is indicated. Throughout the resuscitation effort, keep in mind that a change in the patient's cardiac rhythm or pulse status (i.e., pulseless (PE) to pulse present) usually results in a change in the recommended treatment sequence (i.e., algorithm). For instance, if defibrillation of VF results in a sinus rhythm and the patient has a pulse, the algorithm changes because of the rhythm change as well as the presence of a pulse. If the sinus rhythm on the monitor *does not* produce a pulse, the patient has PEA and treatment continues using the cardiac arrest algorithm; however, the treatment sequence changes from the shockable rhythm segment of the algorithm to the nonshockable rhythm segment. If the sinus rhythm on the monitor *does* produce a pulse, supportive measures must be taken to maintain the perfusing rhythm. This is called postresuscitation support or post–cardiac arrest care. Assess the patient's breathing and blood pressure upon the return of a pulse. If defibrillation of VT results in VF (or vice versa), there is no change in the algorithm since pulseless VT and VF are treated in the same way.

> **ACLS Pearl**
> Pulse oximetry generally does not provide reliable information about oxygen saturation during cardiac arrest because of inadequate blood flow through peripheral tissue beds; however, the existence of a waveform on the pulse oximeter may prove helpful in the resuscitation team's awareness of a return of spontaneous circulation.

When pulseless VT/VF is present, defibrillation is indicated. When the team leader indicates it is time to deliver a shock, all team members with the exception of the person performing chest compressions should *immediately* clear the patient. The airway team member must make sure that oxygen is not flowing near the patient's chest. Once the defibrillator is charged, the chest compressor should clear the patient and a shock should be delivered immediately to the patient. In this way, chest compressions are interrupted for the least amount of time possible during the resuscitation effort. Once the shock is delivered, immediately resume CPR, starting with chest compressions. Continue emergency care according to the appropriate algorithm.

> **ACLS Pearl**
> If the patient's rhythm changes, run a rhythm strip for placement in the patient's medical record.

Establish vascular access. If no IV is in place at the time of the arrest, start a peripheral IV with a large-gauge catheter without interrupting CPR. The antecubital or external jugular veins are preferred. The preferred IV solution for use in cardiac arrest is normal saline or lactated Ringer's. Glucose-containing solutions should be avoided unless documented hypoglycemia exists. If peripheral IV attempts are unsuccessful, IO access should be attempted before trying a central line.

Give medications using the correct algorithm. Drugs given during cardiac arrest should be given during brief pauses for rhythm checks and then followed with a 20-mL flush of IV fluid and brief elevation of the affected extremity. The drug is then circulated when CPR is resumed.

If the decision is made to insert an advanced airway, the procedure should be performed in less than 30 seconds. Make sure that the position of the tube is confirmed and then appropriately secured.

If a pulse returns, repeat the primary survey, ask a team member to obtain the patient's vital signs, and then perform a secondary survey. If there is no response to appropriately performed interventions after a reasonable period, consider termination of efforts after consultation with the members of the resuscitation team.

Phase IV–Maintenance

During the maintenance phase of the resuscitation effort, a spontaneous pulse has returned or the patient's vital signs have stabilized. Efforts of the resuscitation team should be focused on the following:

- Anticipating changes in the patient's condition (and preventing deterioration)
- Repeating the evaluation of the patient's ABCs
- Stabilizing vital signs
- Securing tubes and lines
- Troubleshooting any problem areas
- Preparing the patient for transport or transfer
- Accurately documenting the events that took place during the resuscitation effort
- Drawing blood for laboratory tests and treating the patient as needed on the basis of results

Phase V–Family Notification

Surveys have revealed that most relatives of patients requiring CPR would like to be offered the possibility of being in the resuscitation room.[18,19] According to follow-up surveys with family members who had witnessed a resuscitation effort, most felt that their adjustment to the death or grieving was facilitated by their witnessing the resuscitation and that their presence was beneficial to the dying family member.[20]

If family members are not present during the resuscitation effort, they should be told that resuscitation efforts have begun and they should be periodically updated. The result of the resuscitation effort, whether successful or unsuccessful, should be relayed to the family promptly with honesty and compassion.

When speaking with the family, speak slowly and in a quiet, calm voice. Use simple terms rather than medical terms. Pause every few seconds to ask if they understand what is being said. You may need to repeat information several times. Generally, you should make eye contact with the family members, except where cultural differences may exist. Enlist the assistance of a social worker, a clergy member, or grief support personnel, as needed.

Conveying the News of a Death to Concerned Survivors

Healthcare professionals may not receive sufficient training regarding how the death of a loved one should be conveyed to survivors. Family members often do not remember what was said to them when the news of a death was relayed as much as they remember the attitude of the person who spoke to them.

Assume nothing as to how the news is going to be received. The family's reaction to the disclosure of bad news may be anger, shock, withdrawal, disbelief, extreme agitation, guilt, or sorrow. An expected death may elicit a response of acceptance and relief. The resuscitation efforts may have given the family time to accept the terminal outcome. In some cases, there may be no observable response, or the response may seem inappropriate. No matter what the family's response is, do not personalize the family's expression of emotion.

If the resuscitation effort was unsuccessful, give information that is concise using the words "death," "dying," or "dead" instead of phrases such as "passed on," "no longer with us," "went to another place," or "we lost him," when speaking to the family. Allow time for the shock to be absorbed and as much time as necessary for questions and discussion. Recognize that the initial shock experienced by the family may prevent them from knowing what questions to ask. It may necessary to repeat answers or explanations to make sure they are understood.

A statement such as, "You have my (our) sincere sympathy" may be used to express your feelings. However, there are times that silence is appropriate. Silence respects the family's feelings and allows them to regain composure at their own pace.

Allow the family the opportunity to see their relative. In cases involving severe traumatic cardiac arrest, this may not be advisable. If equipment is still connected to the patient, prepare the family for what they will see. The patient should be gowned before the family views the body. Accompany them if necessary. Some caregivers may prefer not to view the body. If this is their preference, do not attempt to force them to do so.

Offer to contact the patient's attending or family physician and to be available if there are further questions. Arrange for follow-up and continued support during the grieving period.

Phase VI–Transfer

The resuscitation team's responsibility to the patient continues until patient care is transferred to a healthcare team with equal or greater expertise. When transferring care, provide information that is well organized, concise, and complete.

Phase VII–Critique

Regardless of the outcome of the resuscitation effort or its length, the team leader is responsible for making sure that the resuscitation effort is critiqued by the team. A critique of the resuscitation provides the following:

- An opportunity for education ("teachable moment")
- An opportunity to express grieving
- Feedback to hospital and prehospital personnel regarding the efforts of the team
- Review of the events of the resuscitation effort including:
  - Relevant patient history and events preceding the arrest
  - Decisions made during the arrest and any variations from usual protocols
  - Discussion of the elements of the resuscitation that went well, those areas that could be improved, and recommendations for future resuscitation efforts

Immediate Postresuscitation Care

The interval between restoration of spontaneous circulation and transfer to an intensive care unit is called the *postresuscitation period*. After successful resuscitation from cardiac arrest, neurologic impairment and other types of organ dysfunction cause significant morbidity and mortality. The ischemia-reperfusion response that occurs during cardiac arrest and the subsequent restoration of spontaneous circulation results in a series of pathophysiological processes that have been named the *post–cardiac arrest syndrome*. The components of post–cardiac arrest syndrome include post-cardiac arrest brain injury, post–cardiac arrest myocardial dysfunction, systemic ischemia-reperfusion response, and persistent precipitating that caused or contributed to the cardiac arrest.[22] Experts have divided post–cardiac arrest care into four phases[5]:

1. Immediate postarrest phase–the first 20 minutes after ROSC
2. Early postarrest phase–the period between 20 minutes and 6 to 12 hours after ROSC
3. Intermediate phase–between 6 to 12 hours and 72 hours after ROSC4.
4. Recovery phase–beyond 3 days

◌ ACLS Pearl

Post–cardiac arrest care focuses on cardioprotective *and* neuroprotective interventions.

The initial goals of post–cardiac arrest care include the following[21]:

- Provide cardiorespiratory support to optimize tissue perfusion, especially to the heart, brain, and lungs (i.e., the organs most affected by cardiac arrest).
- Transport the out-of-hospital post–cardiac arrest patient to an appropriate facility capable of providing comprehensive post–cardiac arrest care including acute coronary interventions, neurologic care, goal-directed critical care, and therapeutic hypothermia.
- Transport the in-hospital post–cardiac arrest patient to a critical care unit capable of providing comprehensive post–cardiac arrest care.
- Attempt to identify the precipitating cause of the arrest, start specific treatment if necessary, and take actions to prevent recurrence.

Subsequent goals of post–cardiac arrest care include the following[21]:

- Control body temperature to optimize survival and neurological recovery
- Identify and treat acute coronary syndromes
- Optimize mechanical ventilation to minimize lung injury
- Reduce the risk of multiorgan injury and support organ function if required
- Objectively assess prognosis for recovery
- Assist survivors with rehabilitation services when required

Immediately after ROSC, repeat the primary survey. Reassess the patient's mental status. Clinical manifestations of post–cardiac arrest brain injury include coma, seizures, myoclonus, various degrees of neurocognitive dysfunction (ranging from memory deficits to a persistent vegetative state), stroke, and brain death.[22] Seizures after a cardiac arrest may be caused by, as well as worsen, post–cardiac arrest brain injury.[22]

Reassess the effectiveness of initial airway maneuvers and interventions. If tolerated, elevate the head of the bed 30 degrees to reduce the incidence of cerebral edema, aspiration, and ventilatory-associated pneumonia.[21] Apply a pulse oximeter and assess oxygen saturation. Titrate inspired oxygen to achieve an arterial oxygen saturation of 94% or greater.[21] Mechanical ventilation may be necessary for absent or inadequate spontaneous breathing. Begin ventilations at 10 to 12 breaths/min and adjust in concert with a weight-appropriate tidal volume to achieve normal carbon dioxide levels. Assess the effectiveness of ventilations with capnography. Avoid hyperventilation, which increases intrathoracic pressure and lowers cardiac output. Avoid hypoventilation, which can contribute to hypoxia and hypercarbia. Obtain a chest radiograph to confirm advanced airway placement and identify potential breathing complications from resuscitation such as pneumothorax, rib fractures, or sternal fractures.

Perform a thorough physical examination and assess vital signs. Heart rate and blood pressure are extremely variable immediately after ROSC. Normal or elevated heart rate and blood pressure immediately after ROSC can be caused by a transient increase in local and circulating catecholamine concentrations.[23,24]

> **ACLS Pearl**
> Use of a standardized postresuscitation protocol has been shown to improve survival in patients with return of spontaneous circulation after cardiac arrest.[25]

Dysrhythmias, hypotension, and decreased cardiac output caused by intravascular volume depletion, impaired vasoregulation, and/or myocardial dysfunction may occur after ROSC. Ensure continuous ECG monitoring and obtain a 12-lead ECG as soon as possible to determine if interventions are warranted for treatment of an acute coronary syndrome. Obtain cardiac biomarkers, serum electrolytes (including magnesium and calcium), complete blood count, and renal profile. Insert a nasogastric tube and urinary catheter to monitor intake and output.

Establish IV access with normal saline or lactated Ringer's solution if not already done. Hypotonic fluids should be avoided because they may increase edema, including cerebral edema.[21] If IO access was used during the arrest, establish an IV line to replace it when time permits. Administration of IV fluid boluses may be necessary if hypotension is present. Administration of inotropic agents and vasopressors (e.g., epinephrine, dopamine, norepinephrine) should be considered if hypotension (systolic blood pressure lower than 90 mm Hg) persists despite volume expansion. If inadequate organ perfusion persists, mechanical circulatory assistance (e.g., intra-aortic balloon pump, transthoracic ventricular assist devices, etc.) may be considered.

Make certain that the family has been updated regarding events and arrange for patient transfer to a special care unit. Transfer the patient with oxygen, ECG monitoring, and resuscitation equipment and ensure that trained personnel accompany the patient.

Temperature Regulation

Monitor the patient's body temperature closely. Fever can impair brain recovery by creating an imbalance between oxygen supply and demand, and it is associated with worsened neurologic outcome after cardiac arrest.[26] For each degree Celsius higher than 98.6°F (37°C), the risk of an unfavorable neurologic recovery increases.[27]

In 2002, the Hypothermia After Cardiac Arrest (HACA) Study Group demonstrated that the use of postresuscitation therapeutic hypothermia (cooling the body temperature to 89.6° F to 93.2° F (32° to 34° C) for 24 hours in comatose survivors of out-of-hospital cardiac arrest caused by VF improved neurological outcome and overall survival.[28] In the same year, Australian researchers published similar results of improved neurologic outcomes in comatose patients post–cardiac arrest cooled to 91.4° F (33° C) within 2 hours after the ROSC and maintained at that temperature for 12 hours.[29] It is now recognized that therapeutic hypothermia should be part of a standardized treatment strategy for comatose survivors of cardiac arrest.[22]

Therapeutic hypothermia should be considered for any patient who is unable to follow verbal commands after ROSC and the patient should be transported to a facility that reliably provides this therapy in addition to coronary reperfusion (e.g., percutaneous coronary intervention [PCI]) and other goal-directed post–cardiac arrest care therapies.[21]

Glucose Control

Hyperglycemia is common after cardiac arrest. Several studies in post–cardiac arrest patients suggest an association of high glucose levels with mortality or poor neurological outcomes. A 1996 study observed that an elevated initial blood glucose level following either out-of-hospital or in-hospital cardiac arrest was associated with a worse outcome in patients with CPR lasting more than 5 minutes.[30] A 1997 study that was limited to VF cardiac arrest victims observed that elevated blood glucose levels both initially and for the first 24 hours following either in- or out-of-hospital cardiac arrest were associated with worse outcomes.[31] Increased mortality and worse neurological outcome may be related to other factors such as the time to resuscitation, age, delay before ROSC, hypotensive episodes, and epinephrine dose, among others.

The optimum glucose value or range identified in studies has been variable. A 2009 study reported increased mortality in patients treated with intensive glucose control.[32] Studies evaluating tight glucose control versus conventional glucose control in critically ill patients showed no significant difference in mortality but found tight glucose control was associated with a significantly increased risk of hypoglycemia.[33,34]

In summary, current clinical studies have not identified the optimum blood glucose level or interventional strategy to manage glucose levels in the post–cardiac arrest period.[21] Regardless of the optimum glucose level chosen, glucose levels must be measured often, especially when insulin is started and during cooling and rewarming periods.[22]

Helping the Caregivers

An unsuccessful resuscitation effort is difficult for the family as well as the healthcare professionals involved in the resuscitation. Although each healthcare professional may deal with stress differently, reactions suggesting a need for assistance include persistent feelings of anger, self-doubt, sadness, depression, or a desire to withdraw from others. It is important to recognize the warning signs of stress in yourself and others and know how to deal with them. Strategies for dealing with stress may include engaging in exercise, practicing relaxation techniques, talking with family or friends, or meeting with a qualified mental health professional.

STOP AND REVIEW

True/False
Indicate whether the statement is true or false.

_____ 1. During a resuscitation effort, team members should frequently reassess the patient and keep the team leader informed of any changes in the patient's vital signs or condition.

_____ 2. Calcium channel blockers (e.g., verapamil, diltiazem) are recommended in the management of ventricular tachycardia and wide-complex tachycardia of uncertain origin.

_____ 3. A delta wave is often seen with Wolff-Parkinson-White syndrome.

_____ 4. During cardiac arrest, rhythm checks should be brief, and pulse checks should generally be performed only if an organized rhythm is seen on the cardiac monitor.

Multiple Choice
Identify the choice that best completes the statement or answers the question.

_____ 5. The intrinsic rate of the AV junction is:
a. 20 to 40 beats/minute
b. 40 to 60 beats/minute
c. 60 to 100 beats/minute
d. 100 to 180 beats/minute

_____ 6. Examples of irregular tachycardias include which of the following?
a. Sinus tachycardia, accelerated junctional rhythm, and atrial flutter
b. Polymorphic ventricular tachycardia, asystole, and sinus tachycardia
c. Atrial fibrillation, atrial flutter, and polymorphic ventricular tachycardia
d. Accelerated idioventricular rhythm, atrial fibrillation, and accelerated junctional rhythm

_____ 7. The R wave:
a. Is the first positive deflection after the P wave
b. Is the first negative deflection after the P wave
c. Is the second negative deflection after the P wave
d. May be a positive or negative waveform that follows the P wave

_____ 8. The most common type of paroxysmal supraventricular tachycardia is:
a. Atrial tachycardia
b. AV reentrant tachycardia
c. Ventricular escape rhythm
d. AV nodal reentrant tachycardia

_____ 9. Which of the following are the main branches of the left coronary artery?
a. Marginal and oblique arteries
b. Circumflex and marginal arteries
c. Anterior descending and oblique arteries
d. Circumflex and anterior descending arteries

____ 10. A patient is in cardiac arrest. CPR is in progress. Two attempts to establish peripheral IV access have been unsuccessful. To administer medications to this patient, your *best* course of action in this situation will be to:
a. Proceed with insertion of a central line
b. Continue attempts to establish peripheral IV access
c. Intubate the patient and administer drugs via the tracheal tube
d. Establish vascular access by means of an intraosseous infusion

____ 11. Three or more premature ventricular complexes (PVCs) occurring in a row at a rate of more than 100/min is called:
a. Ventricular bigeminy
b. A run of ventricular trigeminy
c. A run of ventricular tachycardia
d. Accelerated idioventricular rhythm

____ 12. Select the INCORRECT statement regarding vagal maneuvers.
a. Simultaneous bilateral carotid pressure is applied to make sure the heart rate slows.
b. Carotid sinus pressure should be avoided in older patients.
c. Carotid sinus pressure should be avoided if carotid bruits are present.
d. An ECG monitor should be used when carotid sinus pressure is performed.

____ 13. Which of the following dysrhythmias has the greatest potential for sudden, third-degree AV block?
a. Junctional rhythm
b. Second-degree AV block, type II
c. First-degree AV block
d. Sinus bradycardia

____ 14. In most adults, the normal QRS complex measures no more than ___ in duration.
a. 0.04 second
b. 0.06 second
c. 0.11 second
d. 0.14 second

____ 15. A 47-year-old man is complaining of dizziness, nausea, and chest discomfort that he rates 4/10. His blood pressure is 74/40, pulse 48, ventilations 16. The patient's breath sounds are clear. The cardiac monitor displays the rhythm below.

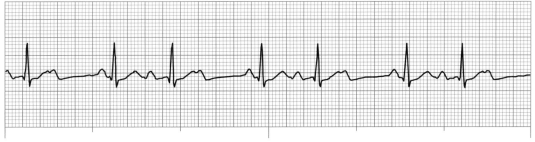

Figure 3-86

Recommended treatment for this patient includes:
a. ABCs, O_2, IV, and atropine IV push
b. ABCs, O_2, IV, and adenosine rapid IV push
c. ABCs, O_2, IV, and morphine titrated to pain relief
d. ABCs, O_2, IV, sublingual nitroglycerin, and transcutaneous pacing

_____ 16. In which of the following situations would an epinephrine IV bolus be indicated?
a. Junctional rhythm, pulseless ventricular tachycardia, and asystole
b. Sinus bradycardia, junctional rhythm, and a ventricular escape rhythm
c. Pulseless electrical activity, pulseless ventricular tachycardia, and asystole
d. Pulseless electrical activity, ventricular fibrillation, and a ventricular escape rhythm

Questions 17 and 18 pertain to the following scenario:

A 72-year-old man is anxious and complaining of palpitations. BP 110/64, P 190 and R 16. The patient denies chest pain. Breath sounds are clear.

_____ 17. The cardiac monitor shows the rhythm below.

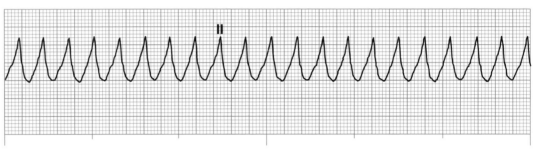

Figure 3-87

This rhythm is:
a. Ventricular fibrillation
b. AV nodal reentrant tachycardia
c. Polymorphic ventricular tachycardia
d. Monomorphic ventricular tachycardia

_____ 18. Recommended treatment in this situation includes:
a. Beginning CPR and defibrillating immediately
b. ABCs, O_2, IV, and vasopressin 40 U rapidly IV
c. ABCs, O_2, IV, and procainamide 20 to 50 mg/min IV
d. ABCs, O_2, IV, sublingual nitroglycerin, and adenosine 6 mg rapidly IV

_____ 19. A 57-year-old man is complaining of chest discomfort and difficulty breathing. He is disoriented and extremely anxious. Examination reveals bibasilar crackles; a weak carotid pulse, and a blood pressure of 60/30. The cardiac monitor displays the rhythm below. The patient has been placed on oxygen and an IV has been established.

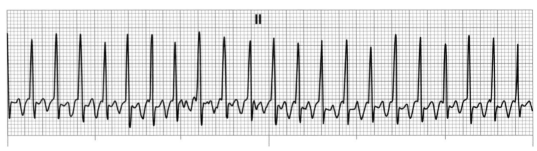

Figure 3-88

Management of this patient should include:
a. Giving sublingual nitroglycerin for pain relief
b. Performing synchronized cardioversion and reassessing the patient
c. Giving 6 mg of adenosine rapid iv bolus and reassessing the patient
d. Giving 2.5 mg of verapamil slow IV bolus and reassessing the patient

_____ 20. A patient has experienced a cardiopulmonary arrest. The cardiac monitor displays the rhythm below.

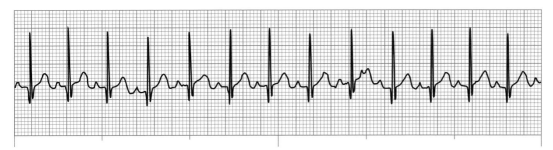

Figure 3-89

Appropriate management of this patient should include:
a. CPR, vascular access, epinephrine, and atropine
b. CPR, defibrillation, IV access, epinephrine, and atropine
c. CPR, transcutaneous pacing, and a search for the cause of the arrest
d. CPR, vascular access, epinephrine, and a search for the cause of the arrest

_____ 21. A rapid, wide-QRS rhythm associated with pulselessness, shock, or heart failure should be presumed to be:
a. Atrial fibrillation
b. Sinus tachycardia
c. Ventricular tachycardia
d. Paroxysmal supraventricular tachycardia

_____ 22. In what type of tachycardia does the impulse begin above the ventricles but travel via a pathway other than the AV node and bundle of His?
a. Sinus tachycardia
b. Atrial tachycardia
c. AV reentrant tachycardia
d. AV nodal reentrant tachycardia

_____ 23. When atropine is used in the management of a symptomatic bradycardia, the correct IV dose is:
a. 40 units, given once
b. 0.5 mg every 3 to 5 minutes to a maximum dose of 3 mg
c. 1 mg every 3 to 5 minutes to a maximum dose of 3 mg
d. 2 to 2.5 mg every 5 to 15 minutes to a maximum dose of 20 mg

_____ 24. Which of the following statements about lidocaine dosing in pulseless VT/VF is correct?
a. Lidocaine is given as a continuous IV infusion of 2 to 10 mcg/min.
b. Lidocaine is given as a continuous IV infusion of 10 to 20 mcg/kg/min.
c. The initial dose is 1 mg IV push which may be repeated twice to a maximum dose of 3 mg.
d. The initial dose is 1 to 1.5 mg/kg IV push; repeat doses of 0.5 to 0.75 mg/kg IV push may be given at 5- to 10-minute intervals, to a maximum dose of 3 mg/kg.

Questions 25 and 26 pertain to the following scenario:

A 69-year-old woman presents with a sudden onset of altered mental status, palpitations, chest pain, and dizziness. The cardiac monitor reveals the rhythm below. Her blood pressure is 77/30 and ventilations are 16. Her SpO₂ on room air is 90%. The patient has been placed on supplemental oxygen and an IV has been started.

_____ 25. The cardiac monitor reveals the following rhythm:

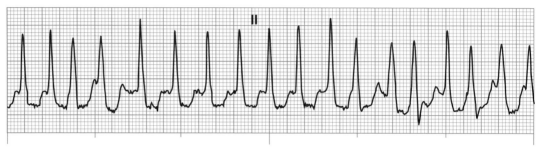

Figure 3-90

This rhythm is:
a. AV nodal reentrant tachycardia
b. Polymorphic ventricular tachycardia
c. Atrial fibrillation with a rapid ventricular response
d. Sinus tachycardia with frequent premature complexes

_____ 26. Your best course of action will be to:
a. Defibrillate immediately
b. Give adenosine 6 mg IV slow IV push over 2 minutes
c. Sedate the patient and perform synchronized cardioversion
d. Begin transcutaneous pacing and then begin a dopamine infusion

_____ 27. A 29-year-old man presents with acute altered mental status. His blood pressure is 50/P, ventilations 14. The cardiac monitor reveals the following:

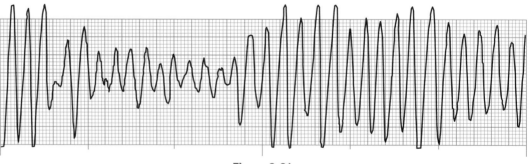

Figure 3-91

Your best course of action in this situation will be to:
a. Give adenosine rapid IV push
b. Give diltiazem IV push over 2 minutes
c. Consider sedation and defibrillate immediately
d. Perform immediate synchronized cardioversion

____ 28.   A 73-year-old woman is found unresponsive with gasping breathing and no pulse.
She was last seen 15 minutes ago. High-quality CPR is in progress. The cardiac
monitor reveals the following:

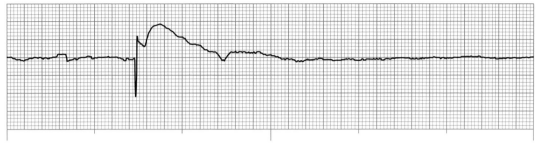

Figure 3-92

You should now:
a. Begin an isoproterenol infusion
b. Establish vascular access and give epinephrine
c. Establish vascular access and give amiodarone
d. Defibrillate immediately, reassess the patient, and administer vasopressin

____ 29.   When administering procainamide, the maximum dose is ____ and the
maintenance infusion dose is ____.
a. 0.25 mg/kg, 5 to 15 mg/hour
b. 0.5 mg/kg, 50 mcg/kg/min
c. 17 mg/kg, 1 to 4 mg/min
d. 150 mg, 0.5 mg/min

Completion

Complete each statement.

30. This rhythm strip is from a 76-year-old woman complaining of back pain. Her medical history
includes a myocardial infarction 2 years ago. Identify the rhythm (lead II).

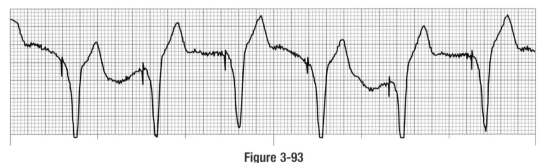

Figure 3-93

Identification: _____

31. Identify the following rhythm (lead II):

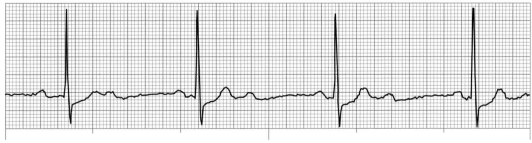

Figure 3-94

Identification: _____

32. Identify the following rhythm (lead II):

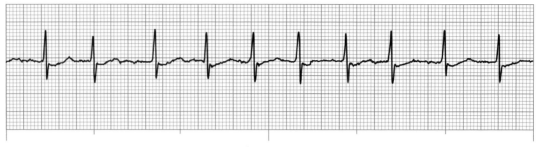

Figure 3-95

Identification: _____

33. Identify the following rhythm:

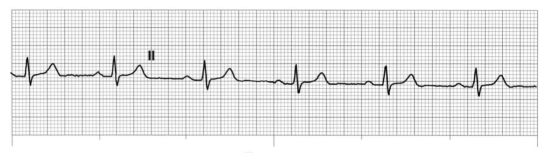

Figure 3-96

Identification: _____

34. Identify the following rhythm:

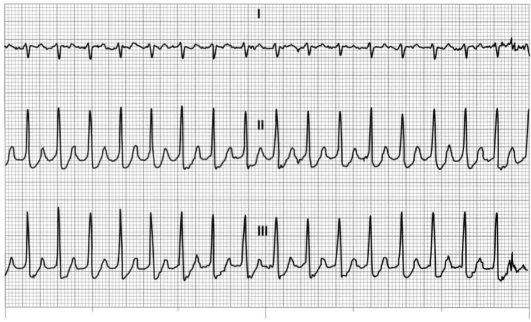

Figure 3-97

Identification: _____

35. Identify the following rhythm:

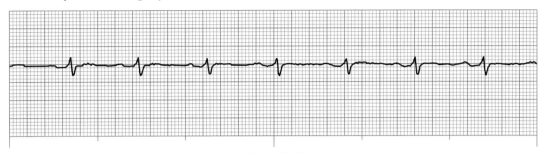

Figure 3-98

Identification: _____

36. Identify the following rhythm:

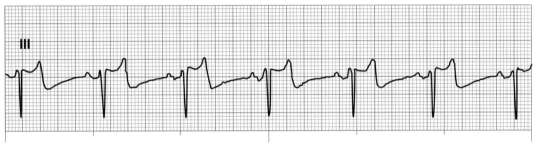

Figure 3-99

Identification: _____

37. Identify the following rhythm:

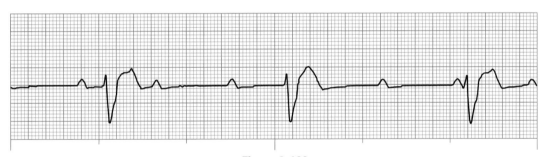

Figure 3-100

Identification: _____

38. Identify the following rhythm:

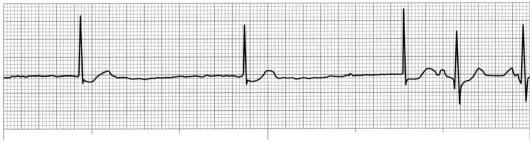

Figure 3-101

Identification: _____

39. Identify the following rhythm:

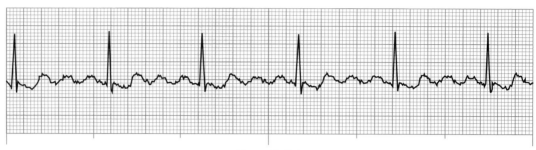

Figure 3-102

Identification: _____

40. These rhythm strips are from a 44-year-old man complaining of dizziness secondary to cocaine use. Identify the rhythm.

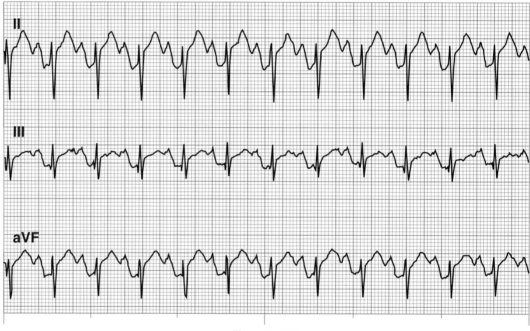

Figure 3-103

Identification: _____

41. Identify the following rhythm (lead II):

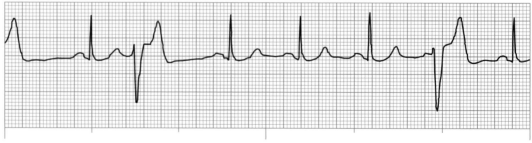

Figure 3-104

Identification: _____

42. This rhythm strip is from an 81-year-old man with weakness and an altered level of responsiveness. Identify the rhythm (lead II).

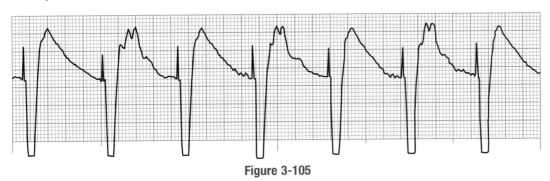

Figure 3-105

Identification: _____

43. Identify the following rhythm:

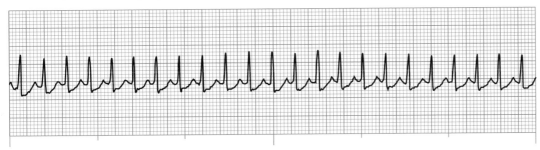

Figure 3-106

Identification: _____

44. Identify the following rhythm (lead II):

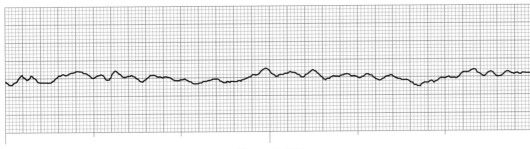

Figure 3-107

Identification: _____

45. Identify the following rhythm:

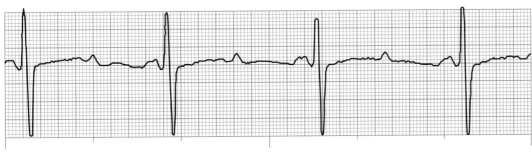

Figure 3-108

Identification: _____

Matching

Match each description below with its corresponding answer.

a. R wave
b. PR segment
c. PR interval
d. ST segment
e. QT interval

f. P wave
g. QRS complex
h. TP segment
i. S wave

_____ 46. Portion of the ECG tracing between the QRS complex and the T wave

_____ 47. Portion of the ECG tracing between the end of the T wave and the beginning of the following P wave

_____ 48. Represents atrial depolarization and the spread of an electrical impulse throughout the right and left atria

_____ 49. Represents the spread of an electrical impulse through the ventricles (ventricular depolarization)

_____ 50. First positive deflection (above the baseline) in the QRS complex

_____ 51. Represents total ventricular activity–the time from ventricular depolarization (stimulation) to repolarization (recovery)

_____ 52. Normally measures 0.12 to 0.20 second in adults

_____ 53. This is *always* negative (below the baseline)

_____ 54. Horizontal line between the end of the P wave and the beginning of the QRS complex

Match each description below with its corresponding answer.

a. Third-degree AV block
b. Polymorphic ventricular tachycardia
c. Ventricular fibrillation
d. Ventricular escape rhythm
e. Second-degree AV block type II
f. Atrial fibrillation

g. AV nodal reentrant tachycardia (AVNRT)
h. Second-degree AV block type I
i. Sinus tachycardia
j. Atrial flutter
k. Monomorphic ventricular tachycardia

_____ 55. Ventricular rhythm may be regular or irregular, waveforms resembling teeth of a saw or picket fence before QRS

_____ 56. Regular ventricular rate between 150 and 250 beats/min; narrow QRS

_____ 57. More P waves than QRSs, P waves occur regularly, irregular ventricular rhythm, lengthening PR intervals, QRS usually narrow

_____ 58. Absent P waves, wide QRS, ventricular rate 40 beats/min or less

_____ 59. Rapid rhythm in which the QRS complex is wide and usually regular; QRS complexes are of same shape and amplitude

_____ 60. Irregularly irregular ventricular rhythm, no identifiable P waves

_____ 61. More P waves than QRSs, P waves occur regularly, regular ventricular rhythm, no pattern to PR intervals, QRS narrow or wide

_____ 62.   Irregularly irregular rhythm with no normal-looking waveforms; chaotic deflections vary in shape and amplitude

_____ 63.   One upright P wave before each QRS, ventricular rate 101 to 180 beats/min

_____ 64.   More P waves than QRSs, P waves occur regularly, irregular ventricular rhythm, constant PR intervals, QRS usually wide

_____ 65.   Rapid rhythm in which the QRS complexes are wide and appear to twist from upright to negative or negative to upright and back

Match each description below with its corresponding answer.

a. Initial dosage of adenosine IV
b. Initial dosage of verapamil IV
c. Atropine dose IV
d. Dosage of vasopressin IV in cardiac arrest
e. Loading dose of IV amiodarone for indications other than cardiac arrest
f. Dopamine IV infusion dosage
g. Initial IV/IO dosage of amiodarone in cardiac arrest

h. Dosage of IV magnesium sulfate for torsades de pointes
i. Epinephrine IV dosage in cardiac arrest
j. Initial dose of diltiazem IV
k. Dosage of procainamide
l. Epinephrine IV infusion dosage
m. Initial IV/IO dosage of lidocaine

_____ 66.   150 mg over 10 min

_____ 67.   20 to 50 mg/min; total dose 17 mg/kg

_____ 68.   40 units

_____ 69.   0.25 mg/kg IV bolus over 2 min

_____ 70.   0.5 mg every 3 to 5 min, total dose 3 mg

_____ 71.   1 mg every 3 to 5 min

_____ 72.   1 to 1.5 mg/kg

_____ 73.   2 to 10 mcg/kg/min

_____ 74.   6 mg rapid IV push

_____ 75.   2 to 10 mcg/min

_____ 76.   1 to 2 g

_____ 77.   2.5 to 5 mg slow IV push

_____ 78.   300 mg

Short Answer

79. Name the four main groups of cardiac rhythms.

80. Is depolarization the same as contraction?

81. Complete the following table.

Lead	Heart Surface Viewed	Lead	Heart Surface Viewed
Lead I		V_1	
Lead II		V_2	
Lead III		V_3	
aVR		V_4	
aVL		V_5	
aVF		V_6	

82. Complete the following table.

Parameter	Sinus Bradycardia	Junctional Rhythm	Ventricular Escape Rhythm
Rate			
Rhythm			
P Waves (lead II)			
PR Interval			
QRS			

83. Describe the sites of first choice for cannulation if no IV is in place at the time of cardiac arrest.

84. Name the primary target organs affected by stimulation of the following receptor sites: $alpha_1$, $beta_1$, and $beta_2$.
    $Alpha_1$:
    $Beta_1$:
    $Beta_2$:

REFERENCES

1. Aehlert B: *ECGs made easy*, ed 4, St Louis, 2010, Mosby.
2. Surawicz B, Childers R, Deal BJ, Gettes LS: AHA/ACCF/HRS recommendations for the standardization and interpretation of the electrocardiogram: part III: intraventricular conduction disturbances: a scientific statement from the American Heart Association Electrocardiography and Arrhythmias Committee, Council on Clinical Cardiology; the American College of Cardiology Foundation; and the Heart Rhythm Society, *J Am Coll Cardiol* 53:976–981, 2009.
3. Rautaharju PM, Surawicz B, Gettes LS: AHA/ACCF/HRS recommendations for the standardization and interpretation of the electrocardiogram: part IV: the ST segment, T and U waves, and the QT interval: a scientific statement from the American Heart Association Electrocardiography and Arrhythmias Committee, Council on Clinical Cardiology; the American College of Cardiology Foundation; and the Heart Rhythm Society, *J Am Coll Cardiol* 53:982–991, 2009.

4. Wagner GS, Macfarlane P, Wellens H, et al: AHA/ACCF/HRS recommendations for the standardization and interpretation of the electrocardiogram: part VI: acute ischemia/infarction: a scientific statement from the American Heart Association Electrocardiography and Arrhythmias Committee, Council on Clinical Cardiology; the American College of Cardiology Foundation; and the Heart Rhythm Society, *J Am Coll Cardiol* 53:1003–1011, 2009.

5. Neumar RW, Otto CW, Link MS, et al: Part 8: adult advanced cardiovascular life support: 2010 American Heart Association guidelines for cardiopulmonary resuscitation and emergency cardiovascular care, *Circulation* 122(suppl 3):S729–S767, 2010.

6. Blomström-Lundqvist C, Scheinman MM, Aliot EM, et al: ACC/AHA/ESC guidelines for the management of patients with supraventricular arrhythmias—executive summary: a report of the American College of Cardiology/American Heart Association Task Force on Practice Guidelines, and the European Society of Cardiology Committee for Practice Guidelines (Writing Committee to Develop Guidelines for the Management of Patients With Supraventricular Arrhythmias,), *J Am Coll Cardiol* 42:1493–1531, 2003.

7. Crawford MV, Spence MI: *Common sense approach to coronary care*, ed 6, St Louis, 1995, Mosby-Year Book.

8. Phalen T, Aehlert B: *12-lead in acute coronary syndromes*, 3e, St Louis, 2011, Mosby.

9. Bernheim A: Atropine often results in complete atrioventricular block or sinus arrest after cardiac transplantation: an unpredictable and dose-independent phenomenon, *Transplantation* 77:1181–1185, 2004.

10. Brunner-La Rocca HP: Atrioventricular block after administration of atropine in patients following cardiac transplantation, *Transplantation* 63(12):1838–1839, 1997. Jun 27.

11. Attaran RR, Ewy GA: Epinephrine in resuscitation: curse or cure? *Future Cardiol* 6(4):473–482, 2010 Jul.

12. Barold SS: Indications for permanent cardiac pacing in first-degree AV block: class I, II, or III? *PACE* 19(5):747–751, 1996.

13. Myerburg RJ, Castellanos A: Cardiac arrest and sudden cardiac death. In Zipes DP, Libby P, Bonow RO, Braunwald EB, editors: *Braunwald's heart disease: a textbook of cardiovascular medicine*, ed 7, 2005, Elsevier-Saunders, pp 865–908.

14. Efrati O, Ben-Abraham R, Barak A, et al: Endobronchial adrenaline: should it be reconsidered? Dose response and haemodynamic effect in dogs, *Resuscitation* 59(1):117–122, 2003 Oct.

15. Manisterski Y, Vaknin Z, Ben-Abraham R, et al: Endotracheal epinephrine: a call for larger doses, *Anesth Analg* 95(4):1037–1041, 2002 Oct.

16. Vaknin Z, Manisterski Y, Ben-Abraham R, et al: Is endotracheal adrenaline deleterious because of the beta adrenergic effect? *Anesth Analg* 92(6):1408–1412, 2001 Jun.

17. Ornato JP, Peberdy MA: The mystery of bradyasystole during cardiac arrest, *Ann Emerg Med* 27:576–587, May 1996.

18. Boyd R: Witnessed resuscitation by relatives, *Resuscitation* 43(3):171–176, 2000 Feb.

19. Meyers TA, Eichhorn DJ, Guzzetta CE: Do families want to be present during CPR? A retrospective survey, *J Emerg Nurs* 24:400–405, 1998.

20. Doyle CJ, Post H, Burney RE, et al: Family participation during resuscitation: an option, *Ann Emerg Med* 16:673–675, 1987.

21. Peberdy MA, Callaway CW, Neumar RW, et al: Part 9: post–cardiac arrest care: 2010 American Heart Association guidelines for cardiopulmonary resuscitation and emergency cardiovascular care, *Circulation* 122(suppl 3):S768–S786, 2010.

22. Neumar RW, Nolan JP, Adrie C, et al: Post–cardiac arrest syndrome: epidemiology, pathophysiology, treatment, and prognostication: a consensus statement from the International Liaison Committee on Resuscitation (American Heart Association, Australian and New Zealand Council on Resuscitation, European Resuscitation Council, Heart and Stroke Foundation of Canada, InterAmerican Heart Foundation, Resuscitation Council of Asia, and the Resuscitation Council of Southern Africa); the American Heart Association Emergency Cardiovascular Care Committee; the Council on Cardiovascular Surgery and Anesthesia; the Council on Cardiopulmonary, Perioperative, and Critical Care; the Council on Clinical Cardiology; and the Stroke Council, *Circulation* 118:2452–2483, 2008.

23. Rivers EP, Wortsman J, Rady MY, et al: The effect of the total cumulative epinephrine dose administered during human CPR on hemodynamic, oxygen transport, and utilization variables in the postresuscitation period, *Chest* 106:1499–1507, 1994.

24. Prengel AW, Lindner KH, Ensinger H, Grünert A: Plasma catecholamine concentrations after successful resuscitation in patients, *Crit Care Med* 20:609–614, 1992.

25. Sunde K, Pytte M, Jacobsen D, et al: Implementation of a standardised treatment protocol for post resuscitation care after out-of-hospital cardiac arrest, *Resuscitation* 73(1):29–39, 2007 Apr. Epub 2007 Jan.

26. Takasu A, Saitoh D, Kaneko N, et al: Hyperthermia: is it an ominous sign after cardiac arrest? *Resuscitation* 49(3):273–277, 2001 Jun.

27. Zeiner A, Holzer M, Sterz F, et al: Hyperthermia after cardiac arrest is associated with an unfavorable neurologic outcome, *Arch Intern Med* 161(16):2007–2012, 2001 Sep 10.

28. Hypothermia after Cardiac Arrest Study Group: Mild therapeutic hypothermia to improve the neurologic outcome after cardiac arrest, *N Engl J Med* 346(8):549–556, 2002 Feb 21.

29. Bernard SA, Gray TW, Buist MD, et al: Treatment of comatose survivors of out-of-hospital cardiac arrest with induced hypothermia, *N Engl J Med* 346(8):557–563, 2002 Feb 21.

30. Steingrub JS, Mundt DJ: Blood glucose and neurologic outcome with global brain ischemia, *Crit Care Med* 24(5):802–806, 1996 May.

31. Müllner M, Sterz F, Binder M, et al: Blood glucose concentration after cardiopulmonary resuscitation influences functional neurological recovery in human cardiac arrest survivors, *J Cereb Blood Flow Metab* 17(4):430–436, 1997 Apr.

32. NICE-SUGAR Study Investigators, Finfer S, Chittock DR, Su SY, Blair D, et al: Intensive versus conventional glucose control in critically ill patients, *N Engl J Med* 360:1283–1297, 2009.

33. Griesdale DE, de Souza RJ, van Dam RM, et al: Intensive insulin therapy and mortality among critically ill patients: a meta-analysis including NICE-SUGAR study data, *CMAJ* 180(8):821–827, 2009 Apr 14. Epub 2009 Mar 24.

34. Wiener RS, Wiener DC, Larson RJ: Benefits and risks of tight glucose control in critically ill adults: a meta-analysis, *JAMA* 300(8):933–944, 2008 Aug 27.

CHAPTER 4

Electrical Therapy

OBJECTIVES

Upon completion of this chapter, you will be able to:

1. Explain defibrillation, its indications, proper pad or paddle relevant placement, relevant precautions, and the steps required to perform this procedure with a manual defibrillator and an automated external defibrillator.
2. Explain synchronized cardioversion, describe its indications, and list the steps required to perform this procedure.
3. For each of the following rhythms, identify the energy levels that are currently recommended, and indicate if the shock delivered should be a synchronized or unsynchronized countershock:
   - Pulseless ventricular tachycardia/ventricular fibrillation (VT/VF)
   - Monomorphic VT
   - Polymorphic VT
   - Narrow-QRS tachycardia
   - Atrial fibrillation
   - Atrial flutter
4. Discuss the procedure for transcutaneous pacing as well as its indications and possible complications.

INTRODUCTION

Electrical therapies used for the management of a cardiac emergency may include defibrillation, synchronized cardioversion, or transcutaneous pacing. Defibrillation may be performed using an automated external defibrillator (AED) or a manual defibrillator. Using an AED is an important part of basic life support that may be performed by nonmedical personnel and healthcare professionals. Knowing how to use a manual defibrillator and performing synchronized cardioversion or transcutaneous pacing are advanced life support skills.

In this chapter we discuss types of electrical therapies, when electrical therapy is indicated, and the steps needed to safely perform each procedure.

DEFIBRILLATION

Definition and Purpose

[Objectives 1, 3]

Defibrillation is the delivery of an electrical current across the heart muscle over a very brief period to terminate an abnormal heart rhythm. Defibrillation is also called *unsynchronized countershock* or *asynchronous countershock*, because the delivery of current has no relationship to the cardiac cycle. Indications for defibrillation include pulseless monomorphic VT, sustained polymorphic VT, and VF.

> **Keeping It Simple**
>
> **Defibrillation Indications**
> • Pulseless monomorphic VT
> • Sustained polymorphic VT
> • VF

Manual defibrillation refers to the placement of paddles or pads on a patient's chest, the interpretation of the patient's cardiac rhythm by a trained healthcare professional, and the healthcare professional's decision to deliver a shock, if indicated. **Automated external defibrillation** refers to the placement of paddles or pads on a patient's chest and the interpretation of the patient's cardiac rhythm by the defibrillator's computerized analysis system. Depending on the type of automated external defibrillator (AED) used, the machine will deliver a shock (if a shockable rhythm is detected) or instruct the operator to deliver a shock. AEDs are discussed in more detail later in this chapter. Defibrillation does not "jump start" the heart. The shock attempts to deliver a uniform electrical current of sufficient intensity to depolarize myocardial cells (including fibrillating cells) at the same time, briefly "stunning" the heart. This provides an opportunity for the heart's natural pacemakers to resume normal activity. When the cells repolarize, the pacemaker with the highest degree of automaticity should assume responsibility for pacing the heart.

> **Keeping It Simple**
>
> Defibrillation and high-quality, effective CPR are the most important treatments for the patient in cardiac arrest due to pulseless VT or VF.

Energy, Voltage, and Current

A **defibrillator** is a device used to deliver a shock to eliminate an abnormal heart rhythm (Figure 4-1). It consists of:

• A **capacitor** that stores energy (electrons) at a particular voltage: Think of voltage as the electrical pressure that drives a flow of electrons (current) through a defibrillator circuit (e.g., the chest).
• An energy select button or dial: The shocks used for defibrillation and cardioversion are expressed in **joules** (J) of energy.
• A charge switch/button that allows the capacitor to charge.
• Discharge buttons that allow the capacitor to discharge.
• Handheld paddles, which require the use of conductive media, or combination pads through which current is delivered from the defibrillator to the patient (Figure 4-2). Combination pads consist of a flexible metal "paddle," a layer of conductive gel, and an adhesive ring that holds them in place on the patient's chest. They are disposable and have multiple functions. Combination pads are applied to a patient's bare chest for electrocardiogram (ECG) monitoring and then used for defibrillation, synchronized cardioversion, and, in some cases, pacing if necessary. Combination pads physically separate the operator from the patient. Instead of leaning over the patient with hand-held paddles, the operator delivers a shock to the patient by means of a discharge button located on a remote cable, an adapter, or on the defibrillator itself.

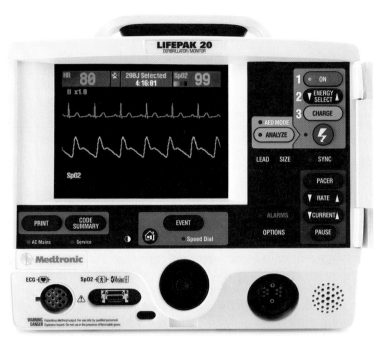

Figure 4-1 A defibrillator is used to deliver an electrical shock to terminate an abnormal heart rhythm.

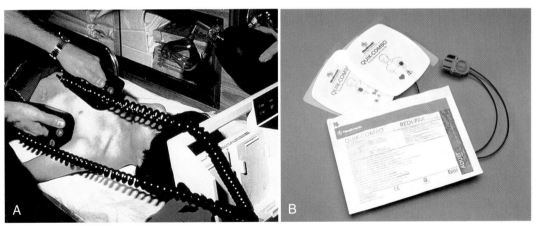

Figure 4-2 A, Hand-held paddles. **B,** Combination pads have multiple functions. They are applied to a patient's bare chest for electrocardiogram (ECG) monitoring and then used for defibrillation and synchronized cardioversion (and in some cases, pacing) if necessary.

Keeping It Simple

Energy (joules) = Current (amperes) × Voltage (volts) × Time (seconds)

When the charge button on the defibrillator is pushed, the capacitor charges. Once the capacitor is charged and the shock control is pressed, voltage pushes a flow of electrons (current) to the patient by means of hand-held paddles or combination pads. Current passes through the heart in "waveforms" that travel from one paddle/pad, through the chest, and back to the other paddle/pad over a brief period.

> **ACLS Pearl**
>
> Combination pads have multiple names including "combo pads," "multi-purpose pads," "multi-function electrode pads," "combination electrodes," "therapy electrodes," and "self-adhesive monitoring/defibrillation pads." Not all combination pads are alike. Some pads can be used for defibrillation, synchronized cardioversion, ECG monitoring, and pacing. Others can be used for defibrillation, synchronized cardioversion, and ECG monitoring, but not for pacing. Be sure you are familiar with the capabilities of the pads you are using.

Monophasic Versus Biphasic Defibrillation

[Objective 1]

There are three general types or classes of defibrillation waveforms: monophasic, biphasic, and triphasic.[1] Waveforms are classified by whether the current flow delivered is in one direction, two directions, or multiple directions.

When a monophasic waveform is used, current passes through the heart in one (i.e., mono) direction (Figure 4-3). Although few monophasic waveform defibrillators are manufactured today, many are still in use. With biphasic waveforms, energy is delivered in two (i.e., bi) phases. The current moves in one direction for a specified period, stops, and then passes through the heart a second time in the opposite direction during a very short period (i.e., milliseconds) (Figure 4-4).

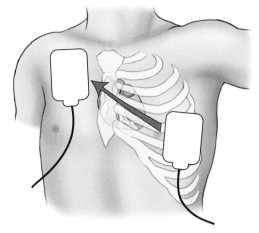

Figure 4-3 When a monophasic waveform is used, current passes through the heart in one direction.

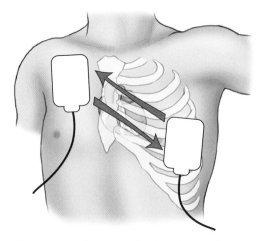

Figure 4-4 With biphasic waveforms, energy is delivered in two phases. The current moves in one direction for a specified period, stops, and then passes through the heart a second time in the opposite direction.

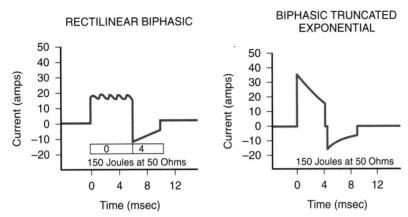

Figure 4-5 Biphasic defibrillators use either a rectilinear biphasic waveform or a biphasic truncated exponential waveform.

Most AEDs and manual defibrillators sold today make use of biphasic waveform technology. Biphasic defibrillators use either a biphasic truncated exponential (BTE) waveform or a rectilinear biphasic waveform (RBW) (Figure 4-5). The BTE waveform has been used in implantable defibrillator-cardioverters (ICDs) for many years; it was approved for use by the U.S. Food and Drug Administration in 1996 as part of the Heartstream AED, which is now a part of Philips Medical Systems (Seattle, WA). In 1999, Zoll Medical Corporation (Burlington, Mass) announced the development of RBW technology, which was subsequently approved for clinical use by the U.S. Food and Drug Administration.

Manufacturers of biphasic defibrillators recommend slightly different energy levels specific for their devices. Both escalating (i.e., increasing energy levels) and nonescalating (i.e., no increase in energy level) biphasic waveform defibrillators are available; however, there are insufficient data to recommend one type of device over another. *When preparing to deliver electrical therapy to a patient, knowledge of the type of device you are using (i.e., monophasic versus biphasic) and the manufacturer's recommended energy levels for the dysrhythmia you are treating is essential.*

Triphasic and quadriphasic waveforms deliver multidirectional shocks. Future generations of defibrillators may implement this technology.

Transthoracic Impedance

Although the energy selected for defibrillation or cardioversion is expressed in joules, it is *current* that delivers energy to the patient and depolarizes the myocardium. The energy delivered through the patient's chest wall is determined by transthoracic impedance. **Impedance** refers to the resistance to the flow of current. **Transthoracic impedance** refers to the natural resistance of the chest wall to the flow of current. Impedance is measured in **ohms**.

When biphasic waveform defibrillation is used, the waveforms compensate for transthoracic impedance to allow for the uniform delivery of energy. The patient's transthoracic impedance is measured through the paddles or combination pads in contact with the patient's chest. Transthoracic impedance varies greatly among individuals. Some of the factors known to affect transthoracic impedance are discussed below.

Body Tissue and Hair

The skin surface, fat, bone, and hair can cause significant increases in resistance. It may be difficult to ensure good electrode-to-skin contact in a patient who has a hairy chest. However, if good contact is not ensured, transthoracic impedance will be high and the effectiveness of defibrillation will be reduced.[3] There is an increased risk of burns from arcing (i.e., sparks) from electrode to skin and from electrode to electrode; ECG identification and analysis may also be inhibited.

If excessive chest hair is present, quickly clip or shave the hair in the areas of intended electrode placement to ensure proper adhesion of the pads. If this is not feasible (or if a razor is not available), check to see if an extra set of electrodes is available. If so, apply one set to the patient's chest and then quickly remove them. This should remove some hair and improve electrode-to-skin contact when you apply a second set of pads. *However, **do not** delay defibrillation.*

Paddle or Pad Size

Optimum pad sizes for defibrillation and pacing on the basis of patient age and weight vary by manufacturer. Carefully follow all manufacturer instructions.

Studies have shown that adult paddles or pads should be used for patients weighing more than 10 kg (22 lb) (i.e., generally older than 1 year).[4-7] For adults, the paddle or pad size ranges from 8 to 12 cm in diameter. Use pediatric paddles or pads for infants and children weighing less than 10 kg (22 lb) or for those whose chests are too small to accommodate standard paddles or pads.[8] Generally, use the largest pads that will fit the patient's chest with at least 1 inch (3 cm) separating the pads. Avoid using pediatric electrodes for adult defibrillation because myocardial injury can occur.[9]

When applying defibrillation paddles or pads, remove the patient's clothing and expose his or her chest. Be sure to look for transdermal patches or disks, which may be used to deliver nitroglycerin, nicotine, analgesics, hormones, or antihypertensives. Do not apply paddles or pads directly over the medication patch or disk because the patch may prevent good electrode contact, hindering the delivery of energy from the defibrillation electrode to the heart. A lack of good contact can cause arcing and may cause skin burns.[10] If a medication patch, disk, or ointment is located at or near the site of paddle or pad placement, remove it and wipe the area clean (do not use alcohol or alcohol-based cleansers) before applying defibrillation paddles or pads.[11]

Because some patients wear jewelry in various body locations, take a moment to look for metal body piercings after the patient's chest is exposed. Although the presence of these materials is not a contraindication to defibrillation, it is possible that their presence can divert the defibrillating current from the myocardium and decrease defibrillation effectiveness. If feasible and if time permits, the metal object should be removed to minimize the potential for burn injuries across the chest.

> **ACLS Pearl**
> When biphasic waveform defibrillation is used, the body weight of the patient does not influence the energy delivered.[12]

Paddle or Pad Position

[Objective 1]

When preparing the skin for paddle or pad placement, do not use alcohol, tincture of benzoin, or antiperspirant. Hand-held paddles or combination pads should be placed on the patient's bare chest according to the manufacturer's instructions. Paddles or pads may be labeled according to their intended position on the chest (e.g., sternum/apex, front/back) or according to their polarity (e.g., positive, negative). Studies have shown that the anterolateral, anteroposterior, anterior-left infrascapular, and anterior-right infrascapular paddle/pad positions are equally effective to treat atrial or ventricular dysrhythmias.[13]

The typical paddle or pad position used during resuscitation is the sternum-apex position, also called the *anterolateral* or *apex-anterior* position. This position is often used because the anterior chest is usually easy to get to and placement of the paddles or pads in this position approximates ECG electrode positioning in lead II. Place the sternum paddle or pad lateral to the right side of the patient's sternum, just below the clavicle. Place the center of the left (apex) paddle or pad in the midaxillary line, lateral to the patient's left nipple (Figure 4-6). If the patient is a woman, elevate the left breast

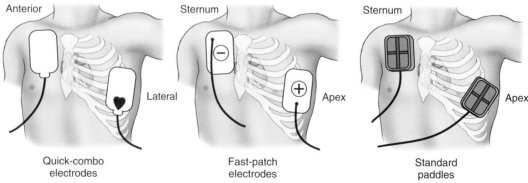

Figure 4-6 Combination pads and standard paddles in a sternum-apex position.

and place the apex paddle or pad lateral to or underneath the breast. Placing defibrillation paddles or pads directly on breast tissue results in higher transthoracic impedance, reducing current flow.[14]

Another common position used for paddle or pad placement is the anterior-posterior position. In this position, one paddle or pad is placed over the patient's left chest with the upper edge of the pad below the nipple. The other is placed on the back, just below the patient's left scapula (Figure 4-7). Alternative positions may be considered based on individual patient characteristics.[13]

> ### Keeping It Simple
>
> In resuscitation situations, precious seconds can be lost when rescuers try to make sure that the "sternum" pad is placed on the sternum and the "apex" pad is placed over the apex of the heart. Delays sometimes occur when rescuers realize that paddles or pads have been placed in reversed positions and then attempt to reposition them to their "proper" location. Reversal of the position of the electrodes is not important during defibrillation, provided the heart is located between them.[15]

Use of Conductive Material

When using hand-held paddles, the use of gels, pastes, or pregelled defibrillation pads aids the passage of current at the interface between the defibrillator paddles/electrodes and the body surface. Failure to use conductive material results in increased transthoracic impedance, a lack of penetration of current, and burns to the skin surface. Combination pads are pregelled and do not require the application of additional gel to the patient's chest.

When applying adhesive pads to the patient's chest, press from one edge of the pad across the entire surface to remove all air and avoid the development of air pockets (Figure 4-8). A hands-free defibrillation cable is used to attach the pads to the monitor/defibrillator.

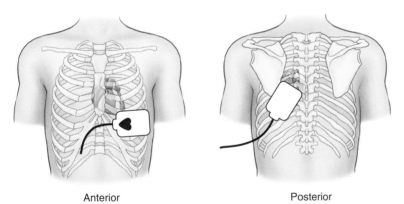

Anterior   Posterior

Figure 4-7 Combination pads in an anterior-posterior position.

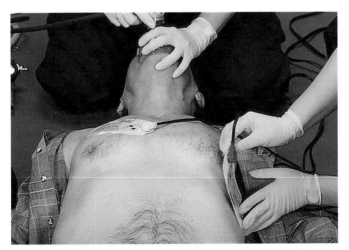

Figure 4-8 When applying adhesive pads to the patient's chest, press from one edge of the pad across the entire surface to remove all air and avoid the development of air pockets.

When using pregelled pads with hand-held paddles, make sure the pads cover the entire paddle surface to avoid arcing current and potential burns. Do not use saline-soaked gauze or alcohol-soaked pads for defibrillation. Excess saline on the chest may cause arcing and burns. Alcohol-soaked pads may ignite. Do not use gels or pastes (e.g., ultrasound gel) that are not specifically made for defibrillation. The use of improper pastes, creams, gels, or pads can cause burns or sparks and may pose a risk of fire in an oxygen-enriched environment.[16] If too much gel is used, the material may spread across the chest wall during resuscitation. This can lead to arcing of the current from one paddle to another and away from the heart, and this can also produce a potentially dangerous spark or burns.

Paddle Pressure

When using hand-held paddles for adult defibrillation, apply firm pressure (i.e., about 25 pounds) to each paddle. This lowers transthoracic impedance by improving contact between the skin surface and the paddles and decreasing the amount of air in the lungs. No pressure is applied when combination pads are used.

Selected Energy

When electrical therapy is used to treat an abnormal heart rhythm, it is important to select the appropriate energy level (i.e., the right amount of joules). If the energy level selected and current delivered are too low, the shock will not eliminate the abnormal rhythm.

Defibrillation Procedure

[Objective 1]
The procedure described below assumes that the patient is an adult and confirmed to be unresponsive, apneic, and pulseless. It also assumes that the patient's cardiac rhythm is pulseless VT or VF and that a four-person team is available to assist with procedures during the resuscitation effort.

Be sure that the cardiopulmonary resuscitation (CPR) team member continues chest compressions as the defibrillator is readied for use (Figure 4-9). The airway team member should coordinate ventilations with the CPR team member until an advanced airway is placed and its position confirmed.

While high-quality CPR continues, instruct the defibrillation team member to expose the patient's chest and remove any transdermal patches or ointment from the patient's chest, if present. If hand-held paddles are used, apply conductive material (e.g., gel) to the defibrillator paddles or apply disposable pregelled defibrillator pads to the patient's bare chest. If combination pads are used, remove the pads from their sealed package. Check the pads for the presence of adequate gel. Attach the pads to the hands-free defibrillation cable, and then attach the combination pads to the patient's chest in the position recommended by the manufacturer.

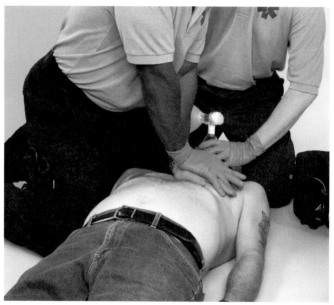

Figure 4-9 Continue chest compressions as the defibrillator is readied for use.

Turn the power to the monitor/defibrillator on and verify the presence of a shockable rhythm on the monitor. Select an appropriate energy level. Use 360 J for all shocks if a monophasic defibrillator is used.[13,17] Use the energy levels recommended by the manufacturer for the initial and subsequent shocks if a biphasic defibrillator is used (i.e., 120 to 200 J). If you do not know what the recommended energy levels are, consider defibrillation at the maximal dose.[13,17]

While the defibrillator is readied, instruct the IV/medication team member to prepare the initial drugs that will be used and start an IV after the first shock is delivered. If hand-held paddles are used, instruct the defibrillation team member to place the paddles in their proper positions on the patient's chest. Be sure that firm downward pressure (about 25 lb) is applied to each paddle. Do not lean on the paddles because they may slip! Charge the defibrillator. If hand-held paddles are used, press the "Charge" button on the machine or the button located on the apex paddle. If combination pads are used, press the "Charge" button on the machine (Figure 4-10).

All team members with the exception of the chest compressor should *immediately* clear the patient as the machine charges. As the airway team member clears the patient, he or she should be reminded to turn off the oxygen flow. Listen as the machine charges. The sound usually changes when it reaches its full charge. To help minimize interruptions in chest compressions, the person who is performing chest compressions should continue CPR while the machine is charging. When the defibrillator is charged, the chest compressor should *immediately* clear the patient.

If a shockable rhythm is still present, call "Clear!" Look around you (360 degrees) to be sure everyone—including you—is clear of the patient, the bed, and any equipment connected to the patient (Figure 4-11). Be sure oxygen is not flowing over the patient's chest. Press the "SHOCK" control to discharge energy to the patient. Release the shock control after the shock has been delivered. Instruct the team to resume chest compressions immediately without pausing for a rhythm or pulse check. Instruct the airway team member to turn on the oxygen and coordinate ventilations with the chest compressor. Instruct the IV/medications team member to establish vascular access and give the patient a vasopressor during CPR. Remember that interruptions in chest compressions must be kept to a minimum throughout the resuscitation effort. Continue CPR for about 2 minutes. After five cycles of CPR (about 2 minutes), recheck the rhythm. If a shockable rhythm is present, charge the defibrillator to a higher dose and then call "Clear!" Check to be certain that everyone is clear and then defibrillate. Resume CPR immediately. While continuing CPR, instruct the IV/medications team member to give an antiarrhythmic (amiodarone or lidocaine if amiodarone is not available). Consider placement of an advanced airway. Use the memory aids PATCH-4-MD or the 5 H's and 5 T's to help identify possible reversible causes of the arrest or factors that may be complicating the resuscitation effort. After 2 minutes of CPR, repeat the sequence, beginning with a rhythm check.

If defibrillation restores an organized rhythm, check for a pulse. If a pulse is present, check the patient's blood pressure and other vital signs and begin post–cardiac arrest care. If you are not sure if a pulse is present, resume CPR.[17] If defibrillation successfully terminates pulseless VT/VF but the rhythm recurs, begin defibrillation at the last energy level used that resulted in successful defibrillation.

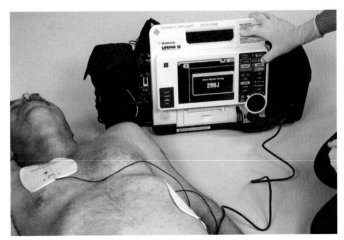

Figure 4-10 Select the appropriate energy level and charge the defibrillator.

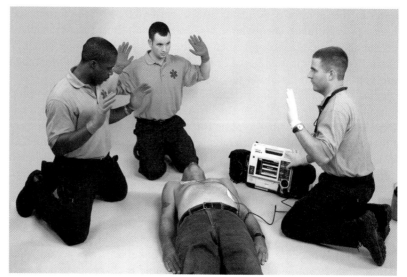

Figure 4-11 Before delivering a shock, call "Clear!" and look around you. Make sure everyone is clear of the patient, bed, and any equipment connected to the patient.

If a rhythm check reveals a nonshockable rhythm, resume CPR, consider possible causes of the arrest, and give medications and other emergency care as indicated. Continue CPR for 2 minutes before performing another rhythm check.

> **YOU SHOULD KNOW**
> - When using a monophasic waveform defibrillator to treat pulseless VT/VF, use 360 J for all shocks.[13,17]
> - When a shockable rhythm is present in cardiac arrest, give *one* shock and then immediately resume CPR, starting with chest compressions. The reason for this is that lengthy interruptions in chest compressions are associated with a decreased probability of conversion of VF to a perfusing rhythm. Resuming CPR immediately after a shock is more likely to be beneficial than another shock.
> - When using a biphasic waveform defibrillator to treat pulseless VT/VF, use the energy levels recommended by the manufacturer for the initial and subsequent shocks. If you do not know what the recommended energy levels are, defibrillation at the maximal dose may be considered. Use at least an equivalent or higher dose for the second or subsequent shocks.[13,17]

What If ...?

What if you charge the defibrillator and the patient spontaneously converts to a rhythm that is not shockable or an organized rhythm before the shock is delivered? Check the operating instructions that accompany the defibrillator you are using for a definitive answer to this question. In most cases, the machine will disarm (i.e., internally remove the stored energy) if the discharge buttons are not pressed within 60 seconds. The machine will also disarm if you change the selected energy or press the energy selector to remove the charge.

What energy should be used if you deliver a shock that eliminates pulseless VT/VF and then the rhythm recurs? If defibrillation terminates pulseless VT/VF that then recurs, defibrillate at the last successful energy setting.[17]

What if the rhythm on the monitor looks like a "flat line?" If the rhythm appears to be asystole, make sure the power to the monitor is turned on, check the lead and cable connections, make sure the correct lead is selected, and turn up the gain (i.e., the ECG size) on the monitor. If the patient is unresponsive, not breathing, or only gasping and has no pulse, begin CPR immediately.

What if the patient has a permanent pacemaker or an ICD? An ICD is typically placed subcutaneously in the left upper quadrant of the patient's abdomen or the left pectoral area (Figure 4-12). It can deliver a range of therapies (also called **tiered-therapy**) including defibrillation, antitachycardia (i.e., "overdrive") pacing, synchronized cardioversion, and bradycardia pacing, depending on the dysrhythmia detected and how the device is programmed (Figure 4-13). A physician determines the appropriate therapies for each patient. Depending on the manufacturer, the ICD may deliver a

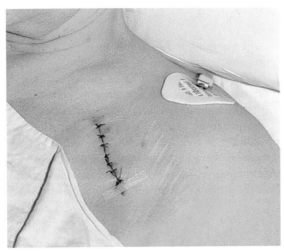

Figure 4-12 Site of implantation of a permanent pacemaker or automatic implantable cardioverter-defibrillator (ICD). The device is usually implanted in the left pectoral region, but it may be placed elsewhere if necessary.

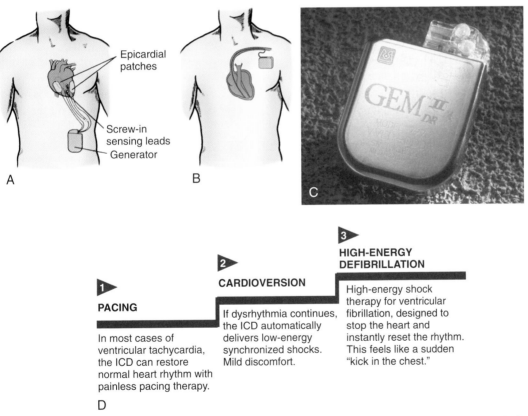

Epicardial patches

Screw-in sensing leads

Generator

A

B

C

> **1**
> **PACING**
>
> In most cases of ventricular tachycardia, the ICD can restore normal heart rhythm with painless pacing therapy.

> **2**
> **CARDIOVERSION**
>
> If dysrhythmia continues, the ICD automatically delivers low-energy synchronized shocks. Mild discomfort.

> **3**
> **HIGH-ENERGY DEFIBRILLATION**
>
> High-energy shock therapy for ventricular fibrillation, designed to stop the heart and instantly reset the rhythm. This feels like a sudden "kick in the chest."

D

Figure 4-13 A, Placement of an implantable cardioverter defibrillator (ICD) and epicardial lead system. The generator is placed in a subcutaneous "pocket" in the left upper abdominal quadrant. The epicardial screw-in sensing leads monitor the heart rhythm and connect to the generator. If a life-threatening dysrhythmia is sensed, the generator can pace-terminate the dysrhythmia or deliver electrical cardioversion or defibrillation through the epicardial patches. With this system, the leads and patches must be placed during an open chest procedure (sternal surgery or thoracotomy). **B,** In the transvenous lead system, open chest surgery is not required. The pacing, cardioversion, and defibrillation functions are all contained in a lead (or leads) inserted into the right atrium and ventricle. New generators are small enough to place in the pectoral region. **C,** An example of a dual-chamber ICD (Medtronic Gem II DR) with tiered therapy and pacing capabilities. **D,** Tiered therapy is designed to use increasing levels of intensity to terminate ventricular dysrhythmias.

maximum of six shocks for VF. About 2 J are delivered at the body surface when the ICD discharges internally. Rescuers in contact with the patient may feel a tingling sensation when the ICD delivers a shock. Although the energy is enough to be felt by the rescuer, it is not enough to cause physiologic harm. If the ICD is delivering shocks, wait 30 to 60 seconds for the ICD to complete the treatment cycle before attaching an AED. When defibrillating or cardioverting a patient with a permanent (implanted) pacemaker or an ICD, be careful to not place the defibrillator paddles or combination pads directly over the device. The anterior-posterior and anterolateral paddle or pad positions are considered acceptable in these patients.[13] Although placement of paddles or pads should not delay defibrillation, defibrillator paddles or combination pads should ideally be placed at least 3 inches (8 cm) from the pulse generator (there will be a bulge under the patient's skin).[13] Because some of the defibrillation current flows down the pacemaker leads, a patient who has a permanent pacemaker or ICD should have the device checked to ensure proper function after defibrillation.

AUTOMATED EXTERNAL DEFIBRILLATORS
Automated External Defibrillator Features

An AED is an external defibrillator that has a computerized cardiac rhythm analysis system. AEDs are easy to use. Voice prompts and visual indicators guide the user through a series of steps that may include defibrillation. When the adhesive electrodes are attached to the patient's chest, the AED examines the patient's cardiac rhythm and analyzes it. Some AEDs require the operator to press an "analyze" control to initiate rhythm analysis whereas others automatically begin analyzing the patient's cardiac rhythm when the electrode pads are attached to the patient's chest. Safety filters check for false signals (e.g., radio transmissions, poor electrode contact, 60-cycle interference, loose electrodes).

When the AED analyzes the patient's cardiac rhythm, it "looks" at multiple features of the rhythm, including the QRS width, rate, and amplitude. If the AED detects a shockable rhythm, it then charges its capacitors. In addition to recommending a shock for VF, AEDs will recommend a shock for monomorphic VT and polymorphic VT. The preset rate for shockable VT varies depending on the AED. For example, some manufacturers set the shockable VT rate for adults at greater than 150 beats/min. Others set the rate at greater than 120 beats/min.

If the machine is a fully automated AED and a shockable rhythm is detected, it will signal everyone to stand clear of the patient and then deliver a shock by means of the adhesive pads that were applied to the patient's chest. If the machine is a semiautomated AED and a shockable rhythm is detected, it will instruct the AED operator (by means of voice prompts and visual signals) to press the shock control to deliver a shock.

Some AEDs:
- Can be configured to allow advanced life support personnel to switch to a manual mode, allowing more decision-making control.
- Are equipped with a small screen allowing the rescuer to view the patient's cardiac rhythm, assisting in identification of shockable versus nonshockable rhythms.
- Have CPR pads available that are equipped with a sensor. The sensor detects the depth of chest compressions. If the depth of chest compressions is inadequate, the machine provides voice prompts to the rescuer.
- Provide voice instructions in adult and infant/child CPR at the user's option. A metronome function encourages rescuers to perform chest compressions at the recommended rate of 100 compressions per minute.
- Are programmed to detect spontaneous movement by the patient or others.
- Have adapters available for many popular manual defibrillators, enabling the AED pads to remain on the patient when patient care is transferred.
- Can detect the patient's transthoracic impedance resistance through the adhesive pads applied to the patient's chest. The AED automatically adjusts the voltage and length of the shock, thus customizing how the energy is delivered to that patient.
- Are equipped with a pediatric attenuator (i.e., a pad-cable system or key). When the attenuator is attached to the AED, the machine recognizes the pediatric cable connection and automatically adjusts its defibrillation energy accordingly (Figure 4-14).

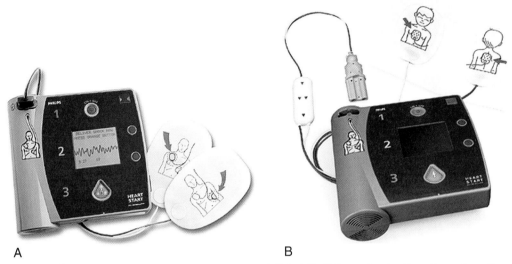

Figure 4-14 A, An automated external defibrillator (AED). **B,** This defibrillation pad and cable system reduces the energy delivered by a standard AED to that appropriate for a child.

Use a standard AED for a patient who is unresponsive, apneic, pulseless, and 8 years old or older. If the patient is between 1 and 8 years old and a pediatric attenuator is unavailable for the AED, use a standard AED. For infants, defibrillation with a manual defibrillator is preferred. If a manual defibrillator is not available, an AED equipped with a pediatric attenuator is desirable. If neither is available, use a standard AED.[13]

Automated External Defibrillator Operation

[Objective 1]
- Assess responsiveness. If the patient is unresponsive, quickly check for breathing. If the patient is not breathing (or only gasping), check for a pulse for up to 10 seconds. If a pulse is absent or if you are not certain that a pulse is present, begin chest compressions.
- Turn on the power to the AED (Figure 4-15A). Depending on the brand of AED, this is achieved by either pressing the "On" button or lifting up the monitor screen or lid.
- Open the package containing the adhesive pads. If the gel in the pads is dried out, use a new set of pads. Connect the pads to the AED cables (if not preconnected), and then apply the pads to the patient's chest in the locations specified by the AED manufacturer (Figure 4-15B). Most models require connection of the AED cable to the AED before use.
- Analyze the ECG rhythm. If several "looks" confirm the presence of a shockable rhythm, the AED will signal that a shock is indicated. Listen for the voice prompts. Artifact due to motion or 60-cycle interference may simulate VF and interfere with accurate rhythm analysis. While the AED is analyzing the patient's cardiac rhythm, all movement (including chest compressions, artificial ventilations, and the movement associated with patient transport) must stop. The chest compressor and ventilator should switch positions during rhythm analysis.
- Clear the area surrounding the patient. Be sure to look around you. Ensure that everyone is clear of the patient, the bed, and any equipment connected to the patient. Make sure oxygen is not flowing over the patient's chest. To help minimize interruptions in chest compressions, the chest compressor should continue CPR while the machine is charging. Once the defibrillator is charged, the chest compressor should *immediately* clear the patient.
- If the area is clear and the AED advises a shock, confirm that all team members are clear and them press the shock control to deliver the energy to the patient when prompted by the AED to do so (Figure 4-15C). After delivering the shock, immediately resume CPR, beginning with chest compressions. After about 2 minutes of CPR, reanalyze the rhythm. Continue to provide care as indicated by the AED's voice and screen prompts.

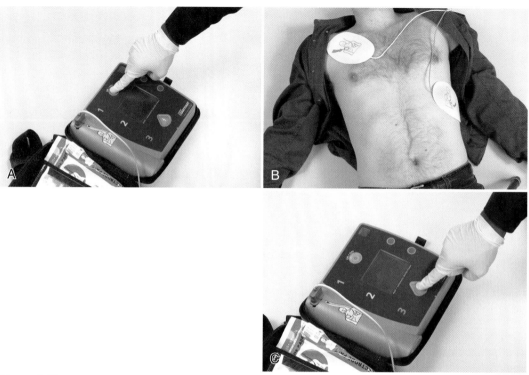

Figure 4-15 AED operation. **A,** Turn on the power to the AED. **B,** Attach the AED pads to the patient's bare chest as directed on the pads. Allow the AED to analyze the patient's rhythm. Do not touch the patient while the rhythm is being analyzed. **C,** If the AED detects a shockable rhythm, clear the area surrounding the patient. Make sure everyone is clear of the patient, the bed, and any equipment connected to the patient. Make sure oxygen is not flowing over the patient's chest. Press the "Shock" button when prompted to do so by the AED.

Keeping It Simple

Automated External Defibrillator Operation
- Turn on the power
- Attach the device
- Analyze the rhythm
- Deliver a shock if indicated and safe

Always follow the AED manufacturer's guidelines for the application, use, and maintenance of the AED.

Special Considerations

If the patient has a pacemaker or ICD, an AED may be used; but the AED pads should be placed at least 3 inches (8 cm) from the implanted device. If an ICD is in the process of delivering shocks to the patient, allow it about 30 to 60 seconds to complete its cycle.

If a transdermal medication patch is present on the patient's chest, do not attempt to defibrillate through it. Remove the patch and wipe the area clean before applying the AED pads if doing so will not delay defibrillation.

AEDs can be used when the patient is lying on snow or ice. If an unresponsive patient is lying in water or the patient's chest is covered with water, it may be reasonable to remove the victim from the water and quickly wipe the chest before applying the AED pads and attempting defibrillation.[13]

If the patient has excessive chest hair, the AED pads may not adhere to the patient's chest resulting in a "check electrodes" message from the AED. If pressing down firmly on each AED pad does not correct the problem, promptly shave the excess hair from the area of the chest where the AED pads will be placed if a razor is available (a razor is often stored in the AED case for this purpose) and then apply a new set of AED pads. If a razor is not available, quickly remove the AED pads, which should also remove some of the chest hair, and apply a second set of AED pads. Ensure that chest compressions are not interrupted and defibrillation is not delayed.

Maintenance

Specific AED maintenance should be performed according to the manufacturer's recommendations. Newer AEDs require minimal maintenance because they perform automated self-checks. AEDs usually self-test their internal circuitry, battery status, ECG electronics, defibrillator electronics, and microprocessor electronics. The frequency with which automatic self-tests occur varies by the device. Some AEDs perform daily self-tests, while others occur weekly. Additional self-tests usually occur when batteries are installed and when the AED is powered on. Manual self-tests can be performed at any time.

SYNCHRONIZED CARDIOVERSION

Description and Purpose

[Objectives 2, 3]

Synchronized cardioversion is a type of electrical therapy during which a shock is timed or programmed for delivery during ventricular depolarization (i.e., QRS complex). When the "sync" control is pressed, a synchronizing circuit in the machine searches for the highest (i.e., R wave deflection) or deepest (i.e., QS deflection) part of the QRS complex and delivers the shock a few milliseconds after this portion of the QRS. The delivery of a shock during this portion of the cardiac cycle reduces the potential for the delivery of current during ventricular repolarization, which includes the vulnerable period of the T wave (i.e., relative refractory period).

Because the machine must be able to detect a QRS complex so that it can "sync," synchronized cardioversion is used to treat rhythms that have a clearly identifiable QRS complex and a rapid ventricular rate (e.g., some narrow-QRS tachycardias, monomorphic VT). Synchronized cardioversion is not used to treat disorganized rhythms (e.g., polymorphic VT) or those that do not have a clearly identifiable QRS complex (e.g., VF).

Keeping It Simple

Synchronized Cardioversion Indications
- Unstable atrial fibrillation
- Unstable atrial flutter
- Unstable monomorphic VT
- Unstable narrow-QRS tachycardia

Procedure

[Objectives 2, 3]

Before performing synchronized cardioversion, take appropriate standard precautions and verify that the procedure is indicated (Figure 4-16). Identify the rhythm on the cardiac monitor. Print an ECG strip to document the patient's rhythm, and assess the patient for serious signs and symptoms from the tachycardia. Make sure suction and emergency medications are available. Give supplemental oxygen, if indicated, and start an IV. If the patient is awake, explain the procedure.

Remove clothing from the patient's upper body (Figure 4-17). With gloves, remove nitroglycerin paste or transdermal patches from the patient's chest if present and quickly wipe away any medication residue. If present, remove excessive hair from the sites where the paddles or electrodes will be placed. Clip or shave hair if necessary (and if time permits). Avoid cutting the skin. Do not apply alcohol, tincture of benzoin, or antiperspirant to the skin.

Turn the power to the defibrillator on. If using standard paddles, you must use defibrillation gel or defibrillation gel pads between the paddle electrode surface and the patient's skin. Place pregelled defibrillation pads on the patient's chest at this time. If using combination pads, place them in proper position on the patient's bare chest.

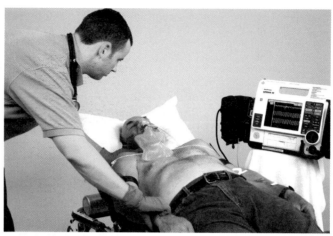

Figure 4-16 Before performing synchronized cardioversion, take appropriate standard precautions and verify that the procedure is indicated.

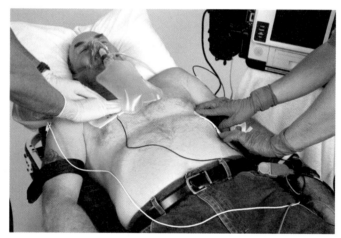

Figure 4-17 Remove clothing, transdermal patches, and medication residue from the patient's upper body. Place pre-gelled defibrillation pads (if using hand-held paddles) on the patient's chest at this time. If using multipurpose adhesive electrodes, place them in proper position on the patient's bare chest according to the defibrillator manufacturer's instructions.

Press the "sync" control on the defibrillator (Figure 4-18). Select a lead with an optimum QRS complex amplitude (either positive or negative) and no artifact. Make sure the machine is marking or flagging each QRS complex and that no artifact is present. The sense marker should appear near the middle of each QRS complex. If sense markers do not appear or are seen in the wrong place (e.g., on a T wave), adjust the ECG size, or select another lead.

If the patient is awake and time permits, administer sedation per local protocol or physician orders, unless contraindicated. Make sure the machine is in "sync" mode and then select the appropriate energy level on the defibrillator (Figure 4-19).

Charge the defibrillator and recheck the ECG rhythm. If using standard paddles, place the paddles on the pregelled defibrillator pads on the patient's chest and apply firm pressure. If the rhythm is unchanged, call "Clear!" and look around you (Figure 4-20). Make sure everyone is clear of the patient, the bed, and any equipment connected to the patient. Make sure oxygen is not flowing over the patient's chest. If the area is clear, press and hold the shock controls until the shock is delivered. A slight delay may occur while the machine detects the next QRS complex. Release the shock control after the shock has been delivered.

Reassess the rhythm and the patient (Figure 4-21). If the tachycardia persists, make sure the machine is in sync mode before delivering another shock. If the rhythm changes to VF, confirm that the patient has no pulse while another team member quickly verifies that all electrodes and cable connections are secure. If no pulse is present, turn off the "sync" control, and defibrillate. See Table 4-1 for a summary of defibrillation and cardioversion.

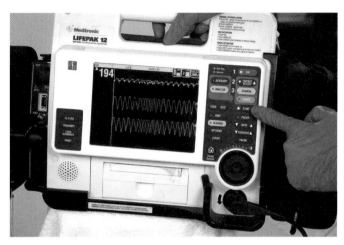

Figure 4-18 Press the "Sync" control on the defibrillator.

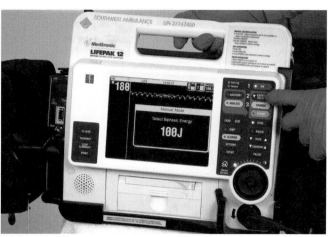

Figure 4-19 Select the appropriate energy level on the defibrillator.

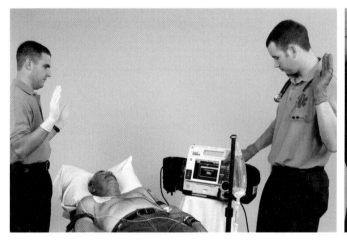

Figure 4-20 Charge the defibrillator, call "Clear!" and look around you.

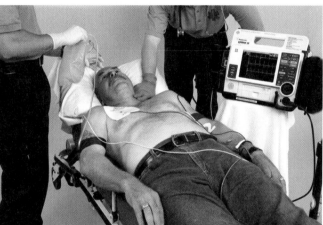

Figure 4-21 Reassess the rhythm and the patient.

ACLS Pearl

- If the patient is unstable and you are unsure if a rhythm is monomorphic VT or polymorphic VT, do not delay shock delivery to definitively identify the rhythm. Instead, provide high-energy *unsynchronized* shocks (e.g., defibrillation doses).[13]
- Some defibrillators revert to the defibrillation (unsynchronized) mode after the delivery of a synchronized shock. This is done to allow immediate defibrillation in case synchronized cardioversion produces VF. Other defibrillators remain in sync mode after a synchronized shock. If VF occurs during synchronized cardioversion, make sure the "Sync" button is off before attempting to defibrillate.

DEFIBRILLATION AND CARDIOVERSION

Special Considerations

Remove supplemental oxygen sources from the area of the patient's bed before defibrillation and cardioversion attempts are made and place them at least 3.5 to 4 feet away from the patient's chest. Examples of supplemental oxygen sources include masks, nasal cannulae, resuscitation bags, and ventilator tubing. Case reports exist that describe instances of fires being ignited by sparks from poorly applied defibrillator paddles that ignited flammable materials in the presence of an oxygen-enriched

TABLE 4-1	Defibrillation and Cardioversion Summary	
Type of Shock	**Rhythm**	**Recommended Energy Levels**[13]
Defibrillation*	Pulseless VT/VF Sustained polymorphic VT	Varies depending on the device used • The biphasic defibrillator effective dose is the typically 120 J to 200 J. • If the effective dose range of the defibrillator is unknown, consider using at the maximal dose. • If using a monophasic defibrillator, use 360 J for all shocks.
Synchronized cardioversion*	Unstable narrow-QRS tachycardia	The biphasic dose is typically 50 J to 100 J initially, increase in a stepwise fashion if the initial shock fails.
	Unstable atrial flutter	The biphasic dose is typically 50 J to 100 J initially, increase in a stepwise fashion if the initial shock fails.
	Unstable atrial fibrillation	The biphasic dose is typically 120 J to 200 J initially (biphasic), increase in a stepwise fashion if the initial shock fails; begin with 200 J if using monophasic energy, and increase if unsuccessful.
	Unstable monomorphic VT	The biphasic dose is typically 100 J initially; it is reasonable to increase in a stepwise fashion if the initial shock fails.

*Use energy levels recommended by the device manufacturer.

atmosphere.[16,18-20] In most cases, fires resulted when high flow oxygen delivery systems (i.e., 10 L/min or more) had been left next to the patient while defibrillation was attempted. There are presently no case reports of fires caused by sparking when defibrillation was performed using adhesive pads.

To enhance safety during defibrillation and cardioversion attempts:
- Be sure to use defibrillator paddles/pads of the appropriate size.
- Make sure there are no air pockets between the paddle or pads and the patient's skin. When applying combination pads to a patient's bare chest, press from one edge of the pad across the entire surface to remove all air.
- Keep monitoring electrodes and wires well away from the area where defibrillator pads or combination pads will be placed. Contact may cause electrical arcing and patient skin burns during defibrillation or cardioversion.
- Remove transdermal patches, bandages, jewelry, and any other materials from the sites that will be used for paddle or pad placement, do not attempt to defibrillate through them. Wipe residue from a medication patch or ointment from the patient's chest. Do not use alcohol or alcohol-based cleansers.
- When using hand-held paddles, use appropriate conductive gel or disposable gel pads and apply firm, even pressure during defibrillation attempts. Do not discharge the defibrillator with the paddles pressed together or into the open air. Discharging the defibrillator with the paddles together may pit or damage the surface of the paddle plates, which may possibly result in patient skin burns during defibrillation.

Possible Complications

Possible complications of electrical therapy include the following:
- Skin burns as a result of lack of conductive material or of gel "bridging" (i.e., the gel forms a "bridge" on the skin)
- Risk of fire from the combination of electrical and oxygen sources
- Myocardial damage or dysfunction
- Embolic episodes
- Dysrhythmias including asystole, atrioventricular (AV) block, bradycardia, or VF after cardioversion
- Injury to the operator or other team members if improper technique is used

Possible Errors

Possible errors that may occur during the delivery of electrical therapy include the following:
- Treating the monitor, rather than the patient
- Operator being unfamiliar with equipment
- Failure to properly maintain equipment (i.e., battery maintenance, paddle cleaning)
- Failure to remove transdermal patches, bandages, jewelry, or other materials from the site used for paddle or pad placement
- Other procedures performed (e.g., establishing an IV, placing an advanced airway) performed before CPR or defibrillation for the patient with pulseless VT/VF
- Prolonged or frequent interruptions of chest compressions
- Improper paddle or electrode position (i.e., insufficient current reaches the left ventricle)
- Excessive use of conductive gel on the patient's chest or on the paddles
- Inappropriate energy level or type of shock (i.e., defibrillation versus synchronized cardioversion) selected for dysrhythmia/clinical situation
- Failure to "clear" self and team members before the delivery of each shock
- Failure to assess for the presence of a pulse when an organized rhythm is observed on the monitor
- Failure to assess the patient's vital signs after the return of a pulse

TRANSCUTANEOUS PACING

Transcutaneous pacing (TCP) is the use of electrical stimulation through pacing pads positioned on a patient's torso to stimulate contraction of the heart. TCP is also called *temporary external pacing* or *noninvasive pacing*.

Although TCP is a type of electrical therapy, the current delivered is considerably less than that used for cardioversion or defibrillation. The energy levels selected for cardioversion or defibrillation are indicated in joules. The stimulating current selected for TCP is measured in milliamperes (mA); the range of output current of a transcutaneous pacemaker varies depending on the manufacturer. For example, the range of output current for one brand of transcutaneous pacemaker is 0 to 140 mA. The range for another brand is 0 to 200 mA. Most transcutaneous pacemakers have a heart rate selection that ranges from 30 to 180 beats/min. You must be familiar with your equipment before you need to use it.

TCP requires attaching two pacing electrodes to the skin surface of the patient's outer chest wall. The pacing pads used during TCP function as a bipolar pacing system. The electrical signal exits from the negative terminal on the machine (and subsequently the negative electrode) and passes through the chest wall to the heart.

Indications

[Objective 1]
TCP is indicated for symptomatic bradycardias unresponsive to atropine therapy or when atropine is not immediately available or indicated. It may also be used as a bridge until transvenous pacing can be accomplished or until the cause of the bradycardia is reversed (as in cases of drug overdose or hyperkalemia). Whether or not TCP is effective, the patient should be prepared for transvenous pacing and expert consultation sought.[17]

Procedure

[Objective 4]
Take appropriate standard precautions and verify that the procedure is indicated (Figure 4-22). Place the patient on oxygen, if indicated. Assess the patient's vital signs, establish IV access, and apply ECG electrodes. Identify the rhythm on the cardiac monitor. Record a rhythm strip and verify the presence of a paceable rhythm. Continuous monitoring of the patient's ECG is *essential* throughout the procedure.

Apply adhesive pacing pads to the patient according to the manufacturer's recommendations (Figure 4-23). Do not place the pads over open cuts, sores, or metal objects. The pacing pads should

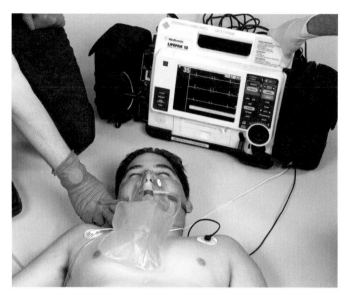

Figure 4-22 Before performing transcutaneous pacing, take appropriate standard precautions and verify that the procedure is indicated.

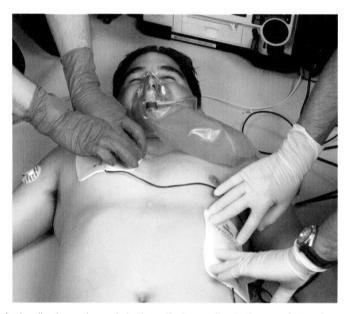

Figure 4-23 Apply adhesive pacing pads to the patient according to the manufacturer's recommendations.

fit completely on the patient's chest. Have a minimum of 1 to 2 inches of space between electrodes or pads, and not overlap bony areas of the sternum, spine, or scapula.

Connect the pacing cable to the pacemaker and to the adhesive pads on the patient. Turn the power to the pacemaker on. Set the pacing rate to the desired number of paced pulses per minute (ppm). In an adult, set the initial rate at a nonbradycardic rate between 60 and 80 pulses/min (Figure 4-24). After the rate has been regulated, start the pacemaker (Figure 4-25). Increase the stimulating current (i.e., output or milliamperes) slowly but steadily until pacer spikes are visible before each QRS complex (i.e., capture). This control is usually labeled "Current," "Pacer output," or "mA." Because transcutaneous pacing is painful in conscious patients, sedation or analgesia may be needed to minimize the patient's discomfort associated with this procedure, particularly with currents of 50 mA or more. Give the patient medications according to local protocol or physician orders.

Watch the cardiac monitor closely for *electrical* capture. This usually is seen in the form of a wide QRS and a broad T wave (Figures 4-26 and 4-27). In some patients, electrical capture is less obvious; it may only be indicated as a change in the shape of the QRS.

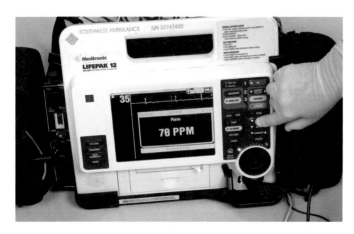

Figure 4-24 Set the pacing rate to the desired number of paced pulses per minute.

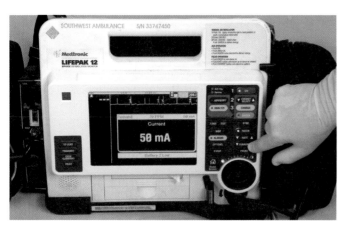

Figure 4-25 After the rate has been regulated, start the pacemaker.

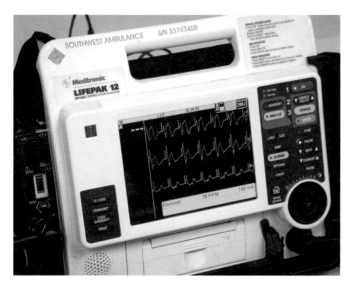

Figure 4-26 Watch the cardiac monitor closely for electrical capture.

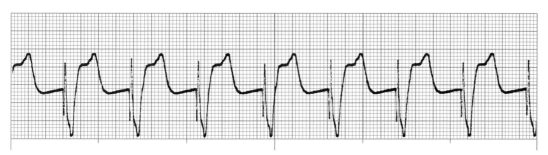

Figure 4-27 One hundred percent ventricular paced rhythm.

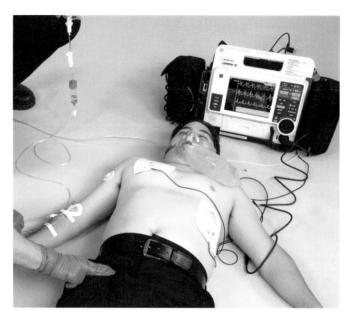

Figure 4-28 Assess mechanical capture by assessing the patient's right upper extremity or right femoral pulses.

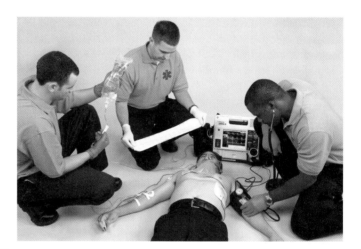

Figure 4-29 Assess the patient's blood pressure, Spo$_2$, and level of responsiveness.

Assess *mechanical* capture (Figure 4-28). Mechanical capture occurs when pacing produces a response that can be measured, such as a palpable pulse and blood pressure. Assess mechanical capture by assessing the patient's right upper extremity or right femoral pulses. Avoid assessment of pulses in the patient's neck or on the patient's left side; this helps minimize confusion between the presence of an actual pulse and skeletal muscle contractions caused by the pacemaker. After capture is achieved, continue pacing at an output level slightly higher (approximately 2 mA) than the threshold of initial electrical capture. For example, if the monitor reveals 100% capture when you reached 80 mA, your final setting would be 82 mA.

Assess the patient's level of responsiveness, SpO$_2$, and blood pressure (Figure 4-29). Closely monitor the patient and assess the skin for irritation where the pacing pads have been applied. Document and record the ECG rhythm. Documentation should include the date and time pacing was initiated (including baseline and pacing rhythm strips), the current required to obtain capture, the pacing rate selected, the patient's responses to electrical and mechanical capture, medications administered during the procedure, and the date and time pacing was terminated, if applicable.

Limitations

The main limitation of TCP is patient discomfort. The discomfort is proportional to the intensity of skeletal muscle contraction and the direct electrical stimulation of cutaneous nerves. The degree of discomfort varies with the device used and the stimulating current required to achieve capture.

Capture may be difficult to achieve or it may be inconsistent for some patients. Increased stimulating current may be required for patients with increased chest wall muscle mass, chronic obstructive pulmonary disease, pleural effusions, dilated cardiomyopathy, hypoxia, or metabolic acidosis because of the extremely high current thresholds required.[21]

ACLS Pearl

Patient Responses to Current with Transcutaneous Pacing

Output (mA)*	Response
20	Prickly sensation on skin
30	Slight thump on chest
40	Definite thump on chest
50	Coughing
60	Diaphragm pacing and coughing
70	Coughing and knock on chest
80	More uncomfortable than 70 mA
90	Strong, painful knock on chest
100	Leaves bed because of pain

*Responses with Zoll-transcutaneous pacemaker.
From Flynn, JB: *Introduction to critical care skills.* St. Louis, 1993, Mosby-Year Book.

Possible Complications

[Objective 4]
Complications of TCP include the following:
- Coughing
- Skin burns
- Interference with sensing from patient agitation or muscle contractions
- Pain as a result of the electrical stimulation of the skin and muscles
- Failure to recognize that the pacemaker is not capturing
- Tissue damage, including third-degree burns (these have been reported in pediatric patients with improper or prolonged TCP)[22]
- When pacing is prolonged, pacing threshold changes, leading to capture failure

Pacemaker Malfunction

Failure to Pace

Failure to pace, which is also referred to as *failure to fire*, is a pacemaker malfunction that occurs when the pacemaker fails to deliver an electrical stimulus or when it fails to deliver the correct number of electrical stimulations per minute. Failure to pace is recognized on the ECG as an absence of pacemaker spikes (although the patient's intrinsic rate is less than that of the pacemaker) and a return of the underlying rhythm for which the pacemaker was implanted. Patient signs and symptoms may include syncope, chest pain, bradycardia, and hypotension.

Causes of failure to pace include battery failure, fracture of the pacing lead wire, displacement of the electrode tip, pulse generator failure, a broken or loose connection between the pacing lead and the pulse generator, electromagnetic interference, and the sensitivity setting being set too high. Treatment may include adjusting the sensitivity setting, replacing the pulse generator battery, replacing the pacing lead, replacing the pulse generator unit, tightening connections between the pacing lead and pulse generator, performing an electrical check, and/or removing the source of electromagnetic interference.

Failure to Capture

Failure to capture is the inability of a pacemaker stimulus to depolarize the myocardium. It is recognized on the ECG by visible pacemaker spikes that are not followed by P waves (i.e., atrial pacing) or QRS complexes (i.e., ventricular pacing) (Figure 4-30). Patient signs and symptoms may include fatigue, bradycardia, and hypotension.

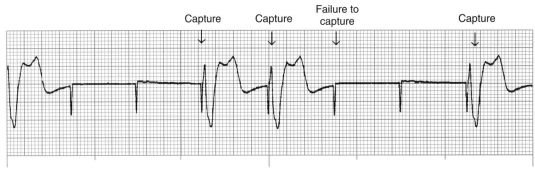

Figure 4-30 Failure to capture.

TABLE 4-2	Electrical Therapy Summary	
Type of Electrical Therapy	**Rhythm**	**Recommended Energy Levels**
Defibrillation*	Pulseless VT/VF Sustained polymorphic VT	Varies depending on the device used: • The biphasic defibrillator effective dose is typically 120 J to 200 J. • If the effective dose range of the defibrillator is unknown, consider using at the maximal dose. If using a monophasic defibrillator, use 360 J for all shocks.
Synchronized cardioversion*	Unstable narrow-QRS tachycardia	The biphasic dose is typically 50 J to 100 J initially; increase in a stepwise fashion if the initial shock fails.
	Unstable atrial flutter	The biphasic dose is typically 50 J to 100 J initially; increase in a stepwise fashion if the initial shock fails.
	Unstable atrial fibrillation	The biphasic dose is typically 120 J to 200 J initially; increase in a stepwise fashion if the initial shock fails; begin with 200 J if using monophasic energy, and increase if unsuccessful
	Unstable monomorphic VT	The biphasic dose is typically 100 J initially; it is reasonable to increase in a stepwise fashion if the initial shock fails
Transcutaneous pacing	Symptomatic bradycardia	• Set the initial rate between 60 and 80 pulses/min. • Increase current (output/mA) until pacer spikes are visible before each QRS complex. Verify electrical and mechanical capture. • Final mA setting should be slightly above (about 2 mA) where capture is obtained to help prevent loss of capture.

*Use energy levels recommended by the device manufacturer.

Causes of failure to capture include battery failure, fracture of the pacing lead wire, displacement of pacing lead wire (this is a common cause), perforation of the myocardium by a lead wire, edema or scar tissue formation at the electrode tip, output energy (mA) being set too low (this is a common cause), and an increased stimulation threshold because of medications, electrolyte imbalance, or increased fibrin formation on the catheter tip.

Treatment may include repositioning the patient, slowly increasing the output setting (mA) until capture occurs or the maximum setting is reached, replacing the pulse generator battery, replacing or repositioning of the pacing lead, or surgery.

Failure to Sense

Sensitivity is the extent to which a pacemaker recognizes intrinsic electrical activity. Failure to sense occurs when the pacemaker fails to recognize spontaneous myocardial depolarization (Figure 4-31). This pacemaker malfunction is recognized on the ECG by pacemaker spikes that follow too closely behind the patient's QRS complexes (i.e., earlier than the programmed escape interval). Because pacemaker spikes occur when they should not, this type of pacemaker malfunction may result in pacemaker spikes that fall on T waves (this is R-on-T phenomenon) and in competition between the pacemaker and the patient's own cardiac rhythm. The patient may complain of palpitations or skipped beats. R-on-T phenomenon may precipitate VT or VF.

Causes of failure to sense include battery failure, fracture of the pacing lead wire, displacement of the electrode tip (this is the most common cause), decreased P wave or QRS voltage, circuitry dysfunction (i.e., the generator is, unable to process the QRS signal), increased sensing threshold as a result of edema or fibrosis at the electrode tip, antiarrhythmic medications, severe electrolyte disturbances, and myocardial perforation. Treatment may include increasing the sensitivity setting, replacing the pulse generator battery, or replacing or repositioning the pacing lead. A summary of the electrical therapies discussed in this chapter is shown in Table 4-2.

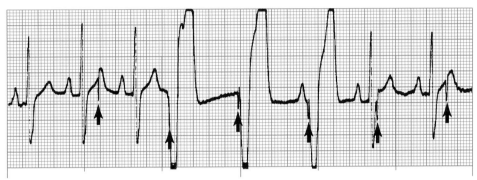

Figure 4-31 Failure to sense.

STOP AND REVIEW

True/False
Indicate whether the statement is true or false.

_____ 1. The anterolateral paddle or pad position is more effective in the treatment of ventricular dysrhythmias than the anteroposterior position.

_____ 2. Transthoracic impedance is significantly increased when defibrillation is performed without the use of conductive material.

Multiple Choice
Identify the choice that best completes the statement or answers the question.

_____ 3. Which of the following statements is true regarding an automated external defibrillator (AED)?
   a. After taking multiple "looks" at the patient's rhythm, an AED will charge its capacitors and then prompt the operator to shock the patient.
   b. AEDs are programmed to recognize VF, monomorphic VT, and asystole as shockable rhythms if the rate exceeds a preset value.
   c. CPR must be performed for at least 5 minutes before pressing the "analyze" control.
   d. To minimize interruptions in chest compressions, CPR should be continued while the device analyzes the patient's cardiac rhythm.

_____ 4. Synchronized cardioversion:
   a. Is used only for atrial dysrhythmias
   b. Delivers a shock during the QRS complex
   c. Delivers a shock between the peak and end of the T wave
   d. Is used only to treat rhythms with a ventricular rate of less than 60 beats/min

_____ 5. Possible complications of transcutaneous pacing include:
   a. Flail chest and burns
   b. Coughing and emboli
   c. Tension pneumothorax and flail chest
   d. Failure to recognize that the pacemaker is not capturing

_____ 6. Defibrillation is indicated in the management of:
   a. Ventricular fibrillation and asystole
   b. Pulseless electrical activity and asystole
   c. Pulseless ventricular tachycardia and ventricular fibrillation
   d. Pulseless ventricular tachycardia and pulseless electrical activity

_____ 7. A 68-year-old man is complaining of chest pain. His level of responsiveness is rapidly decreasing. BP 50/P, P 188, R 6. The cardiac monitor reveals a narrow-QRS tachycardia at 230 beats/min. Your best course of action will be to:
   a. Defibrillate with 360 J
   b. Begin immediate transcutaneous pacing
   c. Sedate and perform synchronized cardioversion with 50 J
   d. Sedate and perform synchronized cardioversion with 120 J

_____ 8. Transcutaneous pacing may be useful in which of the following situations?
   a. Asystole
   b. Ventricular fibrillation
   c. Sinus tachycardia; blood pressure 108/70, unresponsive
   d. Second-degree AV block, type II; blood pressure 64/42, altered mental status

____ 9.   A 49-year-old man is found unresponsive, not breathing, and pulseless. The cardiac monitor reveals monomorphic ventricular tachycardia. The most important actions in the management of this patient are:
a. CPR and defibrillation
b. defibrillation and resuscitation medications
c. CPR and prompt insertion of an advanced airway
d. synchronized cardioversion and resuscitation medications

____ 10.   A 75-year-old man is on the telemetry floor recovering from an inferior wall myocardial infarction. The nursing staff arrive in the patient's room in response to an alarm from his cardiac monitor, which reveals a sinus bradycardia at 40 beats/min. The patient is unresponsive, apneic, and pulseless. An IV is in place. You should now:
a. Defibrillate immediately
b. Begin transcutaneous pacing
c. Begin CPR, ventilate with a bag-mask, and give epinephrine IV
d. Begin CPR, insert an advanced airway, and give atropine IV

____ 11.   A 73-year-old woman is complaining of palpitations and chest pain. Her blood pressure is 72/50, P 188, R 16. The cardiac monitor reveals a wide-QRS tachycardia. Your best course of action will be to:
a. Defibrillate immediately
b. Begin immediate transcutaneous pacing
c. Perform synchronized cardioversion with 100 J
d. Begin CPR and ventilate using a bag-mask device

Matching
Match each description below with its corresponding answer.

a. Recommended initial biphasic energy for monomorphic ventricular tachycardia with pulses
b. When a __ waveform is used for defibrillation, current passes through the heart in one direction.
c. Resistance to the flow of current
d. Another name for sternum-apex paddle or pad position
e. During pacing, assessment of __ capture requires assessment of the patient's pulse.
f. Unstable polymorphic ventricular tachycardia (with or without pulses) should be treated with __.
g. The energy selected for defibrillation or cardioversion is indicated in __.
h. Recommended monophasic energy for ventricular fibrillation
i. Failure to __ is the inability of a pacemaker stimulus to depolarize the myocardium.
j. Recommended initial biphasic energy for atrial fibrillation
k. Failure to __ is a pacemaker malfunction that occurs when the pacemaker fails to deliver an electrical stimulus or when it fails to deliver the correct number of electrical stimulations per minute.
l. When a __ waveform is used for defibrillation, current passes through the heart in two phases.
m. During pacing, assessment of __ capture requires observation of the cardiac monitor.
n. The energy selected for transcutaneous pacing is indicated in __.
o. Recommended initial biphasic energy for unstable narrow-QRS tachycardia
p. Failure to __ occurs when the pacemaker fails to recognize spontaneous myocardial depolarization.

____ 12.   Defibrillation

____ 13.   Electrical

____ 14.   Capture

____ 15.   Defibrillation with 360 J

_____ 16.   Milliamperes

_____ 17.   Impedance

_____ 18.   Biphasic

_____ 19.   Mechanical

_____ 20.   Sense

_____ 21.   Synchronized cardioversion with 100 J

_____ 22.   Synchronized cardioversion with 50 J to 100 J

_____ 23.   Anterolateral

_____ 24.   Synchronized cardioversion with 120 J to 200 J

_____ 25.   Monophasic

_____ 26.   Pace

_____ 27.   Joules

Short Answer

28. What is the purpose of defibrillation?

29. List three indications for defibrillation.
    1.
    2.
    3.

30. Explain the difference between manual defibrillation and automated external defibrillation.

31. Name four possibilities to consider if the cardiac monitor displays a flat line.
    1.
    2.
    3.
    4.

32. Where is the pulse generator of an implantable-cardioverter defibrillator typically located?

33. An 80-year-old man has experienced a cardiac arrest. The cardiac monitor displays ventricular fibrillation. You have exposed the patient's chest and are preparing to defibrillate when you note the patient has a permanent pacemaker in place. What distance from the pacemaker generator should the defibrillator paddles or pads be placed?

34. What are the four main steps in the operation of an AED?
    1.
    2.
    3.
    4.

35. You just delivered a synchronized shock with 50 J to an unstable patient whose cardiac monitor shows AV nodal reentrant tachycardia. The cardiac monitor now shows VF. What course of action should you take at this time?

REFERENCES

1. Huang J, KenKnight BH, Rollins DL, et al: Ventricular defibrillation with triphasic waveforms, *Circulation* 101(11):1324–1328, 2000.
2. White RD: New concepts in transthoracic defibrillation, *Emerg Med Clin N Am* 20:785–807, 2002.
3. Bissing JW, Kerber RE: Effect of shaving the chest of hirsute subjects on transthoracic impedance to self-adhesive defibrillation electrode pads, *Am J Cardiol* 86(5):587–589, A10, 2000.
4. Atkins DL, Sirna S, Kieso R, et al: Pediatric defibrillation: importance of paddle size in determining transthoracic impedance, *Pediatrics* 82(6):914–918, 1988.
5. Atkins DL, Kerber RE: Pediatric defibrillation: current flow is improved by using "adult" electrode paddles, *Pediatrics* 94(1):90–93, 1994.
6. Samson RA, Atkins DL, Kerber RE: Optimal size of self-adhesive preapplied electrode pads in pediatric defibrillation, *Am J Cardiol* 75(7):544–545, 1995.
7. Killingsworth CR, Melnick SB, Chapman FW, et al: Defibrillation threshold and cardiac responses using an external biphasic defibrillator with pediatric and adult adhesive patches in pediatric-sized piglets, *Resuscitation* 55(2):177–185, 2002.
8. Kleinman ME, Chameides L, Schexnayder SM, et al: Part 14: pediatric advanced life support: 2010 American Heart Association guidelines for cardiopulmonary resuscitation and emergency cardiovascular care, *Circulation* 122(Suppl 3):S876–S908, 2010.
9. Dahl CF, Ewy GA, Warner ED, Thomas ED: Myocardial necrosis from direct current countershock. Effect of paddle electrode size and time interval between discharges, *Circulation* 50(5):956–961, 1974 Nov.
10. Panacek EA, Munger MA, Rutherford WF, Gardner SF: Report of nitropatch explosions complicating defibrillation, *Am J Emerg Med* 10(2):128–129, 1992.
11. Wrenn K: The hazards of defibrillation through nitroglycerin patches, *Ann Emerg Med* 19(11):1327–1328, 1990.
12. McGlinch BP, White RD: Cardiopulmonary resuscitation: basic and advanced life support. In Miller RD, editor: Miller's Anesthesia, ed 7, Philadelphia, 2009, Churchill Livingstone.
13. Link MS, Atkins DL, Passman RS, et al: Part 6: electrical therapies: automated external defibrillators, defibrillation, cardioversion, and pacing: 2010 American Heart Association guidelines for cardiopulmonary resuscitation and emergency cardiovascular care, *Circulation* 122(Suppl 3):S706–S719, 2010.
14. Pagan-Carlo LA, Spencer KT, Robertson CE, et al: Transthoracic defibrillation: importance of avoiding electrode placement directly on the female breast, *J Am Coll Cardiol* 27(2):449–452, 1996 Feb.

15. Olsovsky MR, Shorofsky SR, Gold MR: The effect of shock configuration and delivered energy on defibrillation impedance, *Pacing Clin Electrophysiol* 22(1 Pt 2):165–168, 1999.

16. Hummel RS 3rd, Ornato JP, Weinberg SM, Clarke AM: Spark-generating properties of electrode gels used during defibrillation. A potential fire hazard, *JAMA* 25;260(20):3021–3024, 1988.

17. Neumar RW, Otto CW, Link MS, et al: Part 8: adult advanced cardiovascular life support: 2010 American Heart Association guidelines for cardiopulmonary resuscitation and emergency cardiovascular care, *Circulation* 122(Suppl 3):S729–S767, 2010.

18. Miller PH: Potential fire hazard in defibrillation, *JAMA* 221(2):192, 1972.

19. Lefever J, Smith A: Risk of fire when using defibrillation in an oxygen enriched atmosphere, Medical Devices Agency 1995 (Feb). MDA SN95/03.

20. Theodorou AA, Gutierrez JA, Berg RA: Fire attributable to a defibrillation attempt in a neonate, *Pediatrics* 112(3 Pt 1):677–679, 2003 Sep.

21. Wilson JG, Macgregor DC, Goldman BS et al: Factors affecting patient recovery following pacemaker implantation, *Clin Prog Pacing Electrophysiology* 2(6):554, 1984.

22. Beland MJ, Hesslein PS, Finlay CD, et al: Noninvasive transcutaneous cardiac pacing in children, *Pacing Clin Electrophysiol* 10(6):1262–1270, 1987 Nov.

CHAPTER 5

Acute Coronary Syndromes

OBJECTIVES

Upon completion of this chapter, you will be able to:

1. Explain the pathophysiology of acute coronary syndromes (ACSs).
2. Describe the forms of ACSs.
3. Identify key components that should be included in the history and physical examination of the patient with a suspected ACSs.
4. Discuss the typical clinical presentation of the patient with a suspected ACS.
5. Explain and give examples of anginal equivalents.
6. Explain atypical presentation and its significance in ACS.
7. Identify the electrocardiogram (ECG) changes associated with myocardial ischemia, injury, and infarction.
8. Identify the ECG leads that view the anterior wall, inferior wall, lateral wall, septum, inferobasal wall, and right ventricle.
9. Explain the clinical and ECG features of right ventricle infarction (RVI).
10. Describe the initial management of a patient experiencing an ACS.
11. Explain the importance of the 12-lead ECG for the patient with an ACS.
12. Discuss the three groups used when categorizing the 12-lead ECG findings of the patient experiencing an ACS.
13. Identify the most common complications of an acute myocardial infarction (MI).

INTRODUCTION

In 2010, about 785,000 Americans experienced a new heart attack (MI) and about 470,000 had a recurrent attack. An estimated additional 195,000 silent heart attacks occur each year. The average age of an individual having a first heart attack is 64.5 years for men and 70.3 years for women.[1]

This chapter discusses the pathophysiology, history and clinical presentation, patient evaluation, and initial management of the patient experiencing an ACS. Recognition of an ACS and giving appropriate and timely emergency care can have a big impact on patient outcome.

ACLS Pearl
About every 25 seconds, an American will suffer a coronary event and about every minute someone will die as a rusult of one.[1]

PATHOPHYSIOLOGY OF ACUTE CORONARY SYNDROMES

[Objective 1]

Acute coronary syndromes (ACSs) are distinct conditions caused by a similar sequence of pathologic events and that involve a temporary or permanent blockage of a coronary artery. ACSs are characterized by an excessive demand or inadequate supply of oxygen and nutrients to the heart muscle associated with plaque disruption, thrombus formation, and vasoconstriction. The sequence of events that occurs during an ACS results in conditions ranging from myocardial ischemia or injury to death (i.e., necrosis) of heart muscle.

ACLS Pearl
ACSs are also called *acute ischemic coronary syndromes* (AICSs).

Arteriosclerosis is a chronic disease of the arterial system characterized by abnormal thickening and hardening of the vessel walls. **Atherosclerosis** is a form of arteriosclerosis in which the thickening and hardening of the vessel walls are caused by a buildup of fat-like deposits in the inner lining of large and middle-sized muscular arteries. The usual cause of an ACS is the rupture of an atherosclerotic plaque.

ACLS Pearl
Any artery in the body can develop atherosclerosis. If the coronary arteries are involved (i.e., coronary artery disease [CAD]) and if blood flow to the heart is decreased, angina or more serious signs and symptoms may result. If the arteries in the leg are involved (i.e., peripheral vascular disease), leg pain (i.e., claudication) may result. If the arteries supplying the brain are involved (i.e., carotid artery disease), a stroke or transient ischemic attack (TIA) may result.

Research has shown that oxidation and the body's inflammatory response contribute to atherosclerosis and heart disease. A hypothetical sequence of cellular interactions in atherosclerosis is shown in Figure 5-1. Oxidation is a normal chemical process in the body that is caused by the release of free radicals. Free radicals are oxygen atoms created during normal cell metabolism. Too many free radicals can seriously damage cells and impair the body's ability to fight against illness. Examples of conditions that can cause an overproduction of free radicals include stress and exposure to cigarette smoke, pesticides, air pollution, ultraviolet light, and radiation.

Antioxidants, such as Vitamins C and E, work by binding to free radicals and transforming them into nondamaging substances or repairing cellular damage. Oxidation causes injury to the inner (endothelial) layer of arteries. Low-density lipoproteins (LDL) become damaged when they react with free radicals. LDL may be responsible for a buildup of fat-like material on the artery walls.

Injury to the endothelial layer of an artery starts the body's inflammatory response at the injury site. White blood cells are released at the site and oxidize LDL. Cytokines are also released. Cytokines attract even more white blood cells to the site. They also raise blood pressure and increase the tendency for blood to clot. Oxidation converts LDL to a foamy material, which sticks to the smooth muscle cells of the arteries. Over time, the foamy material builds up on artery walls and forms a hard plaque.

Atherosclerotic lesions include the fatty streak, the fibrous plaque, and the advanced (complicated) lesion (Figures 5-2 and 5-3). Fatty streaks are thin, flat yellow lesions composed of lipids (mostly cholesterol) or smooth muscle cells that protrude slightly into the arterial opening. They appear in all populations, even those with a low incidence of coronary artery disease (CAD). Fatty streaks do not obstruct the vessel and are not associated with any clinical symptoms.

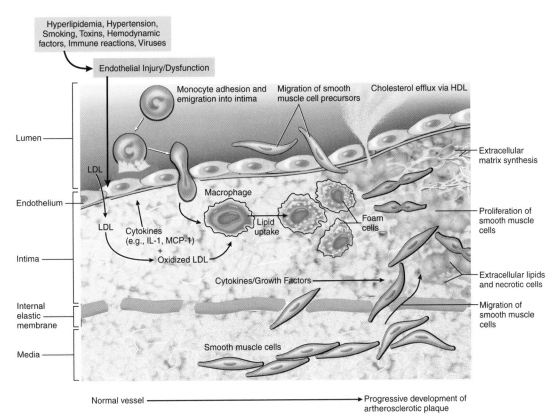

Figure 5-1 Hypothetical sequence of cellular interactions in atherosclerosis. Hyperlipidemia and other risk factors are thought to cause endothelial injury, resulting in adhesion of platelets and monocytes and release of growth factors, including platelet-derived growth factor (PDGF), which lead to smooth muscle cell (SMC) migration and proliferation. Foam cells of atheromatous plaques are derived from both macrophages and SMCs—from macrophages via the very-low-density lipoprotein (VLDL) receptor and low-density lipoprotein (LDL) modifications recognized by scavenger receptors (e.g., oxidized LDL), and from SMCs by less certain mechanisms. Extracellular lipid is derived from insudation from the vessel lumen, particularly in the presence of hypercholesterolemia, and also from degenerating foam cells. Cholesterol accumulation in the plaque reflects an imbalance between influx and efflux, and high-density lipoprotein (HDL) probably helps clear cholesterol from these accumulations. SMCs migrate to the intima, proliferate, and produce extracellular matrix (ECM), including collagen and proteoglycans. IL-1, interleukin 1; MCP-1, membrane cofactor protein 1.

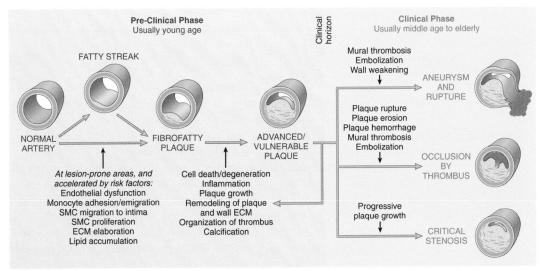

Figure 5-2 The natural history, morphologic features, main pathogenic events, and clinical complications of atherosclerosis. ECM, extracellular matrix; SMC, smooth muscle cell.

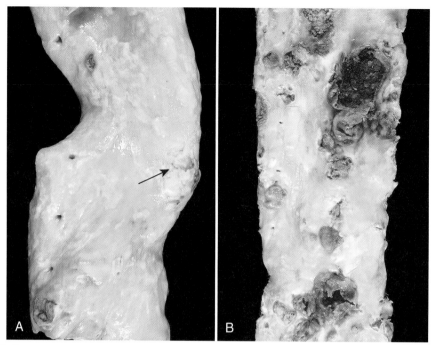

Figure 5-3 Gross views of atherosclerosis in the aorta. **A,** Mild atherosclerosis made up of fibrous plaques, one of which is indicated by the *arrow*. **B,** Severe disease with scattered and complicated lesions.

Progression from a fatty streak to an advanced lesion is associated with injured endothelium that activates the inflammatory response. As the inflammatory response continues, the fatty streak becomes a fatty plaque, then a fibrous plaque, and finally an advanced lesion. Hemorrhage then occurs within the plaque and a thrombus forms.

Initially the walls of the blood vessel outwardly expand (i.e., remodel) as plaque builds up inside of it. This occurs so that the size of the vessel stays relatively constant, despite the increased size of the plaque. When the plaque fills about 40% of the inside of the vessel, remodeling stops because the vessel can no longer expand to make room for the increase in plaque size. As an atherosclerotic plaque increases in size, the vessel becomes severely narrowed (i.e., stenosed). Generally, arterial stenosis of 70% of the vessel's diameter is required to produce anginal symptoms.

> **ACLS Pearl**
> The extent of arterial narrowing and the amount of reduction in blood flow are critical determinants of CAD.

Plaque Rupture

Atherosclerotic plaques differ with regard to their makeup, vulnerability to rupture, and tendency to form a blood clot. A "stable" or "nonvulnerable" atherosclerotic plaque has a relatively thick fibrous cap that separates it from contact with the blood and that covers a core containing a large amount of collagen and smooth muscle cells but a relatively small lipid pool (Figure 5-4). A stable plaque may produce significant luminal obstruction, but has a lower tendency to rupture or erode.[2] Plaques that are prone to rupture are called "vulnerable" plaques because they have a thin cap of fibrous tissue over a large, soft, fatty center that separates it from the opening of the blood vessel. If the fibrous cap erodes or ruptures, the contents of the plaque (i.e., collagen, smooth muscle cells, tissue factor, inflammatory cells, and lipid material) are exposed to flowing blood.

The rupture of a vulnerable plaque may occur after the following: extreme physical activity (especially in someone unaccustomed to regular exercise), severe emotional trauma, sexual activity, exposure to illicit drugs (e.g., cocaine, amphetamines), exposure to cold, or acute infection.[3] Contributing factors to plaque rupture may include shear stress (i.e., the frictional force from blood flow), coronary spasm at the site of the plaque, internal plaque changes, and the effects of risk factors (see Chapter 1).

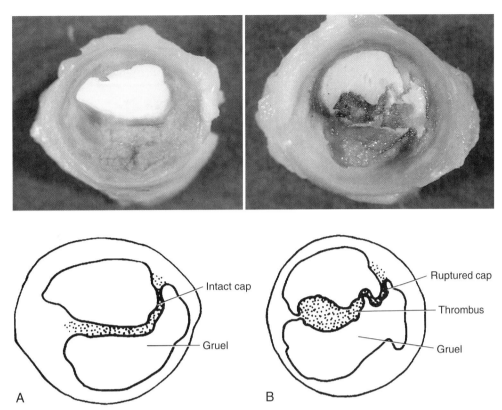

Figure 5-4 Views of stable and vulnerable plaques. **A,** A stable plaque. Yellow, soft fatty material (gruel) is separated from the opening of the vessel by a thin fibrous cap. White radiographic contrast medium is visible in the vessel opening. **B,** A vulnerable plaque. This specimen was just a few millimeters distal to the one shown in A. In this specimen, the thin fibrous cap is ruptured, a big cap fragment and some of the soft atheromatous gruel are missing (from downstream embolization), and a clot has evolved where the fatty gruel has been exposed. White contrast medium has penetrated the soft gruel through the ruptured fibrous cap.

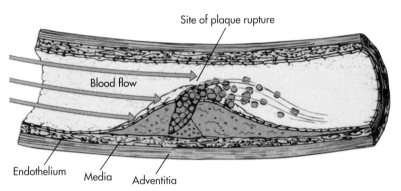

Figure 5-5 Rupture of a vulnerable plaque results in adhesion of platelets at the site and activation of additional platelets (aggregation). The coagulation cascade then begins, resulting in additional platelet aggregation and thrombosis.

Plaque disruption (rupture) is most likely to occur at vessel bifurcations because of the speed of blood flow and turbulence created at these areas. Three vulnerable sites for plaque disruption within the coronary arteries have been identified and include the following[4]:

- The proximal portion of the left anterior descending coronary artery
- Near the origin of the marginal branch on the right coronary artery
- Near the origin of the first obtuse marginal branch on the circumflex coronary artery

Thrombus Development

If the cap of a vulnerable plaque erodes or ruptures, platelets stick to the damaged lining of the vessel and to each other within seconds and form a plug (Figure 5-5). "Sticky platelets" secrete several chemicals, including thromboxane A_2. These substances stimulate vasoconstriction, reducing blood flow at the site. Aspirin, which is an antiplatelet agent, blocks the production of thromboxane A_2, slowing down the clumping (i.e., aggregation) of platelets and lowering the risk of complete blockage of the vessel.

After the platelets are activated, glycoprotein IIb/IIIa receptors that are needed for platelet clumping appear on the surface of the platelet. Fibrinogen molecules bind to these receptors to form bridges (i.e., "cross-links") between nearby platelets, allowing them to clump. Glycoprotein IIb/IIIa receptor inhibitors prevent fibrinogen binding and platelet clumping. As the process continues, fibrinogen cross-links between platelets, thrombin is made, and fibrin is formed; this ultimately produces a clot. Clots can be dissolved by a process called **fibrinolysis**. Fibrinolytics (i.e., "clot-busters") are drugs that stimulate the conversion of plasminogen to plasmin, which dissolves the clot.

Coronary Artery Obstruction

The most common cause of a myocardial infarction is acute plaque rupture. The resultant thrombosis leads to acute closure of coronary arteries. When a temporary or permanent blockage occurs in a coronary artery, the blood supply to the heart muscle is impaired. An impaired blood supply results in a decreased supply of oxygen to the myocardium. When the heart's demand for oxygen exceeds its supply from the coronary circulation, chest discomfort or related symptoms often occur. A decreased supply of oxygenated blood to a body part or organ is called **ischemia**.

Blockage of a coronary artery by a thrombus may be partial or complete. Partial (incomplete) blockage of a coronary artery by a thrombus may result in no clinical signs and symptoms (silent MI), unstable angina, non–ST-segment elevation MI (NSTEMI) or, possibly, sudden death. Complete blockage of a coronary artery may result in ST-elevation MI (STEMI) or sudden death. The patient's signs, symptoms, and outcome depend on factors including the following:
- The amount of heart muscle supplied by the affected artery
- The severity and duration of myocardial ischemia
- The electrical instability of the ischemic myocardium
- The degree and duration of coronary vessel blockage
- The presence and extent or absence of collateral coronary circulation

> **ACLS Pearl**
>
> The complete blockage of a coronary artery may cause an MI. However, because a plaque usually increases in size over months and years, other vascular pathways may enlarge as portions of a coronary artery become blocked. These vascular pathways (i.e., collateral circulation) serve as an alternative route for blood flow around the blocked artery to the heart muscle. Thus the presence of collateral arteries may prevent infarction despite complete blockage of the artery.

Other Causes of Acute Coronary Syndromes

Although a thrombus is the most common cause of blockage of a coronary artery, less commonly, an acute MI may occur as a result of coronary spasm (e.g., with cocaine abuse), abnormalities of coronary vessels, hypercoagulation, trauma to the coronary arteries, or coronary artery emboli (rare).[5]

Cocaine causes myocardial ischemia or MI by (1) increasing myocardial oxygen demand by increasing heart rate, blood pressure, and contractility; (2) decreasing oxygen supply via vasoconstriction; (3) inducing a prothrombotic state by stimulating platelet activation and altering the balance between procoagulant and anticoagulant factors; and (4) accelerating atherosclerosis.[6] Although one study showed that two thirds of MI events occurred within 3 hours of cocaine ingestion,[7] patients may not seek medical attention for hours to days after use.

The patient experiencing a cocaine-associated ACS may deny drug use and have atypical chest discomfort. Common cardiopulmonary complaints among cocaine users appear in Box 5-1.

Although there are no clear predictors for patients at risk of cocaine-associated ACS, the Cocaine-Associated Myocardial Infarction study retrospectively identified 130 patients who sustained a total of 136 cocaine-associated MI events. In this group, the majority of patients were young (mean age 38 years), nonwhite (72%), smokers (91%), and had a history of cocaine use in the preceding 24 hours (88%).[6,8] A 2003 study showed that patients with cocaine-associated chest pain and positive cardiac

| **BOX 5-1** | **Common Cardiopulmonary Complaints among Cocaine Users[6]** |

Anxiety

Chest pain described as pressure-like in
quality (most common symptom)

Diaphoresis

Dizziness

Dyspnea

Nausea

Palpitations

biomarkers for MI had significant angiographic stenosis and of patients without positive serum markers, 18% still had significant disease by angiogram.[9] Cardiac biomarkers are discussed later in this chapter.

Prinzmetal's angina which is also called *Prinzmetal's variant angina* or *variant angina*, is the result of intense spasm of a segment of a coronary artery. This variant angina may occur in otherwise healthy individuals (usually in their 40s or 50s) with no demonstrable coronary heart disease or in patients with a nonobstructive atheromatous plaque. In some studies, coronary arteriography in patients with Prinzmetal's angina showed one-vessel CAD in 39% of patients and multivessel disease in 19%.[10]

Although the episode of coronary artery spasm can be precipitated by exercise, emotional stress, hyperventilation, or exposure to cold, it usually occurs at rest, often occurs between midnight and 8 am, and may awaken the patient from sleep.[11] Episodes may occur in clusters of two or three within 30 to 60 minutes. Although episodes usually last only a few minutes, this may be long enough to produce serious dysrhythmias including atrioventricular (AV) block and ventricular tachycardia (VT), as well as sudden death. If the spasm is prolonged, infarction may result.

It can be difficult to suspect Prinzmetal's angina from the patient's clinical presentation. Patients with Prinzmetal's angina are generally younger and have fewer coronary risk factors (except for smoking) compared with patients with chronic stable angina. Prinzmetal's angina has been associated with other vasospastic conditions such as migraine headache and Raynaud's phenomenon.

The patient with Prinzmetal's angina complains of chest pain that is often described as severe and may be accompanied by syncope. Chest discomfort is usually relieved by nitroglycerin (NTG). However, although typical angina produces ST-segment *depression*, Prinzmetal's angina produces ST-segment *elevation* during periods of chest pain. After the episode of chest discomfort is resolved, ST segments usually return to the baseline. Because NTG is effective at relieving the coronary spasm, the ECG evidence of Prinzmetal's angina may be lost if no pretreatment ECG is obtained.

> **ACLS Pearl**
>
> Obtain a baseline 12-lead ECG before initiating treatment in any patient presenting with a possible ACS.

FORMS OF ACUTE CORONARY SYNDROMES

[Objective 2]

ACSs include unstable angina, NSTEMI, and STEMI.

Unstable Angina

Angina pectoris is chest discomfort that occurs when the heart muscle does not receive enough oxygen (myocardial ischemia). Angina is not a disease. Rather, it is a symptom of myocardial ischemia. Angina most often occurs in patients with CAD involving at least one coronary artery. However, it can be present in patients with normal coronary arteries. Angina also occurs in persons with uncontrolled high blood pressure or valvular heart disease.

The term **angina** refers to squeezing or tightening, rather than pain. The discomfort associated with angina occurs because of the stimulation of nerve endings by lactic acid and carbon dioxide that builds up in ischemic tissue. Common words used by patients experiencing angina to describe the sensation they are feeling are shown in Box 5-2. Some patients have difficulty describing their discomfort.

Chest discomfort associated with myocardial ischemia usually begins in the central or left chest and then radiates to the arm (especially the little finger [ulnar] side of the left arm), wrist, jaw,

BOX 5-2	Common Terms Patients Use To Describe Angina

- "Burning"
- "Bursting"
- "Constricting"
- "Grip-like"
- "Heaviness"
- "Pressing"
- "Squeezing"
- "Strangling"
- "Suffocating"
- "A band across my chest"
- "A vise tightening around my chest"
- "A weight in the center of my chest"

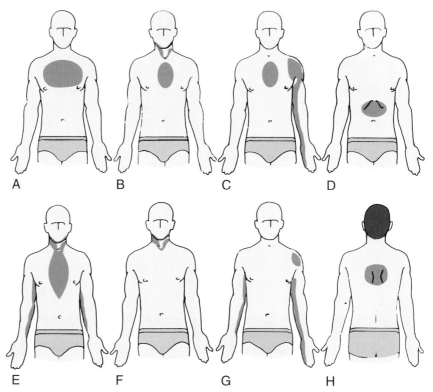

Figure 5-6 Common sites for anginal discomfort. **A,** Upper part of chest. **B,** Beneath the sternum radiating to neck and jaw. **C,** Beneath the sternum radiating down left arm. **D,** Epigastric. **E,** Epigastric radiating to the neck, jaw, and arms. **F,** Neck and jaw (common in women). **G,** Left shoulder and arm (common in older adults and women). **H,** Interscapular. (common in older adults and women).

epigastrium, left shoulder, or between the shoulder blades (Figure 5-6). Ischemic chest discomfort is usually not sharp; it is not worsened by deep inspiration; it is not affected by moving muscles in the area where the discomfort is localized, nor is it positional in nature.

Ischemia can occur because of increased myocardial oxygen demand (i.e., demand ischemia), reduced myocardial oxygen supply (i.e., supply ischemia), or both. If the cause of the ischemia is not reversed and blood flow restored to the affected area of the heart muscle, ischemia may lead to cellular injury and, ultimately, infarction. Ischemia can quickly resolve by reducing the heart's oxygen demand (by resting or slowing the heart rate with medications such as beta-blockers) or by increasing blood flow by dilating the coronary arteries with drugs such as NTG. Early assessment that includes a focused history as well as emergency care are essential to prevent worsening ischemia. Serial ECGs and continuous ECG monitoring should be performed.

Stable (classic) angina remains relatively constant and predictable in terms of severity, signs and symptoms, precipitating events, and response to treatment. It is characterized by brief episodes of chest

BOX 5-3 **Stable Angina**

Common Precipitating Events
Emotional upset
Exercise or exertion
Exposure to cold weather

Related Signs and Symptoms
- Nausea or vomiting
- Palpitations
- Shortness of breath
- Sweating

discomfort related to activities that increase the heart's need for oxygen such as emotional upset, exercise or exertion, and exposure to cold weather. Possible related signs and symptoms are shown in Box 5-3. Symptoms typically last 2 to 5 minutes and occasionally 5 to 15 minutes. Prolonged discomfort (i.e., longer than 30 minutes) is uncommon in stable angina.

ACLS Pearl
Only 18% of MIs are preceded by longstanding angina.[1]

Unstable angina, which is also known as preinfarction angina, is a condition of intermediate severity between stable angina and acute MI. It occurs most often among men and women 60 to 80 years of age who have one or more of the major risk factors for CAD.

Unstable angina is characterized by one or more of the following:
- Symptoms that occur at rest and usually last for more than 20 minutes
- Symptoms that are severe and/or of new onset (i.e., within the last 2 months)
- Symptoms that are increasing in duration, frequency, or both; and intensity in a patient with a history of stable angina

Unlike stable angina, the discomfort associated with unstable angina may be described as painful. Patients with untreated unstable angina are at high risk for a heart attack or death. During their initial presentation, distinguishing patients with unstable angina from those with an acute MI is often impossible because their clinical presentations and ECG findings may be identical. Early assessment, including a focused history, and emergency care are essential to prevent worsening ischemia. Serial ECGs and continuous ECG monitoring should be performed.

The diagnosis of unstable angina versus NSTEMI is made on the basis of the patient's assessment findings and symptoms, history, presence of risk factors, serial 12-lead ECG results, blood test results (i.e., cardiac biomarkers), and other diagnostic tests.

ACLS Pearl
The time from symptom onset to emergency care can be shortened if patients, families, and bystanders are taught to recognize symptoms early and activate the Emergency Medical Services (EMS) system. Teach your patients and their families how to recognize the signs and symptoms of a heart attack. They should be taught to call 9-1-1 within 5 minutes of symptom onset. Let them know that not all heart attacks are accompanied by sudden, crushing chest pain and a loss of responsiveness. Symptoms may begin gradually or may come and go. Patients who have had a previous heart attack should be taught that the signs and symptoms of a second one might differ from those of the first.

Myocardial Infarction

Ischemia prolonged more than just a few minutes results in myocardial *injury*. *Myocardial injury* refers to myocardial tissue that has been cut off from or experienced a severe reduction in its blood and oxygen supply. Injured myocardial cells are still alive but will die (i.e., *infarct*) if the ischemia is not

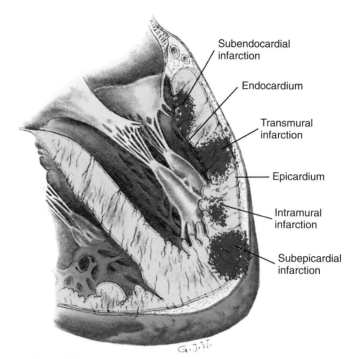

Figure 5-7 Possible locations of infarctions in the ventricular wall.

quickly corrected. If the blocked vessel can be quickly opened to restore blood flow and oxygen to the injured area, no tissue death will occur. Methods to restore blood flow may include giving fibrinolytics, performing a coronary angioplasty, or performing a coronary artery bypass graft (CABG), among others.

An MI occurs when blood flow to the heart muscle stops or is suddenly decreased long enough to cause cell death. The walls of the ventricles consist of an outer layer (the epicardium), middle layer (the myocardium), and an inner layer (the endocardium). The myocardium is subdivided into two areas. The innermost half of the myocardium is called the **subendocardial area** and the outermost half is called the **subepicardial area**. The main coronary arteries lie on the epicardial surface of the heart and feed this area first before supplying the heart's inner layers with oxygenated blood. The endocardial and subendocardial areas of the myocardial wall are the least perfused areas of the heart and the most vulnerable to ischemia because these areas have a high demand for oxygen and are fed by the most distal branches of the coronary arteries. **Transmural** is a term used to describe ischemia, injury, or infarction that extends from the endocardium to the epicardium. For example, an infarction involving the entire thickness of the left ventricular wall is called a **transmural MI**. Possible locations of infarctions in the ventricular wall are shown in Figure 5-7.

In the strictest sense, the term *myocardial infarction* relates to dead heart muscle tissue. In a practical sense, the term *myocardial infarction* is applied to the *process* that results in the death of myocardial tissue. Think of the "process" of MI as a continuum rather than the presence of dead heart tissue (Figure 5-8). Infarcted cells cannot respond to an electrical stimulus or provide any mechanical function. If efforts are made to recognize the process of MI, patients may be identified earlier. If they are promptly treated, the loss of heart tissue may be avoided.[12]

In the past, an MI was classified according to its location (e.g., anterior, inferior), and whether or not it produced Q waves on the ECG (i.e., Q wave versus non-Q wave MI). However, because a pathologic Q wave may take hours to develop (and in some cases, never develops), the patient's history and symptoms, cardiac biomarker results, and the presence of ST-segment elevation provide the strongest evidence for the early recognition of MI. ECG clues that may help to establish the presence, location, extent, and duration of an infarction are discussed in more detail later in this chapter.

Universal Definition of Myocardial Infarction

In 1999, the European Society of Cardiology (ESC) and the American College of Cardiology (ACC) convened a sonference to revise jointly the definition of MI. The definition for MI was examined from seven points of view: pathological, biochemical, electrocardiographic, imaging, clinical trials,

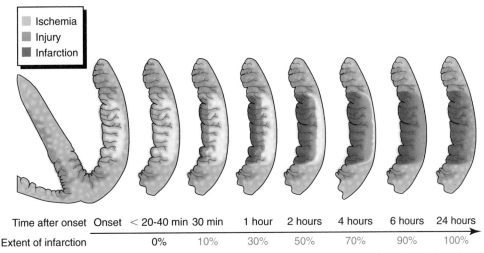

Time after onset | Onset | < 20-40 min | 30 min | 1 hour | 2 hours | 4 hours | 6 hours | 24 hours

Extent of infarction | | 0% | 10% | 30% | 50% | 70% | 90% | 100%

Figure 5-8 Progression of a myocardial infarction (MI). When a coronary artery is blocked (usually by a thrombus), ischemia occurs immediately in the area supplied by the culprit artery, and subendocardial injury occurs within 20 to 40 minutes. Death of subendocardial tissue occurs in about 30 minutes and necrosis extends to about half of the myocardial wall by 2 hours. By 6 hours, necrosis involves about 90% of the myocardial wall and is complete by 24 hours. Healing begins within 24 to 72 hours. Within 2 to 8 weeks of the infarction, the necrotic tissue has been replaced by fibrous tissue.

BOX 5-4   Criteria for Acute Myocardial Infarction[13]

The term myocardial infarction should be used when there is evidence of myocardial necrosis in a clinical setting consistent with myocardial ischemia. Under these conditions any one of the following criteria meets the diagnosis for MI:

- Detection of rise and/or fall of cardiac biomarkers (preferably troponin) with at least one value above the 99th percentile of the upper reference limit (URL) together with evidence of myocardial ischemia with at least one of the following:
  - Symptoms of ischemia
  - ECG changes indicative of new ischemia (new ST-segment or T wave changes or new left bundle branch block [LBBB])
  - Development of pathological Q waves in the ECG
  - Imaging evidence of new loss of viable myocardium or new regional wall motion abnormality
- Sudden, unexpected cardiac death, involving cardiac arrest, often with symptoms suggestive of myocardial ischemia, and accompanied by presumably new ST elevation, or new LBBB, and/or evidence of fresh thrombus by coronary angiography and/or at autopsy, but death occurring before blood samples could be obtained, or at a time before the appearance of cardiac biomarkers in the blood.
- For percutaneous coronary interventions (PCI) in patients with normal baseline troponin values, elevations of cardiac biomarkers above the 99th percentile URL are indicative of peri-procedural myocardial necrosis. By convention, increases of biomarkers greater than 3 × 99th percentile URL have been designated as defining PCI-related MI. A subtype related to a documented stent thrombosis is recognized.
- For CABG in patients with normal baseline troponin values, elevations of cardiac biomarkers above the 99th percentile URL are indicative of peri-procedural myocardial necrosis. By convention, increases of biomarkers greater than 5 × 99th percentile URL plus either new pathological Q waves or new LBBB, or angiographically documented new graft or native coronary artery occlusion, or imaging evidence of new loss of viable myocardium have been designated as defining CABG-related MI.
- Pathological findings of an acute MI.

epidemiological, and public policy. The consensus committee findings were published in 2000 in the European Heart Journal and Journal of the American College of Cardiology. The ESC, ACC, and the American Heart Association (AHA) convened, together with the World Heart Federation (WHF), a Global Task Force to update the 2000 document and an updated expert consensus document was published in 2007.[13] Classifications of MI are shown in Table 5-1 and the criteria for acute MI appear in Box 5-4.

TABLE 5-1 Myocardial Infarction—Classifications

Anatomic Classification[14]	Description
Transmural	Ischemic necrosis of the full thickness of the affected muscle segment(s), extending from the endocardium through the myocardium to the epicardium
Nontransmural	Area of ischemic necrosis is limited to the endocardium or endocardium and myocardium, it does not extend through the full thickness of myocardial wall segment(s)

Classification by Size[13]	Description
Microscopic	Focal necrosis
Small	Less than 10% of the left ventricular (LV) myocardium
Moderate	10% to 30% of the LV myocardium
Large	More than 30% of the LV myocardium

Pathological Classification[13]	Time Frame	Description
Evolving	Less than 6 hours	Minimal or no polymorphonuclear leukocytes may be seen
Acute	6 hours to 7 days	Presence of polymorphonuclear leukocytes
Healing	7 to 28 days	Presence of mononuclear cells and fibroblasts, absence of polymorphonuclear leukocytes
Healed	29 days or more	Scar tissue without cellular infiltration

Classification by Location		
Anterior	Inferior	Septal
Lateral	Inferobasal (posterior)	Right ventricular

Clinical Classification[13]	Description
Type 1	Spontaneous myocardial infarction (MI) related to ischemia due to a primary coronary event such as plaque erosion and/or rupture, fissuring, or dissection
Type 2	MI secondary to ischemia due to either increased oxygen demand or decreased supply such as coronary artery spasm, coronary embolism, anemia, arrhythmias, hypertension, or hypotension
Type 3	Sudden unexpected cardiac death, including cardiac arrest, often with symptoms suggestive of myocardial ischemia, accompanied by presumably new ST elevation, or new left bundle branch block, or evidence of fresh thrombus in a coronary artery by angiography and/or at autopsy, but death occurring before blood samples could be obtained, or at a time before the appearance of cardiac biomarkers in the blood
Type 4a	MI associated with percutaneous coronary intervention
Type 4b	MI associated with stent thrombosis as documented by angiography or at autopsy
Type 5	MI associated with coronary artery bypass graft

Data from Thygesen K, Alpert JS, White HD; Joint ESC/ACCF/AHA/WHF Task Force for the Redefinition of Myocardial Infarction: Universal definition of myocardial infarction. *J Am Coll Cardiol* 2007;50:2173–2195.[13]
Data from Bolooki HM, Bajzer CT: Acute myocardial infarction. In *Cleveland Clinic: current clinical medicine,* Philadelphia, 2009, Elsevier.[14]

Criteria for Prior Myocardial Infarction[13]

Any one of the following criteria meets the diagnosis for prior MI:
- Development of new pathological Q waves with or without symptoms.
- Imaging evidence of a region of loss of viable myocardium that is thinned and fails to contract, in the absence of a nonischemic cause.
- Pathological findings of a healed or healing MI.

HISTORY AND CLINICAL PRESENTATION[12]

[Objective 3]
Patient History

The average patient experiencing an ACS does not seek medical attention for 2 hours or more after the onset of ischemic chest pain symptoms.[10,15] Women often delay longer than men do when seeking medical help. Common reasons that individuals delay in seeking medical care for ischemic-type chest discomfort are shown in Box 5-5.

Not all chest discomfort is cardiac-related. Obtaining an accurate history is important to help determine if a patient's signs and symptoms are most likely related to ischemia as a result of CAD. Because time is muscle when caring for patients with an ACS, it is important to ask targeted questions to determine the patient's probability of an ACS and to not delay reperfusion therapy, if indicated. Important information to obtain when eliciting a targeted history is shown in Table 5-2.

> **ACLS Pearl**
>
> When obtaining the patient's history, use the patient's words for the discomfort. For example, the patient may not consider their symptom "discomfort" or "pain" but instead have another appropriately descriptive term to describe their symptom. Whatever term the patient uses, continue to use that term when interacting with the patient.

> **ACLS Pearl**
>
> Patients with possible symptoms of ischemic chest discomfort should be taught the importance of calling 9-1-1, rather than arranging for their own transport to the hospital. Teach your patients that EMS professionals can provide life-saving care if complications develop en route to the hospital.

Predisposing Factors

Studies have shown that the peak incidence of acute cardiac events is between 6 am and noon.[16-19] The early morning hours are associated with increases in blood pressure, heart rate, sympathetic nervous system activity, cortisol, and platelet aggregability. Some studies have shown that an MI is more likely to occur on Monday (as the patient transitions from weekend to work week) and during the winter months.[16,20-22]

A predisposing factor (i.e., trigger) is present in about 50% of patients experiencing an acute cardiac event.[23] Examples include moderate to heavy physical exertion, unusual emotional stress, lack of sleep, overeating or use of alcohol, acute respiratory infection, or pulmonary embolism.[19,24-27] Cocaine use may be a factor, particularly in patients younger than 40 years of age.

BOX 5-5	**Common Reasons for Delays in Seeking Medical Care for Ischemic-type Chest Discomfort[10,15]**

- Unaware of the importance of calling EMS or 9-1-1 for symptoms
- Unaware of the need for rapid treatment
- Mild discomfort began slowly rather than abruptly and with severe pain as depicted on television or in the movies
- Believed symptoms would go away or were not serious
- Believed symptoms were caused by another chronic condition (e.g., arthritis, muscle strain, influenza)
- Did not want to "bother" EMS personnel, physicians, or other healthcare professionals unless they were "really sick"
- Afraid of embarrassment if symptoms turned out to be a false alarm
- Wanted family approval before seeking medical care
- Felt they were not at risk for a heart attack (especially common among women or young, healthy men)
  Note: Although these responses from 2004 and 2007 are still true today, the economy (i.e., lack of employment or medical benefits) is another common reason for delays in seeking care (i.e., "I can't afford it").

TABLE 5-2 Acute Coronary Syndromes—Targeted History

Historical Information to Obtain	Notes
Patient age, gender	Important risk factors

SAMPLE History

Signs and Symptoms	*What prompted you to seek medical assistance today?*
Allergies	Ask the patient about allergies to medications, food, environmental elements (e.g., pollen), and products (e.g., latex).
Medications	• *What prescription and over-the-counter medications are you currently taking?* • *Do you take your medicine as prescribed?* • *Have you missed any doses or taken extra doses of any medicine?* • *Have you taken any medication for erectile dysfunction in the past 24 to 48 hours?* • *Do you take any herbal supplements or use recreational drugs such as cocaine?* Ask about the use of cocaine in patients with suspected acute coronary syndromes, particularly in patients younger than 40 years of age.
Past medical history	• *Are you currently under a physician's care?* • *Do you have a history of a heart attack, angina, heart failure, high blood pressure, or abnormal heart rhythm?* If the patient answers yes to this question, ask how his or her current symptoms compare to the previous episode. • *Have you ever had a heart-related medical procedure such as a bypass (open-heart surgery), cardiac catheterization, angioplasty, transplant, valve replacement, or pacemaker?* • *Do you have a history of stroke; diabetes; lung, liver, or kidney disease; or other medical condition?* Find out the patient's risk factors for heart disease. Ask the patient if he or she smokes. If the answer is yes, ask how many packs per day. Ask the patient if a history of heart disease is in the family. If the answer is yes, ask whether anyone died of heart disease and at what age. Ask about a family history of high blood pressure, diabetes, and high cholesterol. • *Have you been hospitalized recently? Any recent surgery?*
Last oral intake	Ask the patient when he or she last had anything to eat or drink and if any recent changes in eating patterns or fluid intake (or output) have occurred.
Events leading to the incident	*What were you doing when your symptoms began?* Try to find out what precipitated the patient's current symptoms. For example, did an event or activity cause the patient's symptoms, such as strenuous exercise, sexual activity, or unusual stress?

OPQRST (Pain Presentation)

Onset	• *When did your symptoms begin?* • *Did it begin suddenly or gradually?* • *Have you ever had this discomfort before? When? How long did it last? Were you seen, evaluated, or treated for it? If so, what was the diagnosis? How does the discomfort you are feeling right now compare with that?*
Provocation/ **P**alliation/ **P**osition	• *What were you doing when your symptoms started?* • *What makes the discomfort better or worse?* • *What have you tried to relieve the problem?* • *Does a change in position lessen the discomfort?*
Quality	• *What does your discomfort feel like?* Document the words the patient uses to describe discomfort.
Region/ **R**adiation/ **R**eferral	• *Where is your discomfort?* Ask the patient to point to it. • *Does it stay in one area? Do you have symptoms in a different area of your body?*
Severity	• *On a scale of 0 to 10, with 0 being the least and 10 being the worst, what number would you assign your discomfort?*

TABLE 5-2	**Acute Coronary Syndromes—Targeted History—cont'd**
Historical Information to Obtain	**Notes**
Timing	• *Is your discomfort still present? Is it getting better, worse, or staying about the same?* • *Does it come and go or is it constant?*
Presence of associated symptoms?	Nausea, vomiting, difficulty breathing, sweating, weakness, fatigue
Special considerations	• Consider the possibility of potentially lethal conditions that mimic acute MI such as aortic dissection, acute pericarditis, acute myocarditis, and pulmonary embolism • Consider conditions that can produce ST elevation on the ECG (mimicking STEMI) including acute pericarditis, early repolarization, hyperkalemia, left ventricular hypertrophy, and bundle branch blocks

Typical Symptoms

[Objective 4]

Chest discomfort is the most common symptom of infarction. It is present in 75% to 80% of patients with acute MI. Patients experiencing a heart attack may describe the sensation they are feeling as similar to angina, or use words such as "heartburn," "indigestion," "dull," "squeezing," "gnawing," "aching," "tightness," or "pressure." The patient may describe his or her discomfort with a clenched fist held against the sternum (Levine's sign). The discomfort typically lasts longer than 30 minutes. It may be constant or come and go, and occasionally may be relieved with belching.[15]

The ACC/AHA guidelines list the following as pain descriptions that are *not* characteristic of myocardial ischemia[10]:

- Pleuritic pain (i.e., sharp or knife-like pain brought on by respiratory movements or cough)
- Primary or sole location of discomfort in the middle or lower abdominal region
- Pain that may be localized at the tip of one finger, particularly over the left ventricular apex
- Pain reproduced with movement or palpation of the chest wall or arms
- Constant pain that persists for many hours
- Very brief episodes of pain that last a few seconds or less
- Pain that radiates into the lower extremities

Anginal Equivalents

[Objective 5]

Anginal equivalent symptoms are symptoms of myocardial ischemia other than chest pain or discomfort. Examples of anginal equivalents include the following:

- Difficulty breathing
- Dizziness
- Dysrhythmias
- Excessive sweating
- Fatigue
- Generalized weakness
- Isolated arm or jaw pain
- Palpitations
- Syncope or near-syncope
- Unexplained nausea or vomiting

Atypical Presentation

[Objective 6]

Not all patients experiencing an ACS present similarly. **Atypical presentation** refers to uncharacteristic signs and symptoms that are experienced by some patients. Atypical chest discomfort is localized to the chest area but may have musculoskeletal, positional, or pleuritic features. Examples of atypical presentations of STEMI are listed in Box 5-6.

BOX 5-6 **Atypical ST-Elevation Myocardial Infarction Signs and Symptoms**

Atypical presentations of STEMI include the following[28]:

- Acute indigestion
- Apprehension and nervousness
- Atypical location of the pain
- Central nervous system manifestations, resembling those of stroke as a result of a sharp reduction in cardiac output in a patient with cerebral arteriosclerosis
- Classic angina pectoris without a particularly severe or prolonged episode
- Heart failure
- Overwhelming weakness
- Peripheral embolization
- Sudden mania or psychosis
- Syncope

Patients experiencing an ACS who are most likely to present atypically include older adults, diabetic individuals, women, patients with prior cardiac surgery, and patients during the immediate postoperative period after noncardiac surgery.[5]

Older adults may have atypical symptoms such as dyspnea, shoulder or back pain, weakness, fatigue, a change in mental status, syncope, unexplained nausea, and abdominal or epigastric discomfort. They are also more likely to present with more severe preexisting conditions, such as hypertension, heart failure, or a previous acute MI than a younger patient. Individuals with diabetes may present atypically due to autonomic dysfunction. Common signs and symptoms include generalized weakness, syncope, lightheadedness, or a change in mental status.

Women who experience an ACS report acute symptoms including prodromal chest discomfort, unusual fatigue, sleep disturbances, dyspnea, nausea or vomiting, indigestion, dizziness or fainting, sweating, arm or shoulder pain, and weakness. When chest discomfort is present, it is often described as "aching," "tightness," "pressure," "sharpness," "burning," "fullness," or "tingling." The location of the discomfort is often in the back, arm, shoulder, or neck. Some women have vague chest discomfort that tends to come and go with no known aggravating factors.

ACLS Pearl

Researchers compared African-American, Hispanic, and Caucasian women's prodromal and acute symptoms of MI.[29] Symptom severity and frequency were compared among racial groups. Among the women, 96% reported prodromal symptoms. Unusual fatigue (73%) and sleep disturbance (50%) were the most frequent. Eighteen symptoms differed significantly by race. African-American women reported higher frequencies of 10 symptoms than did Hispanic or Caucasian women. Thirty-six percent reported prodromal chest discomfort. Hispanic women reported more pain/discomfort symptoms than did African-American or Caucasian women. Minority women reported more acute symptoms. The most frequent symptom, regardless of race, was shortness of breath (63%); 22 symptoms differed by race. In total, 28% of Hispanic, 38% of African-American, and 42% of Caucasian women reported no chest pain/discomfort. These researchers concluded that prodromal and acute symptoms of MI differed significantly according to race.

Physical Examination

[Objective 3]

Although the physical examination for patients being evaluated for possible ACS is often normal, performing a physical examination is important to identify potential precipitating causes of myocardial ischemia (e.g., such as uncontrolled hypertension, gastrointestinal [GI] bleeding), assess the hemodynamic impact of the ischemic event, and identify coexisting conditions (e.g., pulmonary disease, malignancies) that could influence treatment decisions.[10] Because the goals of reperfusion therapy are to give fibrinolytics within 30 minutes of patient arrival or provide percutaneous coronary intervention (PCI) within 90 minutes of arrival, the targeted history and focused physical examination must be performed quickly and efficiently. The physical examination should include the following:

- Measurement of vital signs (obtain blood pressure readings in both arms if dissection is suspected)
- Auscultation of breath sounds for crackles (i.e., rales)
- Auscultation of cardiac sounds for murmurs, gallops, and friction rubs
- Assessment for jugular venous distention (JVD), peripheral pulse deficits, and the presence of bruits
- Neurologic evaluation
- Identification of contraindications to antiplatelet or fibrinolytic therapy

PATIENT EVALUATION

Electrocardiogram Findings[12]

[Objective 7]

The sudden blockage of a coronary artery may result in ischemia, injury, or death of the area of the myocardium supplied by the affected artery. The area supplied by the blocked artery goes through a sequence of events that has been identified as "zones" of ischemia, injury, and infarction. Each zone is associated with characteristic ECG changes (Figure 5-9).

The positive electrode of each ECG lead is like an eye looking in at the heart. Therefore, the ECG changes associated with ischemia, injury, or infarction will not be seen in every lead. They appear in the leads "looking" at the area fed by the culprit (i.e., blocked) vessels; these are indicative changes. Indicative changes are significant when they are seen in two anatomically contiguous leads. Two leads are contiguous if they look at the same or adjacent areas of the heart or they are numerically consecutive chest leads. Contiguous leads are discussed in more detail later in this chapter.

ECG changes associated with ischemia, injury, or infarction will usually be associated with reciprocal (i.e., "mirror image") ECG changes in leads opposite (i.e., about 180 degrees away from) the leads that show the indicative change. For example, ST elevation in lead III (i.e., the indicative change) will show ST depression in lead aVL (i.e., the reciprocal change).

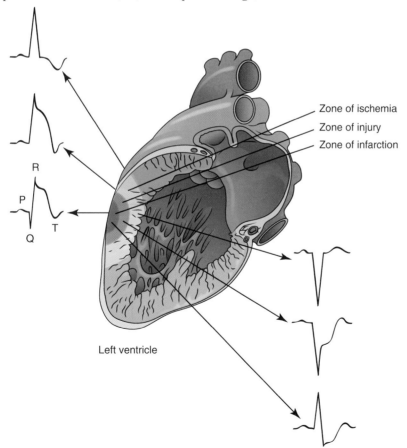

Left ventricle

Zone of ischemia
Zone of injury
Zone of infarction

Figure 5-9 Zones of ischemia, injury, and infarction showing indicative electrocardiogram (ECG) changes and reciprocal changes corresponding to each zone.

ACLS Pearl
The 12-lead ECG is an essential part of the diagnostic work-up of patients with a suspected ACS.

Myocardial Ischemia[12]

[Objective 7]

Ischemia affects the heart's cells responsible for contraction as well as those responsible for generation and conduction of electrical impulses. Because ischemia affects repolarization, its effects can be viewed on the ECG as brief changes in ST segments and T waves in the leads facing the affected area of the ventricle.

ST-segment depression of more than 0.5 mm in leads V_2 and V_3 and more than 1 mm in all other leads is suggestive of myocardial ischemia when it is viewed in two or more anatomically contiguous leads.[35-37] Negative (i.e., inverted) T waves may also be present (Figure 5-10).

These ECG changes and the chest pain or discomfort that accompanies myocardial ischemia usually resolve when the demand for oxygen is reduced to a level that can be supplied by the coronary artery or when increasing blood flow is supplied by dilating the coronary arteries with medications such as NTG. After the episode of chest discomfort is resolved, ST segments usually return to the baseline.

Myocardial Injury[12]

[Objective 7]

The term **myocardial injury** refers to myocardial tissue that has been cut off from or experienced a severe reduction in its blood and oxygen supply. Injured myocardium does not function normally because depolarization is incomplete and repolarization is impaired. Myocardial injury can be extensive enough to produce a decrease in pump function or electrical conductivity in the affected cells. However, the tissue is not yet dead and may be salvageable if the blocked vessel can be quickly opened, restoring blood flow and oxygen to the injured area.

ECG evidence of myocardial injury in progress can be seen on the ECG as ST elevation in the leads facing the affected area (see Figure 5-10). In leads opposite the affected area, ST depression (i.e., reciprocal changes) may be seen.

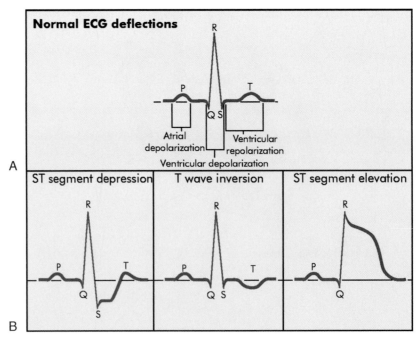

Figure 5-10 Electrocardiogram (ECG) changes and myocardial ischemia and injury. **A,** A normal ECG. **B,** ECG changes associated with ischemia include ST-segment depression and T wave inversion. ECG changes associated with myocardial injury include ST-segment elevation.

For men 40 years of age and older, the threshold value for abnormal J-point elevation is 2 mm in leads V_2 and V_3 and 1 mm in all other leads. For men younger than 40 years of age, the threshold value for abnormal J-point elevation in leads V_2 and V_3 is 2.5 mm. For women, the threshold value for abnormal J-point elevation is 1.5 mm in leads V_2 and V_3 and greater than 1 mm in all other leads. For men and women, the threshold for abnormal J-point elevation in V_3R and V_4R is 0.5 mm, except for males younger than 30 years of age, for whom 1 mm is more appropriate. For men and women, the threshold value for abnormal J-point elevation in leads V_7 through V_9 is 0.5 mm.[30-32]

Myocardial Infarction[12]
[Objective 7]
The recognition of infarction on the ECG relies on the detection of morphologic changes (i.e., changes in shape) of the QRS complex, the ST segment, and the T wave. These changes occur in relation to certain events during the infarction. The ECG changes described below appear in leads looking at the area fed by the blocked (culprit) vessel. These changes are referred to as the indicative changes of MI.

- *Hyperacute phase.* The first change you might notice on the ECG is the development of a tall T wave. Hyperacute T waves are sometimes called "tombstone" T waves and typically measure more than 50% of the preceding R wave. In addition to an increase in height, the T wave becomes more symmetric and may become pointed (Figure 5-11A). These changes are often not recorded on the ECG because they have typically resolved by the time the patient seeks medical assistance.
- *Early acute phase.* Over time, ST-segment elevation may develop, indicating myocardial injury is in progress (Figure 5-11B). ST-segment elevation may occur within the first hour or first few hours of infarction.
- *Later acute phase.* During the later acute phase of the infarction, you may see the presence of T wave inversion, suggesting the presence of ischemia (Figure 5-11C). In fact, T-wave inversion may precede the development of ST-segment elevation, or they may occur at the same time.
- *Fully evolved phase.* A few hours later, the ECG may show the first signs that tissue death has occurred. That evidence comes with the development of abnormal (i.e., pathologic) Q waves (Figure 5-11D). A Q wave that is 0.04 second or more wide (i.e., one small box or more) or is more than one third of the amplitude of the R wave in that lead is suggestive of infarction. An abnormal Q wave indicates the presence of dead myocardial tissue and, subsequently, a loss of electrical activity. These can appear within hours after blockage of a coronary artery, but they more commonly appear several hours or days after the onset of signs and symptoms of an acute MI. However, when combined with ST-segment or T wave changes, the presence of abnormal Q waves suggests an acute MI.
- *Healed phase.* In time, the T wave regains its normal shape and the ST segment returns to the baseline. However, the Q wave often remains as evidence that tissue death has occurred (Figures 5-11E and 5-12). When this pattern is seen, establishing the time of the infarction is impossible; it is only possible to recognize the presence of a previous MI. T-wave inversion, which may occur simultaneously with ST-segment elevation, suggests the presence of ischemia.

As the name NSTEMI implies, patients experiencing the condictinon do not show signs of myocardial injury (ST elevation) on their ECGs. The diagnosis of NSTEMI is made on the basis of the

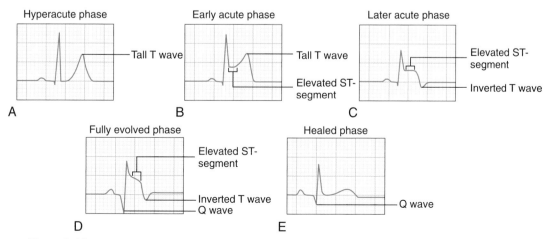

Figure 5-11 The evolving pattern of ST-elevation myocardial infarction (STEMI) on the electrocardiogram (ECG).

patient's signs and symptoms, history, and cardiac biomarker results that confirm the presence of an infarction. If cardiac biomarkers are not present in the patient's circulation on the basis of two or more samples collected at least 6 hours apart, the diagnosis is unstable angina.[10] If elevated biomarker levels are present, indicating evidence of myocardial necrosis, then the diagnosis is NSTEMI.

Localization of a Myocardial Infarction[12]
[Objective 8]
To localize the site of infarction, note which leads are displaying changes in the shape of the QRS complex, the ST segment, and the T wave, and consider which part of the heart those leads "see." When the infarction has been recognized and localized, an understanding of coronary artery anatomy makes it possible to predict which coronary artery is affected.

The left ventricle has been divided into regions where an MI may occur: septal, anterior, lateral, inferior, and inferobasal (i.e., posterior) (Figure 5-13). If an ECG shows changes in leads II, III, and aVF, then the inferior wall is affected. Because the inferior wall of the left ventricle is supplied by the right coronary artery in most people, it is reasonable to suppose that these ECG changes are due to partial or complete blockage of the right coronary artery. When indicative changes are seen in the leads viewing the septal, anterior, or lateral walls of the left ventricle (i.e., V_1-V_6, I, aVL), it is reasonable to suspect that these ECG changes are the result of partial or complete blockage of the left coronary artery (LCA).

One way to gauge the relative extent or size of an infarction is to evaluate how many leads are showing indicative changes. An ECG showing changes in only a few leads suggests a smaller infarction than one that produces changes in many leads. In general, the more proximal the blockage in the vessel, the larger the infarction and the greater the number of leads showing indicative changes. Table 5-3 summarizes the pattern in which coronary arteries most commonly supply the myocardium.

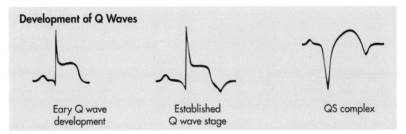

Development of Q Waves

Eary Q wave development   Established Q wave stage   QS complex

Figure 5-12 The development of abnormal Q waves provides evidence that tissue death has occurred.

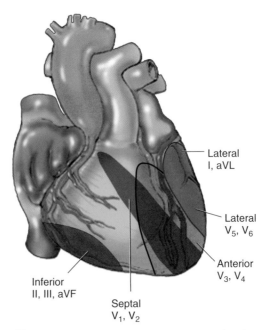

Lateral
I, aVL

Lateral
V_5, V_6

Anterior
V_3, V_4

Inferior
II, III, aVF

Septal
V_1, V_2

Figure 5-13 The surfaces of the heart. The posterior surface is not shown.

TABLE 5-3 Localization of a Myocardial Infarction

Location of MI	Indicative Changes (Leads Facing Affected Area)	Reciprocal Changes (Leads Opposite Affected Area)	Affected (Culprit) Coronary Artery
Anterior	V_3, V_4	V_7, V_8, V_9	Left coronary artery • LAD–diagonal branch
Anteroseptal	V_1, V_2, V_3, V_4	V_7, V_8, V_9	Left coronary artery • LAD–diagonal branch • LAD–septal branch
Anterolateral	I, aVL, V_3, V_4, V_5, V_6	II, III, aVF, V_7, V_8, V_9	Left coronary artery • LAD–diagonal branch and/or • Circumflex branch
Inferior	II, III, aVF	I, aVL	Right coronary artery (most common)–posterior descending branch or left coronary artery (circumflex branch)
Lateral	I, aVL, V_5, V_6	II, III, aVF	Left coronary artery • LAD–diagonal branch and/or • Circumflex branch Right coronary artery
Septum	V_1, V_2	V_7, V_8, V_9	Left coronary artery • LAD–septal branch
Inferobasal (posterior)	V_7, V_8, V_9	V_1, V_2, V_3	Right coronary or circumflex artery
Right ventricle	V_1R-V_6R	I, aVL	Right coronary artery • Proximal branches

TABLE 5-4 Localizing ECG Changes

I	Lateral	aVR	---------	V_1	Septum	V_4	Anterior
II	Inferior	aVL	Lateral	V_2	Septum	V_5	Lateral
III	Inferior	aVF	Inferior	V_3	Anterior	V_6	Lateral

> **ACLS Pearl**
>
> It is important to remember that some areas of the heart are not shown on a standard 12-lead ECG. It is also essential to recall that some infarctions do not show changes on the 12-lead ECG. Therefore, if infarct changes are seen on the 12-lead ECG, the greater the number of leads showing indicative changes, the larger the infarction. However, if the patient presents with signs and symptoms suggestive of an ACS and the 12-lead ECG does not show indicative changes, an MI cannot be ruled out solely on the basis of ECG findings.[12]

Indicative changes are significant when they are seen in two anatomically contiguous leads. Two leads are contiguous if they look at the same or adjacent areas of the heart or they are numerically consecutive chest leads. To better understand this, look at Table 5-4, which shows the area viewed by each lead of a standard 12-lead ECG. The colors in the table were added so that you can quickly see the areas of the heart viewed by the same leads. For example, leads II, III, and aVF appear the same color in the table because they view the inferior wall of the left ventricle. Because these leads "see" the same part of the heart, they are considered contiguous leads.

Leads I, aVL, V_5, and V_6 are contiguous because they all look at adjoining tissue in the lateral wall of the left ventricle. Leads V_1 and V_2 are contiguous because both leads look at the septum. Leads V_3 and V_4 are contiguous because both leads look at the anterior wall of the left ventricle.

TABLE 5-5	**Localizing ECG Changes with Right Chest Leads**							
I	Lateral	aVR	----------	V_1	Septum	V_4	Anterior	V_4R	Right ventricle
II	Inferior	aVL	Lateral	V_2	Septum	V_5	Lateral	V_5R	Right ventricle
III	Inferior	aVF	Inferior	V_3	Anterior	V_6	Lateral	V_6R	Right ventricle

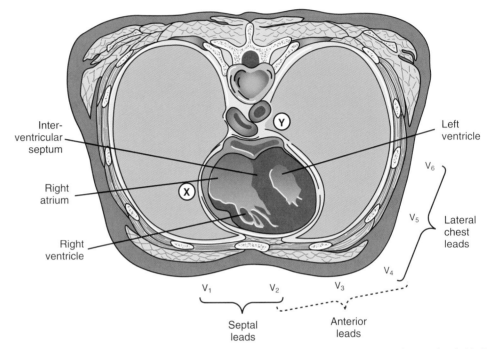

Figure 5-14 The areas of the heart as seen by the chest leads. Leads V_1, V_2, and V_3 are contiguous. Leads V_3, V_4, and V_5 are contiguous as well as V_4, V_5, and V_6. Note that neither the right ventricular wall *(X)* nor the inferobasal (posterior) surface of the left ventricle *(Y)* is well visualized by any of the usual six chest leads.

If right chest leads such as V_4R, V_5R, and V_6R are used, they are contiguous because they view the right ventricle (Table 5-5). Leads V_7, V_8, and V_9 are contiguous because they look at the inferobasal (i.e., posterior) surface of the heart.

Are leads II and V_2 contiguous? No, leads II and V_2 are not contiguous. Remember that two leads are contiguous if they look at the same or adjacent areas of the heart or they are numerically consecutive *chest* leads. Lead II is a *limb* lead that looks at the inferior wall, whereas V_2 is a *chest* lead that looks at the septum.

Now look at Figure 5-14. We have already determined that V_1 and V_2 are contiguous leads. Are leads V_2 and V_3 contiguous? Yes. V_2 and V_3 are right next to each other on the patient's chest. When each of these positive electrodes "looks in" at tissue, they see adjoining tissue in the heart as well. Leads V_3, V_4, and V_5 are contiguous, and so are V_4, V_5, and V_6.

Look at the 12-lead ECG in Figure 5-15. Note the leads in which ST-segment elevation is observed and those in which ST-segment depression is seen. You will find that ST-segment elevation is present in leads II, III, and aVF. Are these leads contiguous? Yes, leads II, III, and aVF view the inferior wall of the left ventricle. Which coronary artery is most likely affected? The right coronary artery (in the majority of the population). To recap, ST-segment elevation is seen in leads II, III, and aVF, which view the inferior wall of the left ventricle, an area supplied by the right coronary artery in most people. Reciprocal changes (ST-segment depression) are seen in leads I and aVL.

ACLS Pearl

The ECG is nondiagnostic in approximately 50% of patients with chest discomfort. A normal ECG does not rule out an acute MI, particularly during the early hours of a coronary artery occlusion.

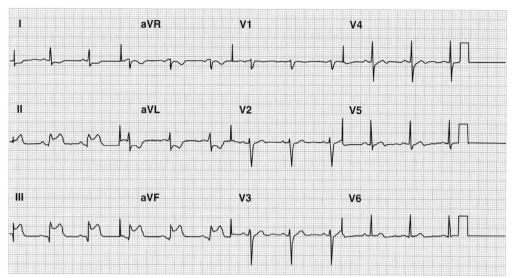

Figure 5-15 ST-segment elevation in leads II, III, and aVF suggests an inferior wall injury pattern. Reciprocal changes are seen in leads I and aVL.

Anterior Wall Infarctions[33]
[Objective 8]

Leads V_3 and V_4 face the anterior wall of the left ventricle. The left main coronary artery supplies the left anterior descending (LAD) artery and the circumflex artery. Blockage of the left main coronary artery (i.e., the "widow maker") often leads to cardiogenic shock and death without prompt reperfusion. Because the LAD artery supplies approximately 40% of the heart's blood and a critical section of the left ventricle, a blockage in this area can lead to complications such as left ventricular dysfunction, including heart failure and cardiogenic shock. Increased sympathetic nervous system activity is common with anterior MIs with resulting tachycardia, high blood pressure, or both. An anterior MI may cause dysrhythmias including premature ventricular complexes (PVCs), atrial flutter, or atrial fibrillation (AFib). Although some portions of the bundle branches are supplied by the right coronary artery (RCA), the LCA supplies most of the bundle branch tissue. Thus bundle branch blocks (BBBs) may occur if the LCA is blocked. This is why it is important to identify new left BBB.

Blockage of the midportion of the LAD artery results in an anterior infarction (Figure 5-16). However, an infarction involving the anterior wall is usually not localized only to this area. For example, proximal occlusion of the LAD may become an anteroseptal infarction if the septal branch is involved or an anterolateral infarction if the marginal branch is involved. If the blockage occurs proximal to both the septal and diagonal branches, an extensive anterior infarction (i.e., anteroseptal-lateral MI) will result. Reciprocal changes of injury in an anterior or anteroseptal MI appear in leads V_7, V_8, and V_9. Reciprocal changes with an anterior or anteroseptal MI do not appear in the limb leads because they are in a different plane. An example of an infarction involving the anterior wall is shown in Figure 5-17.

Inferior Wall Infarctions[33]
[Objective 8]

Leads II, III, and aVF view the inferior surface of the left ventricle. In most individuals, the inferior wall of the left ventricle is supplied by the posterior descending branch of the RCA ("right dominant system") (Figure 5-18). Blockage of the RCA proximal to the marginal branch will result in an inferior wall MI and RVI. Blockage of the RCA distal to the marginal branch will result in an inferior infarction, sparing the right ventricle. Reciprocal changes are observed in leads I and aVL.

In some individuals, the circumflex artery supplies the inferior wall through the posterior descending artery ("left dominant system") (Figure 5-19). Blockage of the posterior descending artery will result in an inferior infarction; however, a proximal occlusion of the circumflex may result in infarction in the lateral and posterior walls. ST elevation in lead II that is equal to or greater than the ST elevation in lead III has been used to predict the circumflex as the culprit artery with some success.[34,35]

Parasympathetic nervous system hyperactivity is common with inferior wall MIs, resulting in bradydysrhythmias. Conduction delays such as first-degree AV block and second-degree AV block type

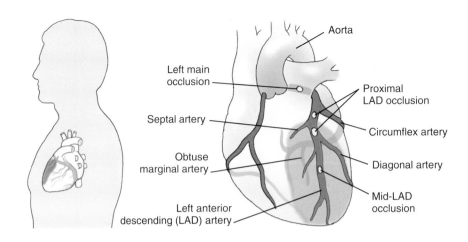

I Lateral	aVR	V$_1$ Septum	V$_4$ Anterior
II Inferior	aVL Lateral	V$_2$ Septum	V$_5$ Lateral
III Inferior	aVF Inferior	V$_3$ Anterior	V$_6$ Lateral

Figure 5-16 Anterior wall infarction. Occlusion of the midportion of the left anterior descending (LAD) artery results in an anterior infarction. Proximal occlusion of the LAD may become an anteroseptal infarction if the septal branch is involved or an anterolateral infarction if the marginal branch is involved. If the occlusion occurs proximal to both the septal and diagonal branches, an extensive anterior infarction will result.

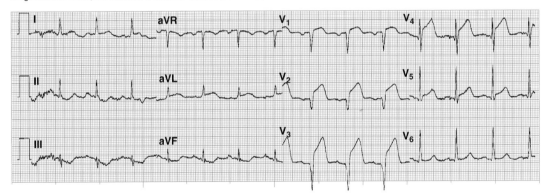

Figure 5-17 Anteroseptal infarction.

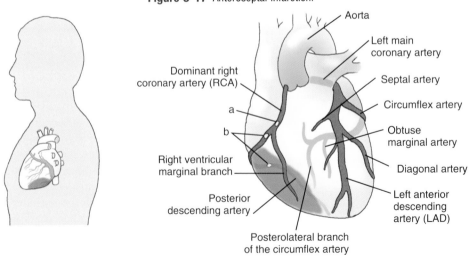

Figure 5-18 Inferior wall infarction. Coronary anatomy shows a dominant right coronary artery (RCA). A blockage at point *a* results in an inferior infarction and right ventricular infarction. A blockage at point *b* involves only the inferior wall, sparing the right ventricle.

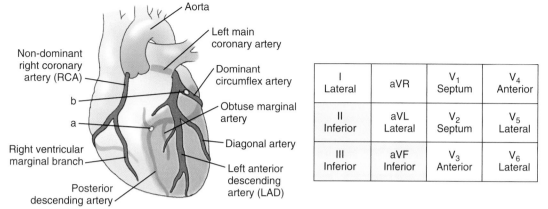

I Lateral	aVR	V₁ Septum	V₄ Anterior
II Inferior	aVL Lateral	V₂ Septum	V₅ Lateral
III Inferior	aVF Inferior	V₃ Anterior	V₆ Lateral

Figure 5-19 Inferior wall infarction. Coronary anatomy shows a dominant circumflex artery. A blockage at point *a* results in an inferior infarction. A blockage at *b* may result in a lateral and inferobasal infarction.

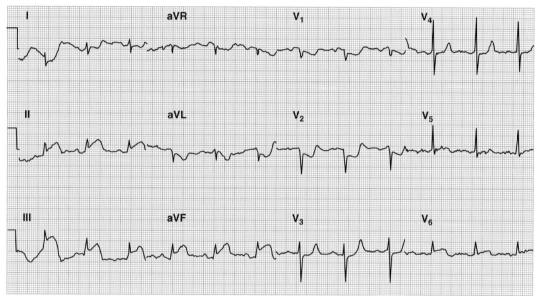

Figure 5-20 Acute inferior wall infarction. Note the ST-segment elevation in leads II, III, and aVF and the reciprocal ST depression in leads I and aVL. Abnormal Q waves are also present in leads II, III, and aVF.

I are common and usually transient. An example of an infarction involving the inferior wall is shown in Figure 5-20.

Lateral Wall Infarctions[33]
[**Objective 8**]

Leads I, aVL, V₅, and V₆ view the lateral wall of the left ventricle. The lateral wall of the left ventricle may be supplied by the circumflex artery, the LAD artery, or a branch of the RCA (Figure 5-21).

Lateral wall infarctions often occur as extensions of anterior or inferior infarctions. Isolated lateral wall infarctions usually involve occlusion of the circumflex artery and are frequently missed. More commonly, the lateral wall is involved with proximal occlusion of the LAD artery (i.e., anterolateral MI) or a branch of the RCA (i.e., inferolateral MI). Blockage of the marginal branches of the circumflex artery may cause a posterolateral MI. An example of an infarction involving the lateral wall is shown in Figure 5-22.

Septal Infarctions[33]
[**Objective 8**]

Leads V₁ and V₂ face the septal area of the left ventricle. The septum, which contains the bundle of His and bundle branches, is normally supplied by the LAD artery (Figure 5-23). A blockage in this area may result in right BBB, left BBB (more common), second-degree AV block type II, and third-degree AV block.

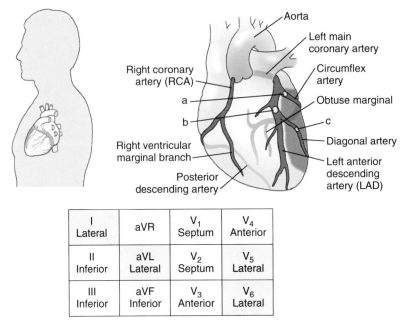

I Lateral	aVR	V$_1$ Septum	V$_4$ Anterior
II Inferior	aVL Lateral	V$_2$ Septum	V$_5$ Lateral
III Inferior	aVF Inferior	V$_3$ Anterior	V$_6$ Lateral

Figure 5-21 Lateral wall infarction. Coronary artery anatomy shows blockage of the circumflex artery at point *a*, blockage of the proximal left anterior descending artery at point *b*, and blockage of the diagonal artery at point *c*.

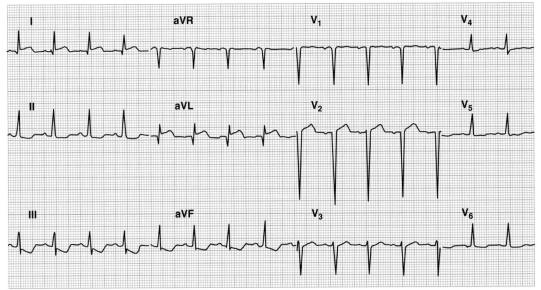

Figure 5-22 Lateral wall infarction. Lead I shows a small Q wave with ST-segment elevation. A larger Q wave with ST-segment elevation can be seen in lead aVL. This patient had an anterior non-ST-elevation infarction 4 days earlier with ST-segment elevation and T wave inversion in leads V$_2$ through V$_6$. A coronary arteriogram at that time showed a blocked left anterior descending artery distal to its first large septal perforator. The ST-segment elevation evolved and the T waves in all of the chest leads had become upright the day before this tracing was recorded. The patient then had another episode of chest pain associated with the appearance of signs of acute lateral infarction as shown in this tracing. A repeat coronary arteriogram showed new blockage of the obtuse marginal branch of the circumflex artery.

If the site of infarction is limited to the septum, ECG changes are seen in V$_1$ and V$_2$. If the entire anterior wall is involved, ECG changes will be visible in V$_1$, V$_2$, V$_3$, and V$_4$. An example of a septal infarction is shown in Figure 5-24.

Inferobasal Wall Infarctions[33]
[Objective 8]
Posterior wall MIs usually occur in conjunction with an inferior or lateral infarction. Current expert opinion recommends the term *inferobasal wall* be used instead of posterior wall.[13] The inferobasal wall of the left ventricle is supplied by the circumflex coronary artery in most patients; however, in some

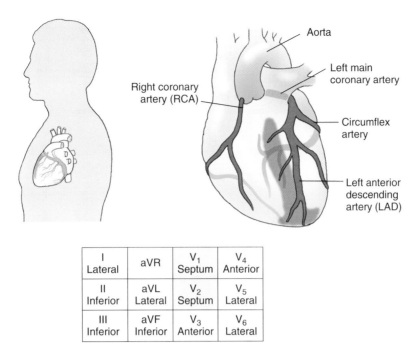

I Lateral	aVR	V₁ Septum	V₄ Anterior
II Inferior	aVL Lateral	V₂ Septum	V₅ Lateral
III Inferior	aVF Inferior	V₃ Anterior	V₆ Lateral

Figure 5-23 Septal infarction.

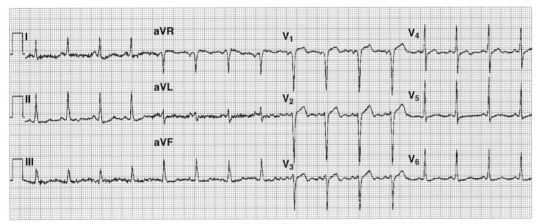

Figure 5-24 Septal infarction. Poor R wave progression.

patients it is supplied by the RCA (Figure 5-25). If the inferobasal wall is supplied by the right coronary artery, complications may include dysrhythmias involving the sinoatrial (SA) node, AV node, and bundle of His.

Because no leads of a standard 12-lead ECG directly view the inferobasal wall of the left ventricle, additional chest leads should be used to view the heart's posterior surface. Indicative changes of an inferobasal infarction include ST elevation in these leads.

If placement of posterior chest leads is not feasible, changes in the opposite (anterior) wall of the heart can be viewed as reciprocal changes. An inferobasal MI usually produces tall R waves and ST-segment depression in leads V_1, V_2, and to a lesser extent in lead V_3. To assist with the recognition of ECG changes suggesting an inferobasal MI, the "mirror test" is helpful. Flip over the ECG to the blank side and turn it upside down. When the tracing is then held up to the light, the tall R waves become deep Q waves and ST depression becomes ST elevation; these are the "classic" indicative changes associated with MI (Figure 5-26). An example of an inferobasal infarction is shown in Figure 5-27.

ACLS Pearl

If a patient presents with a possible ACS and the only ST-segment change seen on a standard 12-lead ECG is depression (particularly in leads V_1-V_4), strongly consider obtaining posterior chest leads V_7-V_9 to assess for a possible inferobasal (i.e., posterior) infarction.

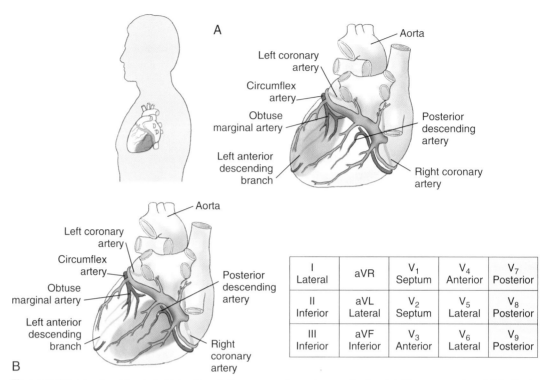

I Lateral	aVR	V$_1$ Septum	V$_4$ Anterior	V$_7$ Posterior
II Inferior	aVL Lateral	V$_2$ Septum	V$_5$ Lateral	V$_8$ Posterior
III Inferior	aVF Inferior	V$_3$ Anterior	V$_6$ Lateral	V$_9$ Posterior

Figure 5-25 Inferobasal (posterior) infarction. **A,** Coronary anatomy shows a dominant right coronary artery (RCA). Blockage of the RCA commonly results in an inferior and inferobasal infarction. **B,** Coronary anatomy shows a dominant circumflex artery. Blockage of a marginal branch is the cause of most isolated inferobasal infarctions.

Figure 5-26 Application of the mirror test. This test is most helpful in assessing a patient with an acute inferior infarction, in whom you suspect an acute inferobasal infarction. **A,** Schematic 12-lead electrocardiogram (ECG) with indicative changes of inferior infarction in lead III. Note the tall R wave in lead V$_1$ and the ST-segment depression in leads V$_1$, V$_2$, and V$_3$. **B,** The tracing in A is now flipped over. Looking through the paper (as it is held up to the light), you now see Q waves and ST-segment elevation in leads V$_1$, V$_2$, and V$_3$. This is a positive mirror test and suggests that the lead changes observed in A may reflect associated acute inferobasal infarction.

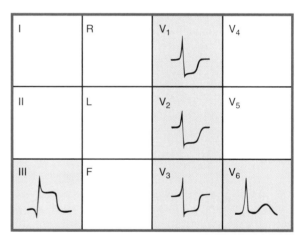

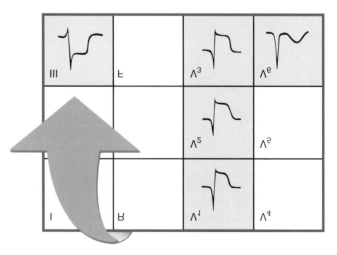

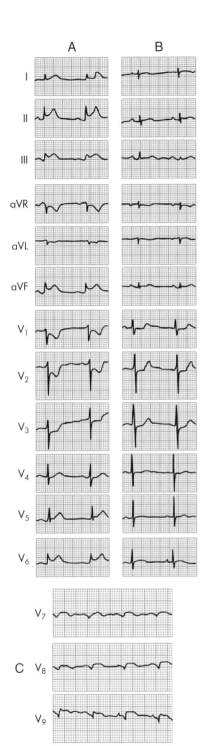

Figure 5-27 Evolutionary changes in inferior and inferobasal myocardial infarction (MI). **A,** Acute inferior and apical injury. **B,** At 24 hours. Note the tall R wave in lead V_1 that is not present in A, suggesting inferobasal MI. **C,** (V_7 through V_9) Inferobasal infarction confirmed.

Right Ventricular Infarctions[12]
[Objective 9]

RVI should be suspected when ECG changes suggesting an inferior infarction (i.e., ST elevation in leads II, III, and/or aVF) are observed. The right ventricle is supplied by the right ventricular marginal branch of the RCA (Figure 5-28). A blockage of the right ventricular marginal branch results in an isolated RVI. Blockage of the RCA proximal to the right ventricular marginal branch results in an inferior and right ventricular infarction.

To view the right ventricle, right chest leads are used. These leads then "look" directly at the right ventricle, and they can show the ST elevation created by the infarction. If time does not permit the acquisition of all six right-sided chest leads, the lead of choice is V_4R. An example of an infarction involving the right ventricle is shown in Figure 5-29.

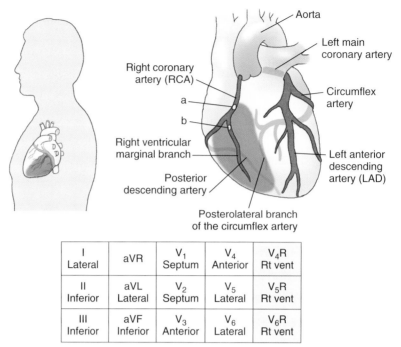

I Lateral	aVR	V$_1$ Septum	V$_4$ Anterior	V$_4$R Rt vent
II Inferior	aVL Lateral	V$_2$ Septum	V$_5$ Lateral	V$_5$R Rt vent
III Inferior	aVF Inferior	V$_3$ Anterior	V$_6$ Lateral	V$_6$R Rt vent

Figure 5-28 Right ventricular infarction (RVI). At *a*, blockage of the right coronary artery proximal to the right ventricular marginal branch results in an inferior infarction and RVI. At *b*, blockage of the right ventricular marginal branch results in an isolated RVI.

In addition to ECG evidence, certain clinical signs also support the suspicion of RVI. The clinical evidence of RVI involves three main areas: hypotension (of varying degrees), JVD, and clear breath sounds. However, this triad of signs is estimated to be present in only 10% to 15% of patients with RVI.[36]

In the setting of RVI, the right ventricle may lose some of its ability to pump blood into the pulmonary circuit. When this happens, blood stalls in the right ventricle and may begin to back up. (Technically, the blood does not back up; rather the venous return exceeds the ventricular output and blood begins to build up). This stalling and backing up produce the hypotension, JVD, and absence of pulmonary edema (i.e., clear lung sounds) considered the clinical triad of RVI. As blood backs up from the right ventricle, the jugular veins become enlarged. Hypotension results from the decrease in blood volume moving into the lungs and left ventricle. The left ventricle can only pump as much blood as it receives; if less blood reaches the left ventricle, less blood is pumped into the systemic circulation. The net effect of this reduction in left ventricular output is a decrease in blood pressure.

Complications associated with RVI include hypotension, cardiogenic shock, AV blocks, atrial flutter or fibrillation, and premature atrial complexes. AV blocks are particularly common, and they occur in about half of all patients with RVI.

Cardiac Biomarkers

As myocardial cells die, intracellular substances pass through broken cell membranes and leak substances into the bloodstream. The presence of these substances in the blood can subsequently be measured by means of blood tests to verify the presence of an infarction. These substances, which are called **cardiac biomarkers**, **serum cardiac markers**, **serum biomarkers**, or **inflammatory markers**, include creatine kinase (CK), creatine kinase myocardial band (CK-MB), myoglobin, troponin I (TnI), and troponin T (TnT).

Cardiac biomarkers are useful for confirming the diagnosis of MI when patients present without ST-segment elevation on their ECG, when the diagnosis may be unclear, and to distinguish patients with unstable angina from those with NSTEMI. Because there is no tissue death, there is no cardiac biomarker release in patients with stable or unstable angina. Cardiac biomarkers are also useful for confirming the diagnosis of MI for patients with STEMI. Because the ranges of normal biomarker levels vary among laboratories, the ACC/AHA guidelines require that any level that can be interpreted as positive for infarction must be elevated by more than 99% compared with a normal reference population.[10]

Example of an acute inferior wall and right ventricular wall MI. Shows ST elevation in leads II, III, aVF and reciprocal changes (ST depression) in anterior and lateral leads.

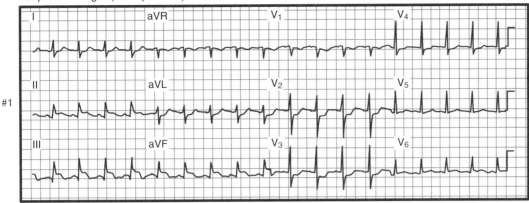

Reciprocal changes seen in V_1, V_2, V_3, V_4, I, and aVL, which provides a clue as to the extent of the MI. Angiographic changes associated with an occlusion of the RCA.
These findings can range from:
  - Proximal occlusion (near origin of RCA), which will produce inferior MI, posterior MI, and RVI
  - Middle RCA occlusion, which will produce posterior and inferior MI
A - Distal RCA occlusion, which will produce inferior wall MI

Example of an acute right ventricular MI in right precordial leads.

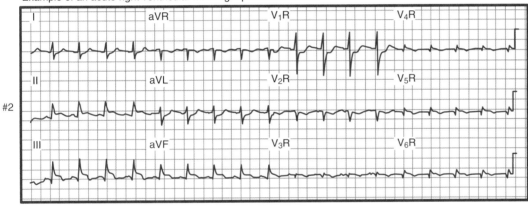

ECG shows ST elevation in right chest leads (V_3R to V_6R) indicating RV wall injury/infarct.
    Note limb leads are identical in both ECGs.

B   **These two 12-lead ECGs are from the same patient with RVI**

Figure 5-29 A, Example of an acute inferior/right ventricular (RV) wall myocardial infarction (MI) with a standard 12-lead electrocardiogram (ECG). **B,** Example of an acute RV wall MI with a right-sided 12-lead ECG. Both 12-lead ECGs are taken from the same patient. RCA, right coronary artery.

The cardiac-specific troponins (i.e., TnI and TnT) are the biomarkers of choice because they are both highly sensitive and specific for myocardial necrosis, although their elevation may be delayed for up to 8 to 12 hours after onset of patient symptoms. Troponin levels remain elevated after myocardial necrosis (i.e., 4 to 7 days for TnI, 10 to 14 days for TnT). The use of cardiac troponins is preferred for patients with possible ACS and cocaine use because troponins are considered the most sensitive and specific markers for the diagnosis of cocaine-associated MI.[6,37]

CK-MB is less sensitive and less specific than the cardiac troponins and may show elevated levels in healthy individuals and in processes involving skeletal muscle damage. Myoglobin is released by necrotic myocardium more rapidly than CK-MB and the cardiac troponins and may be detected as early as 2 hours after MI. However, myoglobin is found in both cardiac and skeletal muscle, thus it is not specific to cardiac tissue (cannot distinguish cardiac muscle injury from skeletal muscle injury).

Ischemia-modified albumin (IMA) has been recognized as a marker of inflammation and myocardial ischemia but has been less well studied than those previously mentioned. Studies have shown that measurement of beta-type natriuretic peptide (BNP), which is expressed after ventricular wall stress and myocardial hypoxia, has potential as an independent prognostic indicator in ACSs.

Troponin levels should be obtained at the patient's initial presentation to rule out infarction and again between 6 and 12 hours after symptom onset. If the ST segments are elevated and elevated cardiac biomarkers are present, the diagnosis is STEMI. If the ST segments are not elevated and cardiac biomarkers are not present in the patient's circulation on the basis of two or more samples collected at least 6 hours apart, the diagnosis is unstable angina.[10] If ST elevation is not present but biomarker levels are elevated, the diagnosis is NSTEMI. Treatment decisions for patients with an ACS should not be delayed pending cardiac biomarker test results.

Imaging Studies

A portable chest radiograph should be obtained for patients with a suspected ACS within 30 minutes of patient presentation. Echocardiography is useful for the evaluation of left and right ventricular function, including assessment of myocardial thickness, thickening, and motion at rest, and for the diagnosis of mechanical complications. Other imaging studies such as transesophageal echocardiography, a contrast-enhanced computed tomography scan of the chest, or magnetic resonance imaging are mainly useful for excluding some of the nonischemic causes of acute chest pain such as valvular heart disease, aortic dissection, pulmonary embolism, myocarditis, and cardiomyopathy.

INITIAL MANAGEMENT OF ACUTE CORONARY SYNDROMES

[Objectives 10, 11, 12]
The primary goals of therapy for patients with ACS include the following[32]:
- Reduce the amount of myocardial necrosis that occurs in patients with MI, preserving left ventricular function and preventing heart failure
- Prevent major adverse cardiac events, such as death, nonfatal MI, and the need for urgent revascularization
- Treat acute, life-threatening complications of ACS, such as ventricular fibrillation (VF)/pulseless VT, symptomatic bradycardias, unstable tachycardias, pulmonary edema, cardiogenic shock, and mechanical complications of acute MI

Although only a physician can make a final diagnosis of an ACS, as an advanced cardiac life support (ACLS) provider you must take responsibility for recognizing an ACS and take steps to speed the process of data collection, physician evaluation, and, when appropriate, reperfusion therapy. The reality of this expectation is that nurses, paramedics, and all other cardiac care professionals must be able to develop a "working diagnosis" of infarction. Although this working diagnosis must be confirmed by a physician before definitive treatment may begin, it has been clearly demonstrated that early recognition of infarction by a nonphysician can greatly reduce the time to treatment.[12]

General Measures

The initial management of all ACSs is generally the same, and management of the patient must be done efficiently. The patient experiencing ischemic chest discomfort should be placed on bedrest in a position of comfort while symptoms are present and may be moved to a chair after symptoms have subsided. In the prehospital setting, make sure that the patient does not walk up or down stairs or to the stretcher.

Assess the patient's vital signs and determine oxygen saturation levels. Supplemental oxygen is warranted if the patient is cyanotic, having difficulty breathing, having obvious signs of heart failure or shock, or if his or her oxygen saturation level declines to less than 94%.[32] Establish IV access and obtain a targeted history and physical examination. This can be done at the same time as other procedures. Consider the possibility of other conditions that mimic acute MI, such as aortic dissection, acute pericarditis, acute myocarditis, and pulmonary embolism. Assess and document the degree of the patient's pain or discomfort using a 0-to-10 scale.

Continuous ECG monitoring is essential during the prehospital, emergency department, and early hospital phases of care because sudden, unexpected VF is the major preventable cause of death during

BOX 5-7 **Recommended use of continuous ST-segment monitoring[38]**

The use of continuous ST-segment monitoring is recommended in the following situations:
- Patients with ACSs: monitor for a minimum of 24 hours and until the patient remains event-free for 12 to 24 hours
- Patients who present to the emergency department or observational unit with chest pain or angina-equivalent symptoms: monitor for 8 to 12 hours in combination with serum biomarkers to assess for new, transient, or resolving ischemia
- Patients who have undergone nonurgent PCI with suboptimal angiographic results: monitor immediately after the procedure and continue for 24 hours or longer if ST events occur
- Patients with the potential for vasospasm (e.g., Prinzmetal's angina, cocaine); monitor until therapy has been started and the patient has been ST-event–free for 12 to 24 hours

this early period.[10]Continuous 12-lead ST-segment monitoring can be helpful for detecting ST-segment changes that confirm the diagnosis of an ACS as well as for detecting silent or unrecognized myocardial ischemia. The microprocessor-controlled device used for continuous 12-lead monitoring is fully programmable. An initial 12-lead ECG is obtained and considered the "pretrigger" ECG. A new 12-lead ECG is then automatically obtained about every 20 seconds and the ST segments analyzed. Depending on programming parameters, an alarm sounds when subsequent ST-segment changes of 2 mm in a single lead or 1 mm in two leads (as compared by the machine with the pretrigger ECG) are present. Recommendations for the use of continuous ST-segment monitoring appear in Box 5-7.

ACLS Pearl

Monitoring of ST-segment changes can provide useful diagnostic and predictive information in the patient experiencing an ACS.

Obtaining and reviewing a 12-lead ECG is part of the initial assessment of the patient presenting with ischemic chest discomfort, and it is important when determining an appropriate treatment plan. Obtain the first 12-lead ECG with 10 minutes of patient contact. Obtain a repeat 12-lead ECG with each set of vital signs, when the patient's symptoms change, and as often as necessary.

After the 12-lead has been obtained, it should be reviewed carefully. Look at each lead for the presence of ST-segment displacement (i.e., elevation or depression). Patients experiencing a STEMI are considered the most emergent, followed by those with unstable angina (UA)/NSTEMI, and then persons experiencing chest pain of probable cardiac origin.

If ST-segment elevation is present, note its elevation in millimeters. Examine the T waves for any changes in orientation, shape, and size. Examine each lead for the presence of a Q wave. If a Q wave is present, measure its duration. Assess the areas of ischemia or injury by assessing lead groupings. Remember that ECG evidence must be found in at least two contiguous leads. On the basis of the 12-lead ECG findings, categorize the patient into one of three groups:

1. *ST-segment elevation.* ST elevation in two or more contiguous leads or new-onset left BBB suggests myocardial injury. This patient is classified as having a STEMI. Patients with obvious ST elevation in leads II, III, and/or aVF should also be evaluated for a possible right ventricular infarction. Patients with ST elevation in two or more contiguous leads should be evaluated for immediate reperfusion therapy.
2. *ST-segment depression.* ST depression or transient ST-segment/T wave changes that occur with pain or discomfort suggest myocardial ischemia. This patient is classified as having high-risk UA/NSTEMI. Patients with obvious ST depression in leads V_1 and V_2 should be evaluated for possible posterior MI. The patient with high-risk UA/NSTEMI should be admitted to a monitored bed for further evaluation.
3. *Normal* **or** *nondiagnostic ECG.* A normal ECG or nonspecific ST- and T wave changes are nondiagnostic and should prompt consideration for further evaluation. Consider admission of the patient with signs and symptoms suggesting an ACS and a nondiagnostic ECG to the emergency department chest pain unit or to an appropriate bed. Obtain cardiac biomarkers at the patient's initial presentation and again between 6 and 12 hours after symptom onset.

Obtaining serial ECGs at 5- to 10-minute intervals or continuous monitoring of the ST segment should be performed to detect the potential development of ST elevation if the initial ECG is not diagnostic of STEMI but the patient remains symptomatic and there is a high clinical suspicion of STEMI. If there is no evidence of ischemia or infarction and clinical suspicion is low, the patient is usually discharged with follow-up instructions.

> **ACLS Pearl**
> Distinguishing between NSTEMI and STEMI is valuable because the prognosis and treatment for these conditions differ.

Treatment options for UA/NSTEMI include conservative management (which includes analgesic, anti-ischemic, antiplatelet, and anticoagulant therapy), early intervention with PCI, or surgical revascularization (i.e., angioplasty, stenting, or bypass surgery). For STEMI, fibrinolytic therapy is an additional option but is generally not recommended for patients presenting between 12 and 24 hours after symptom onset unless persistent ischemic pain is present with continuing ST elevation. The AHA recommendations for the initial treatment of ACS are summarized in Figure 5-30.

Analgesic and Anti-ischemic Therapy

Relief of cardiac-related discomfort is a priority for the management of a patient experiencing an ACS and often requires a combination of oxygen, nitroglycerin, and narcotic analgesics. Relief of pain decreases anxiety, myocardial oxygen demand, and the risk of dysrhythmias.

Nitroglycerin

NTG relaxes smooth muscle, thereby dilating peripheral arteries and veins. This causes a pooling of venous blood and decreased venous return to the heart, which decreases preload. NTG also dilates normal and atherosclerotic epicardial coronary arteries,[10] and reduces left ventricular systolic wall tension, which decreases afterload.

Before giving NTG, assess the degree of the patient's pain or discomfort using a 0-to-10 scale. Also record the pain's duration, time of onset, the activity that was being done, and the pain quality. Reassess and document the patient's vital signs and level of discomfort after each dose. Common adverse effects of NTG administration include headache, flushing, tachycardia, dizziness, and orthostatic hypotension. Hypotension usually responds to supine positioning and administration of IV fluids.

Make sure that the patient has not used a phosphodiesterase inhibitor such as sildenafil (e.g., Viagra) within 24 hours or tadalafil (e.g., Cialis) within 48 hours before NTG administration. The combination of a phosphodiesterase inhibitor and nitrates may result in severe hypotension. NTG should be avoided in inferior wall MI with a possible associated RVI. Consider the presence of RVI if the patient with an inferior wall MI becomes hypotensive after nitrate administration.

Morphine

Morphine sulfate is a potent narcotic analgesic and anxiolytic. It causes venodilation and can lower heart rate (through increased vagal tone) and systolic blood pressure, reducing myocardial oxygen demand. The adverse effects of morphine administration include nausea and vomiting, which occurr in about 20% of patients, as well as respiratory depression. Hypotension may occur, particularly in patients who are volume depleted or have received vasodilators. Supine positioning or IV boluses of normal saline are used to restore blood pressure. Respiratory or circulatory depression may require administration of a narcotic antagonist. Other narcotics may be considered for patients allergic to morphine.

Morphine is the preferred analgesic for patients with STEMI who experience persistent chest discomfort unresponsive to nitrates.[32] A study published in the American Heart Journal in 2005 reviewed the use of morphine in patients with non-ST elevation ACS and demonstrated an increase in mortality among patients who received morphine, either alone or in combination with NTG.[39] Because these findings raise a safety concern, the strength of the recommendation for the use of morphine for uncontrolled ischemic chest discomfort was downgraded in the 2007 ACC/AHA UA/NSTEMI guidelines from a Class I to a Class IIa recommendation for non-ST elevation ACS.[10,32]

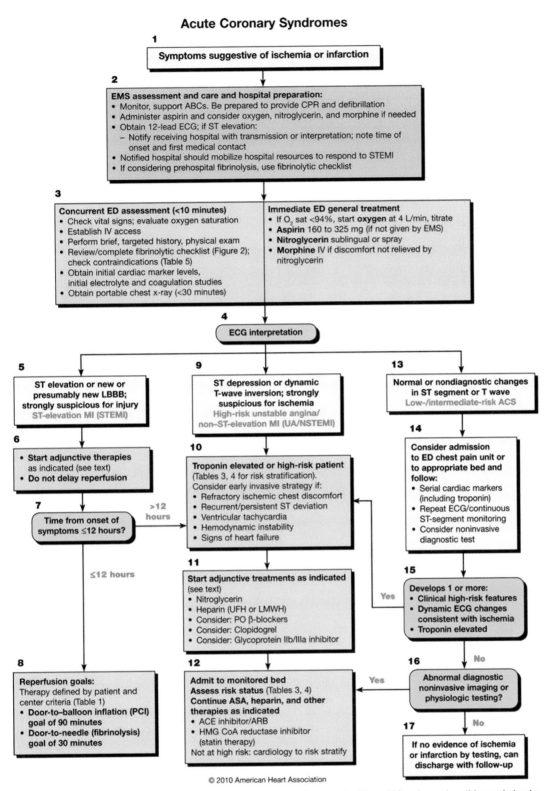

Figure 5-30 The American Heart Association acute coronary syndromes algorithm. ABCs, airway, breathing and circulation; ACE, angiotensin-converting enzyme; ACS, acute coronary syndrome; ARB, angiotensin receptor blocker; ASA, aspirin; CPR, cardiopulmonary resuscitation;, ECG, electrocardiogram; ED, emergency department; EMS, Emergency Medical Services; HMG CoA, hydroxymethylglutaryl coenzyme A; LMWH, low-molecular-weight heparins; PCI, percutaneous coronary intervention; PO, oral; UFH, unfractionated heparin.

Before giving morphine, assess the degree of the patient's pain or discomfort using a 0-to-10 scale. Also determine the pain's duration, time of onset, the activity that was being done, and the pain quality. Reassess and document the patient's vital signs and level of discomfort after each morphine dose.

> **ACLS Pearl**
>
> Pain increases sympathetic response, increasing heart rate, systemic vascular resistance, and blood pressure, which, in turn, increases myocardial oxygen consumption. This is why pain relief is a priority for the management of the patient with an ACS. When treating a patient with an ACS, it is not enough to simply reduce the patient's degree of pain or discomfort. The goal is to ensure that the patient is free of pain, while closely monitoring his or her vital signs.

> **YOU SHOULD KNOW**
>
> Many healthcare professionals are using fentanyl (i.e., Sublimaze) for pain relief as well as vasodilation in place of morphine for patients experiencing an ACS. Fentanyl is a lipid-soluble synthetic opioid that has minimal cardiovascular effects, and a more rapid onset and shorter duration of action than morphine. Unlike morphine, which is dosed in milligrams, fentanyl is dosed in micrograms. Typically, an initial dose of 50 to 100 mcg (1 mcg/kg) is given slowly IV.[42] Although protocols for administration vary, a generally accepted repeat dose is half the initial dose every 5 to 10 minutes, titrated to effect. The total maximum dose is 3 mcg/kg. The adverse effects of fentanyl are similar to those of morphine.

Beta-Blockers

Inhibition of beta$_1$-adrenergic receptor sites reduces myocardial contractility, SA node rate, and AV node conduction velocity, decreasing cardiac work and reducing myocardial oxygen demand. The choice of beta-blocker for an individual patient is based primarily on how the body absorbs, distributes, breaks down, and eliminates the drug; the drug's adverse effects; and physician familiarity. It is essential to closely monitor the patient's heart rate, blood pressure, pulmonary status, and ECG rhythm during treatment with a beta-blocker. Simultaneous IV administration with IV calcium channel blockers (e.g., verapamil, diltrazem) can cause severe hypotension.

The Clopidogrel and Metoprolol in Myocardial Infarction Trial/Second Chinese Cardiac Study (COMMIT/CCS-2) demonstrated that beta-blocker use increased the risk of cardiogenic shock, heart failure, heart block, and symptomatic bradycardia–with most of these complications occurring on the first day of the patient's infarction.[40] Because the results of the COMMIT-CCS 2 trial raised questions about the safety of early use of IV beta-blockers (particularly in high-risk populations), the ACC/AHA STEMI guideline recommendations were revised and are shown in Table 5-6.

Angiotensin-Converting Enzyme Inhibitors

Angiotensin-converting enzyme (ACE) inhibitors produce vasodilation by blocking the conversion of angiotensin I into angiotensin II. Because angiotensin is a potent vasoconstrictor, limiting its production decreases peripheral vascular resistance, reducing the pressure that the heart must pump against and decreasing the myocardial workload. ACE inhibitors also increase renal blood flow, which helps rid the body of excess sodium and fluid accumulation. ACE inhibitors have been shown to be most beneficial for patients with anterior infarction, pulmonary congestion, or left ventricular ejection fraction less than 40%. A summary of analgesic and anti-ischemic therapy in ACSs is shown in Table 5-6.

> **Keeping It Simple**
>
> **MONA**
>
> MONA is a memory aid that may be used to recall medications used for the management of ACSs (although not in the order they are given).
> **M** = Morphine
> **O** = Oxygen (if indicated)
> **N** = Nitroglycerin
> **A** = Aspirin

TABLE 5-6 Analgesic and Anti-ischemic Therapy in Acute Coronary Syndromes

Analgesic and Anti-ischemic Therapy	UA/NSTEMI	STEMI	Comments
Medication	**Indications and Dose**	**Indications and Dose**	
Nitroglycerin (NTG) Class: organic nitrate, vasodilator, antianginal Nitrostat, Nitrobid (Sublingual forms); Tridil (IV)	NTG sublingual tablets or spray may be given at 5-minute intervals to a maximum of three doses. Intravenous NTG can benefit patients whose symptoms are not relieved with three sublingual NTG tablets taken 5 minutes apart.[10]	Patients with ongoing ischemic discomfort should receive sublingual NTG (0.4 mg) every 5 minutes for a total of three doses, after which an assessment should be made about the need for IV NTG.[15]	Establish an IV before giving sublingual NTG. Nitrates should not be administered to patients with a systolic BP less than 90 mm Hg or 30 mm Hg or more below baseline, severe bradycardia (slower than 50 beats/min), or tachycardia in the absence of heart failure (faster than 100 beats/min), or suspected right ventricular infarction.[15,32]
Morphine sulfate Class: narcotic (opioid) analgesic	Morphine sulfate (1 to 5 mg IV) is reasonable for patients whose symptoms are not relieved despite NTG (e.g., after three serial sublingual NTG tablets) or whose symptoms recur despite adequate anti-ischemic therapy.[10]	Morphine sulfate (2 to 4 mg IV with increments of 2 to 8 mg IV repeated at 5- to 15-minute intervals) is the analgesic of choice for patients with STEMI who experience persistent chest discomfort unresponsive to nitrates.[15,32]	Ensure that a narcotic antagonist and airway equipment is readily available before administration.
Beta-blockers atenolol (Tenormin); metoprolol (Lopressor); propranolol (Inderal)	Oral beta-blockers should be started within the first 24 hours after hospitalization in the absence of contraindications to beta blockade (signs of heart failure, evidence of a low output state [such as oliguria], increased risk for cardiogenic shock, or other relative contraindications to beta blockade [PR interval greater than 0.24 seconds, second- or third-degree heart block, active asthma, or reactive airway disease]).[10,32] IV administration may be warranted at the time of presentation to patients who have severe hypertension or tachydysrhythmias in the setting of ACS and who do not have contraindications to beta blockade.[32]	Same as for UA/NSTEMI	Risk factors for cardiogenic shock (the greater the number of risk factors present, the higher the risk of developing cardiogenic shock) are age greater than 70 years, systolic blood pressure less than 120 mm Hg, sinus tachycardia greater than 110 beats/min or heart rate less than 60 beats/min, and increased time since onset of symptoms of STEMI.[43]

Continued

TABLE 5-6	Analgesic and Anti-ischemic Therapy in Acute Coronary Syndromes—cont'd		
Analgesic and Anti-ischemic Therapy	UA/NSTEMI	STEMI	Comments
Angiotensin-converting enzyme (ACE) inhibitors captopril (Capoten); enalapril (Vasotec); lisinopril (Prinivil, Zestril); ramipril (Altace)	There is insufficient evidence to support the routine administration of ACE inhibitors and angiotensin receptor blockers in the prehospital or emergency department setting in patients with an MI.[41]	Recommended within the first 24 hours after onset of STEMI symptoms in patients with pulmonary congestion or left ventricular ejection fraction less than 40% in the absence of hypotension.[32]	May cause a profound drop in BP following the first dose or if used with diuretics.

ACS, Acute coronary syndrome; BP, blood pressure; NSTEMI, non-ST-elevation myocardial infarction; STEMI, ST-elevation myocardial infarction; UA, unstable angina.

Antiplatelet Therapy

Antiplatelet and anticoagulant therapies are important components of ACS patient management because exposure of a ruptured plaque's contents triggers activation of the coagulation cascade.

Aspirin and Clopidogrel

Aspirin should be administered to patients experiencing an ACS as soon as possible after presentation and continued indefinitely unless contraindicated (Table 5-7). Clopidogrel (Plavix) is an antiplatelet agent that helps prevent platelets from sticking together and forming clots. Platelets exposed to clopidogrel are affected for the remainder of their lifespan. A loading dose of clopidogrel followed by a daily maintenance dose should be administered to patients who are unable to take aspirin because of hypersensitivity or major GI intolerance.[10]

Patients routinely taking nonsteroidal antiinflammatory drugs (NSAIDs) (except for aspirin), both nonselective as well as cyclooxygenase-2 (COX-2) selective agents, before STEMI should have those agents discontinued at the time of presentation with STEMI because of the increased risk of mortality, reinfarction, hypertension, heart failure, and myocardial rupture associated with their use.[43]

Glycoprotein IIb/IIIa Inhibitors

Glycoprotein (GP) IIb/IIIa inhibitors are potent antiplatelet medications that are given intravenously. They act on the GP IIb/IIIa receptors on the platelet membrane to inhibit platelet aggregation and prevent platelets from binding with fibrinogen. When the use of any of these medications is planned, minimize arterial and venous punctures; intramuscular injections; and use of urinary catheters, nasotracheal intubation, and nasogastric tubes. When establishing IV access, avoid noncompressible sites (e.g., the subclavian or jugular veins).

Anticoagulant Therapy

Anticoagulants prevent new clots from forming, but do not dissolve previously formed clots. Unfractionated heparin (UFH) is the oldest anticoagulant available (Table 5-8). It indirectly inhibits thrombin, acting at multiple sites in the normal coagulation system. Heparin can be given intravenously or subcutaneously. The anticoagulant effect of low-molecular-weight heparins (LMWH), such as enoxaparin and dalteparin, is mostly due to Factor Xa inhibition. Fondaparinux is a synthetic anticoagulant that inhibits Factor Xa. It is administered subcutaneously. The half-life of UFH is about 1 hour, LMWH about 2 to 4 hours, and fondaparinux about 17 to 21 hours. Bivalirudin is a synthetic direct thrombin inhibitor that is given intravenously. It has a half-life of 25 minutes in patients with normal renal function.

TABLE 5-7	Antiplatelet Therapy in Acute Coronary Syndromes		
Antiplatelet Therapy	UA/NSTEMI	STEMI	Comments
Medication	**Indications and Dose**	**Indications and Dose**	
Aspirin Class: Nonnarcotic analgesic, antipyretic, anti-inflammatory agent, salicylate	Give 162 to 325 mg orally as soon as possible after patient presentation followed by 75 to 162 mg/day indefinitely (if no history of aspirin allergy or signs of active or recent GI bleeding).[10,32]	Aspirin should be chewed by patients who have not taken aspirin before presentation with STEMI and who have no history of aspirin allergy or signs of active or recent GI bleeding. The initial dose should be 162 mg to 325 mg and continued indefinitely at a daily dose of 75 to 162 mg.[15,32]	Consider an aspirin suppository for patients with severe nausea, vomiting, or upper GI disorders.[32]
Clopidogrel (Plavix) Class: Antiplatelet agent	In patients younger than 75 years of age, an oral loading dose of 300 to 600 mg is recommended for NSTEMI regardless of whether the patient undergoes reperfusion with fibrinolytic therapy or does not receive reperfusion therapy.[32] No data are available to guide decision making regarding an oral loading dose in patients older than 75 years.[43]	Same as for UA/NSTEMI	Platelet aggregation and bleeding time gradually return to baseline values after treatment is discontinued, generally in about 5 days.
Glycoprotein (GP) IIb/IIIa inhibitors abciximab (ReoPro); eptifibatide (Integrilin); tirofiban (Aggrastat)	There is insufficient data to support the routine use of GP IIb/IIIa inhibitors in the prehospital or emergency department settings.[41] For selected high-risk patients with NSTEMI, abciximab, eptifibatide, or tirofiban administration may be acceptable, provided PCI is planned.[41]	The usefulness of GP IIb/IIIa receptor antagonists (as part of a preparatory pharmacological strategy for patients with STEMI before their arrival in the cardiac catheterization laboratory for angiography and PCI) is uncertain.[32,44]	

CABG, coronary artery bypass graft; GI, gastrointestinal; NSTEMI, non-ST-elevation myocardial infarction; PCI, percutaneous coronary intervention; STEMI, ST-elevation myocardial infarction; UA, unstable angina.

UFH requires frequent dosing adjustments to achieve an activated partial thromboplastin time (aPTT) of 1.5 to 2 times the control value. In contrast, the dosing for LMWH is determined by the patient's weight without monitoring aPTT and dose titration; however, periodic complete blood counts, including platelet count, and stool occult blood tests are recommended during the course of treatment. Bleeding is the major adverse effect of all anticoagulants.

Percutaneous Coronary Intervention

Angiography can be used to identify ACS patients who do not have CAD and can be discharged; patients who have a coronary artery lesion that is amenable to PCI and who can have the procedure performed immediately; and patients with left main CAD and those with multivessel disease and left ventricular dysfunction who need bypass surgery.

TABLE 5-8 Anticoagulant Therapy and Acute Coronary Syndromes

Anticoagulant Therapy	UA/NSTEMI	STEMI	Comments
Medication	**Indications**	**Indications**	
Unfractionated heparin Class: Anticoagulant, indirect thrombin inhibitor	Reasonable for NSTEMI patients selected for early invasive treatment May be considered for patients with NSTEMI and renal insufficiency[32] May be considered for patients with NSTEMI and who are at high risk of bleeding, where anticoagulant therapy is not contraindicated[32]	STEMI patients undergoing PCI (similar or improved outcomes have been demonstrated when enoxaparin was compared to UFH in patients undergoing contemporary PCI [use of GP IIb/IIIa inhibitors and a thienopyridine])[32] Administration may be necessary to avoid catheter thrombi in patients on fondaparinux	Risk of developing heparin-induced thrombocytopenia. Effects may be reversed with protamine sulfate.
enoxaparin sodium (Lovenox) Class: Anticoagulant, low-molecular-weight heparin, indirect thrombin inhibitor	Reasonable for NSTEMI patients and early conservative treatment Reasonable for NSTEMI patients selected for early invasive treatment	Reasonable to administer instead of UFH for patients with STEMI managed with fibrinolysis in the hospital setting[32] May consider instead of UFH for prehospital STEMI patients managed with fibrinolysis[32] Considered a safe and effective alternative to UFH for STEMI patients undergoing contemporary PCI	Cannot be used interchangeably (unit for unit) with heparin or other low molecular weight heparins. Adjust dose in patients with renal impairment.
fondaparinux (Arixtra) Class: Synthetic anticoagulant, Factor Xa inhibitor	Reasonable for NSTEMI patients and early conservative treatment May be used in the setting of PCI Requires co-administration of UFH Reasonable for patients with NSTEMI and who are at high risk of bleeding, where anticoagulant therapy is not contraindicated[32]	May be considered for in-hospital STEMI patients treated with nonfibrin-specific fibrinolytics (e.g., streptokinase)[32]	Adjust dose in patients with renal impairment.
bivalirudin (Angiomax, Hirulog) Class: Anticoagulant, synthetic direct thrombin inhibitor	May be considered for patients with NSTEMI and renal insufficiency[32] Reasonable for patients with NSTEMI and who are at high risk of bleeding, where anticoagulant therapy is not contraindicated[32]	Insufficient evidence to provide recommendation for use in STEMI patients undergoing fibrinolysis[32] In STEMI patients undergoing PCI who are at high risk of bleeding, bivalirudin anticoagulation is reasonable[44]	

GP, Glycoprotein; NSTEMI, non–ST-elevation myocardial infarction; PCI, percutaneous coronary intervention; STEMI, ST-elevation myocardial infarction; UA, unstable angina; UFH, unfractionated heparin.

ACLS Pearl
Angiography has shown that about 10% to 20% of patients with UA/NSTEMI have no significant coronary artery stenosis and approximately 20% have three-vessel disease with left ventricular dysfunction or left main CAD.[10] Three-vessel disease or left main CAD is more common in men (35%) than women (23%).[45]

A PCI is a procedure in which a catheter is used to open a coronary artery that has been blocked or narrowed by CAD. PCI procedures include percutaneous transluminal coronary angioplasty (PTCA), which is also called **angioplasty** or **balloon angioplasty**; percutaneous transluminal coronary rotational atherectomy; directional coronary atherectomy; laser atherectomy; and intracoronary stent implantation (Figure 5-31). The term **primary PCI** is used when PCI is done alone as the primary treatment after diagnostic angiography. The term **facilitated PCI** refers to a combination of medications (e.g., fibrinolytics, GP IIb/IIIa inhibitors) and PCI. The administration of fibrinolytics before PCI is intended to improve patency of the coronary artery before the procedure.[43] The term **contemporary PCI** refers to the use of GP IIb/IIIa inhibitors and a thienopyridine (e.g., clopidogrel). The term **rescue PCI** is used if the procedure is performed after an unsuccessful reperfusion attempt with fibrinolytics.

Of the patients experiencing ACSs, those who are experiencing a STEMI are most likely to benefit from reperfusion therapy. The benefits of reperfusion therapy are often time-dependent; remember that "time is muscle." If the patient has a STEMI, time targets to minimize *total ischemic time*, which is defined as the time from onset of symptoms of STEMI to initiation of reperfusion therapy, are to give fibrinolytics within 30 minutes of patient contact or provide primary PCI within 90 minutes of arrival (i.e., door-to-balloon inflation [D2B]).[32,43] Optimally, PCI should be performed at a high-volume facility with surgical backup. Although mechanical catheter-based intervention has been proven to produce better outcomes when performed in a timely manner, fibrinolytic therapy continues to play a major role in the treatment of acute MI because it is estimated that only 25% of U.S. hospitals have PCI capabilities.[46] As a result, a system of referral to a PCI-capable hospital is necessary.

ACLS Pearl
When prehospital professionals have the ability to perform 12-lead ECGs, the door-to-drug or door-to-balloon inflation time begins on arrival of the EMS professionals, which can decrease the door-to-reperfusion therapy time on arrival at the hospital.

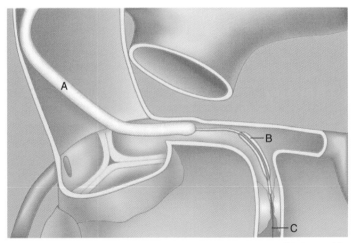

Figure 5-31 Schematic view of coronary angioplasty technique. A guide catheter *A* is inserted into the coronary artery (in this figure, the left main); a balloon catheter *B* is advanced over a thin guidewire *C* into the lesion. Balloon inflation dilates the stenotic region.

STEMI alert programs have been implemented in many EMS systems and hospitals across the country in an attempt to minimize total ischemic time. Total ischemic time is comprised of four key intervals:

1. Onset of symptoms to arrival of EMS personnel
2. Arrival of EMS personnel to hospital arrival
3. Hospital arrival to 12-lead ECG
4. Twelve-lead ECG to drug/balloon

EMS personnel quickly obtain a diagnostic-quality 12-lead ECG when they arrive on the scene of a patient complaining of chest discomfort or an anginal equivalent (e.g., difficulty breathing, weakness or nausea). In some EMS systems, the paramedic manually reads the 12-lead ECG; in other EMS systems the 12-lead ECG machine's computer reads and interprets the ECG. If the computer reads, "Acute MI Suspected" and the paramedic agrees with the computer's interpretation, the patient is transported by EMS to a hospital with an interventional cardiac catheterization (cath) lab. In some EMS systems, the paramedic must transmit the 12-lead ECG to the hospital for physician interpretation.

 YOU SHOULD KNOW A 12-lead ECG machine's computer interpretation is not always accurate and should not be relied upon as 100% correct. Evaluation of the patient and the healthcare professional's assessment of the patient's ECG findings should always take precedence over the machine's analysis.

When EMS personnel recognize that they have a patient with STEMI, they should alert the receiving hospital and begin completing a reperfusion checklist. Information that should be relayed by paramedics to the hospital before their arrival includes the following:

- Patient age, gender
- Time of symptom onset
- ECG and assessment findings (including initial and repeat vital signs)
- Do not resuscitate status
- Reperfusion checklist findings (including presence or absence of surgeries in the last 3 months)
- Patient's primary physician and cardiologist (obtaining this information enables retrieval of the patient's medical records and previous ECGs before arrival at the receiving facility)
- Past history of MI, PCI, stent, or CABG; renal failure, allergy to contrast dye
- Current medications, including whether or not the patient is taking warfarin (Coumadin)

Early activation of the cath lab is an important factor in minimizing total ischemic time, but methods to accomplish this vary. In many areas, the cath lab is activated by an emergency department physician. In the most progressive EMS systems, when a prehospital 12-lead ECG clearly shows evidence of STEMI, the cath lab team is activated by paramedics and the patient is taken directly to the cath lab, bypassing the emergency department. En route, additional IV lines are established and medications are given for pain control per local or system protocol. Closer hospitals are sometimes bypassed to transport the patient with STEMI to a hospital with interventional cath lab capability. Air medical transport is sometimes used to transport patients with STEMI from rural areas to an urban heart center.

Fibrinolytic Therapy

Fibrinolytics ("clot-busters") work by altering plasmin in the body, which then breaks down fibrinogen and fibrin clots. At present, fibrinolytic therapy is only indicated for patients with UA/NSTEMI who also have a true posterior MI as evidenced by ST depression in two contiguous anterior chest leads or isolated ST elevation in posterior chest leads.[10]

For EMS systems that have fibrinolytic capabilities, prehospital fibrinolysis should be started within 30 minutes of the arrival of EMS on the scene if the patient meets the criteria for fibrinolytic therapy. For EMS systems that do not have fibrinolytic capability and if the patient is transported to a non–PCI-capable hospital, the door-to-needle time should be within 30 minutes for patients for whom fibrinolysis is indicated. For EMS systems that are not capable of administering prehospital fibrinolysis and the patient is transported to a PCI-capable hospital, the EMS arrival-to-balloon time should be within 90 minutes.[43]

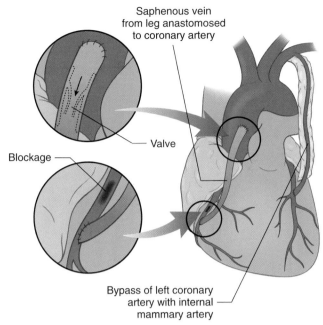

Saphenous vein
from leg anastomosed
to coronary artery

Valve

Blockage

Bypass of left coronary
artery with internal
mammary artery

Figure 5-32 Coronary artery bypass graft (CABG) surgery. The saphenous vein, radial artery, or internal mammary artery is harvested from the patient's leg, arm, or chest and grafted to the coronary artery.

Before starting fibrinolytic therapy, choose an ECG monitoring lead that shows clear evidence of ST elevation. During fibrinolytic therapy, monitor the ECG and the patient's vital signs closely. Watch for ST changes, dysrhythmias, hypotension, and question the patient about chest discomfort. When reperfusion occurs, the patient's chest discomfort typically stops abruptly as blood flow to the ischemic myocardium is restored. Watch for reperfusion dysrhythmias (e.g., such as premature ventricular complexes, bradycardias, heart block, VT, VF) as blood flow is reestablished through the infarct-related artery. Previously elevated ST segments should quickly return to baseline as blood flow is restored to the affected myocardium. Reocclusion may occur. Pay careful attention to all potential bleeding sites (including catheter insertion sites, arterial and venous puncture sites, cutdown sites, and needle puncture sites).

Coronary Artery Bypass Graft Surgery

A CABG is a surgical procedure in which blood flow is rerouted around one or more blocked coronary arteries by means of a blood-vessel graft to create new pathways for blood to flow to the heart muscle tissue. The grafts usually are harvested from the patient's own internal mammary artery, radial artery, or saphenous vein (Figure 5-32). Internal mammary artery grafts have better long-term patency than saphenous vein grafts.[48,49]

Although a traditional CABG requires open-chest surgery, newer and less invasive techniques can be used instead of open-chest surgery in some cases. For example, minimally invasive coronary artery bypass (MIDCAB) surgery is an option for some patients who require a left internal mammary artery bypass graft to the LAD artery. Benefits of the less invasive procedures include a smaller incision and smaller scars. Although these techniques have not been well studied and may not be available in all medical centers, additional benefits may include a reduced risk of infection, less bleeding, less pain and trauma, decreased length of hospital stay, and shorter recovery time.

COMPLICATIONS OF ACUTE MYOCARDIAL INFARCTION

[Objective 13]

Ischemic, electrical, mechanical, inflammatory, and embolic complications may result after an MI (Box 5-8).

BOX 5-8 | Complications Associated with Myocardial Infarction

Electrical Complications
- Bradydysrhythmias (sinus bradycardia most common)
- Tachydysrhythmias
- AV blocks
- Bundle branch and fascicular blocks
- Sudden cardiac death

Embolic Complications
- Stroke
- Deep vein thrombosis
- Pulmonary embolism

Inflammatory Complications
- Pericarditis

Ischemic Complications
- Angina
- Reinfarction
- Infarct extension

Mechanical Complications
- Ventricular aneurysm
- Ventricular septal rupture
- Papillary muscle disorders
- Cardiac wall rupture
- Left ventricular failure/cardiogenic shock
- Right ventricular failure

Dysrhythmias

Dysrhythmias are the most common electrical complication in the first few hours following MI. Dysrhythmias that originate from the SA node can occur if the blood supply to the SA node is disrupted or as a result of the administration of certain medications (e.g., beta-blockers, calcium channel blockers). Sinus bradycardia is the most common SA node dysrhythmia, and it is common with inferior wall infarctions, particularly in the first hour of inferior STEMI.[15] In the setting of an MI, sinus bradycardia is often transient. A slow heart rate can be beneficial for the patient who has had an MI and has no symptoms caused by the slow rate; this is because the heart's demand for oxygen is less when the heart rate is slow. If the patient is symptomatic because of the slow rate, treatment options include oxygen, IV access, and the administration of atropine. Transcutaneous pacing is rarely required.

Sinus tachycardia most often occurs with an anterior wall MI. Sinus tachycardia that is present in a patient who has experienced an acute MI may be an early warning signal for heart failure, cardiogenic shock, or more serious dysrhythmias.

Premature atrial complexes (PACs), AFib, atrial flutter, and supraventricular tachycardia (SVT) can occur in patients who sustain an acute MI. AFib occurs more frequently than atrial flutter or paroxysmal supraventricular tachycardia (PSVT) in patients with STEMI.[15]

AFib may occur spontaneously or may be preceded by PACs. AFib that develops during hospitalization is associated with an increased in-hospital and long-term mortality. Because of its rapid rate, sustained PSVT *without* signs of hemodynamic compromise should initially be treated with vagal maneuvers and, if these are unsuccessful, IV adenosine. Synchronized cardioversion is warranted if AFib, atrial flutter, or SVT are sustained and cause hemodynamic compromise. Short-acting anesthetic medications or drugs that produce conscious sedation should be used to avoid the discomfort related to delivery of the electric shock.[15]

An accelerated junctional rhythm is more often associated with inferior wall MI than anterior MI and may indicate digitalis toxicity. Antiarrhythmic therapy for an accelerated junctional rhythm generally is not indicated.

Varying degrees of AV block may occur in patients with acute MI. It has been estimated that AV blocks may develop in about 6% to 14% of patients with STEMI.[15] Ischemia of the AV node can result in first-degree or second-degree type 1 AV block. These dysrhythmias are relatively common with an inferior infarction. However, they are usually transient (resolving within 2 to 3 days), generally do not warrant treatment, and have a low mortality rate unless associated with hypotension or heart failure.[15] Second-degree AV block type II and complete AV block with slow, wide QRS complexes are often unstable rhythms with a moderate to high risk of ventricular asystole and may require treatment with transcutaneous or possibly transvenous, pacing.[15] Because most patients receive fibrinolysis or undergo PCI to open the occluded vessel, the development of sudden AV block in the setting of an anterior STEMI has become much less common.

ACLS Pearl

Complete AV block occurs in about 20% of patients with acute right ventricular infarction.[49]

PVCs are seen in about 90% of patients within the first few hours after an MI.[49] For many years, PVCs observed in patients experiencing an acute MI were thought to be "warning" dysrhythmias of impending VF, particularly when they were multiform PVCs, R-on-T PVCs, couplets, and frequent (i.e., more than 6/min) PVCs. Careful monitoring has disproved this idea and suppression of PVCs with antiarrhythmics is no longer recommended unless they lead to hemodynamic compromise.[15] It is now considered prudent clinical practice to closely observe these premature beats, consider the reason for their occurrence (e.g., hypoxemia, acid-base disturbance, electrolyte imbalance, heart failure), and correct the underlying cause. An accelerated idioventricular rhythm commonly occurs during the first 12 hours of infarction but antiarrhythmic therapy is not indicated because suppression of the rhythm may lead to hemodynamic compromise.[15]

Sustained (i.e., more than 30 seconds) monomorphic VT that is associated with hemodynamic compromise (e.g., angina, pulmonary edema, hypotension) should be treated with synchronized cardioversion. Sustained monomorphic and polymorphic VT that is not associated with hemodynamic compromise is treated with antiarrhythmics. Sustained polymorphic VT that is associated with hemodynamic compromise should be treated with defibrillation.

Primary VF is VF that occurs during the acute phase of an MI. Secondary VF occurs in the presence of severe heart failure or cardiogenic shock.[15] The incidence of VF is highest during the first 4 hours after the onset of symptoms and remains an important contributing factor to death during the first 24 hours after STEMI. Ventricular fibrillation or pulseless VT should be treated with cardiopulmonary resuscitation and defibrillation.

Ventricular Aneurysm

When a section of the heart's muscular wall dies as a result of an MI, scar tissue forms in response to the inflammatory changes of the infarction. The presence of scar tissue weakens the affected wall of the myocardium. To maintain cardiac output, the unaffected part of the heart wall must continue pumping blood and compensate for the dead muscle.

A true ventricular aneurysm involves bulging of the full thickness of the ventricular wall.[50] It may develop in a few days, weeks, or months after a large (usually anterior) acute MI and may affect cardiac output (Figure 5-33). The affected area may contract poorly (i.e., hypokinetic), consist of noncontractile (i.e., akinetic) scar tissue, or consist of scar tissue that moves in the opposite direction of the normal contractile myocardium (i.e., dyskinetic). The rupture of a true ventricular aneurysm is rare. A false ventricular aneurysm (i.e., pseudoaneurysm) is an incomplete rupture of the ventricular wall in which the wall of the aneurysm is not myocardium but rather an external border (e.g., pericardium). False aneurysms almost always contain a thrombus and rupture is common.

Acute heart failure, systemic emboli, angina, and recurrent ventricular dysrhythmias are the most common complications of a ventricular aneurysm. The most frequent symptom of left ventricular

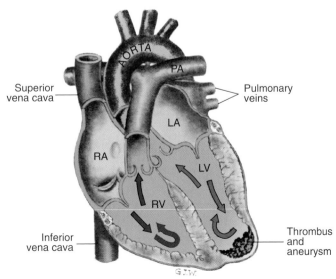

Figure 5-33 Ventricular aneurysm after acute myocardial infarction. LA, left atrium; LV, left ventricle; PA, pulmonary artery; RA, right atrium; RV, right ventricle.

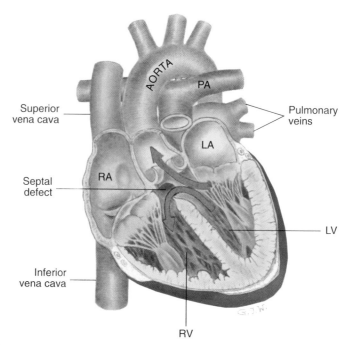

Figure 5-34 Ventricular septal rupture after acute myocardial infarction. LA, left atrium; LV, left ventricle; PA, pulmonary artery; RA, right atrium; RV, right ventricle.

aneurysm is angina and 60% or more of these patients have three-vessel coronary disease.[51] Dyspnea is the second most common symptom of ventricular aneurysm and often develops when 20% or more of the ventricular wall is infarcted.[50]

When a ventricular aneurysm is present, the patient's ECG will show evidence of persistent ST elevation. Echocardiography is performed to determine whether a thrombus is present. Left ventriculography is performed to confirm the diagnosis of left ventricular aneurysm. Surgical removal may be indicated when left ventricular failure or dysrhythmias persist and are unresponsive to conventional therapy.

Ventricular Septal Rupture

Ventricular septal rupture (VSR), which is also known as **acquired ventricular septal defect** (VSD), is an abnormal communication that develops in an area of dead myocardial tissue between the right and left ventricles after an acute MI (Figure 5-34). This potentially lethal complication typically occurs within the first 10 to 14 days after an acute MI and often precipitates cardiogenic shock. Before the use of fibrinolytic therapy, VSR occurred in 1% to 2% of patients after acute MI and is now estimated to occur in less than 1% of all MIs.[15]

The most consistent physical finding of postinfarction VSR is a new loud systolic murmur that is best heard at the left lower sternal border. The murmur is accompanied by a thrill in 50% of cases.[49] Before development of the murmur, the patient may appear relatively comfortable, with no clinically significant cardiopulmonary symptoms. Onset of the murmur is generally accompanied by sudden worsening of the patient's condition caused by shunting of blood from the high-pressure left ventricle into the low-pressure right ventricle through the new septal opening. The ECG may show AV nodal or infranodal conduction delay abnormalities in about 40% of patients.[49] Methods used to diagnose VSR include echocardiography and assessment of oxygen saturation levels in the right ventricle and pulmonary artery (PA) with PA catheterization. An intra-aortic balloon pump (IABP) is inserted and vasodilators (e.g., nitroprusside) are administered to decrease afterload, reduce the amount of blood being shunted to the right side of the heart, and consequently to increase the flow of blood into the systemic circulation until surgery can be accomplished.[52]

Papillary Muscle Rupture

Papillary muscle rupture is a rare consequence of acute MI. An inferior wall infarction can lead to rupture of the posteromedial papillary muscle that supports the mitral valve (Figure 5-35). An

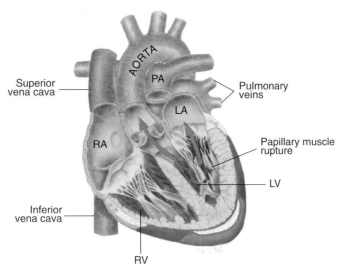

Figure 5-35 Papillary muscle rupture after acute myocardial infarction. LA, left atrium; LV, left ventricle; PA, pulmonary artery; RA, right atrium; RV, right ventricle.

anterolateral MI can lead to rupture of the anterolateral papillary muscle that supports the mitral valve. The posteromedial papillary muscle is most frequently involved (i.e., in 75% of cases) because of its single blood supply through the posterior descending coronary artery, making it more susceptible to ischemia.[53] By contrast, the anterolateral papillary muscle has a dual blood supply, because it is perfused by the left anterior descending and circumflex coronary arteries.[49] In 50% of patients with papillary muscle rupture, the infarction is relatively small.[53]

Dysfunction of a papillary muscle results in ineffective valve closure, which allows blood to flow from the affected ventricle backward into the atrium during ventricular systole. Papillary muscle rupture may be partial or complete. Partial rupture of a papillary muscle that supports the mitral valve is more common. This results in mitral regurgitation and can cause fatigue, shortness of breath, palpitations, peripheral edema, and complaints of lightheadedness. Complete papillary muscle rupture is rare and usually precipitates severe acute mitral regurgitation, an abrupt onset of shortness of breath and pulmonary edema, and cardiogenic shock. Because complete rupture leads to death in 75% of patients within 24 hours,[36] urgent mitral valve repair (if possible) or replacement is required. Insertion of an IABP and the administration of nitroprusside (to lower preload and improve peripheral perfusion) and medications to improve contractility (e.g., dobutamine, dopamine) are used to help stabilize the patient until surgery can be undertaken.

Cardiac Wall Rupture

Cardiac wall rupture, which is also called **free wall rupture**, occurs in 1% to 6% of patients admitted with STEMI. It most commonly occurs in the lateral wall of the left ventricle, although any wall can be involved (Figure 5-36).[49] Patients most likely to experience cardiac rupture include those with their first MI, those with anterior infarction, women, and older adults.[15] Additional risk factors include hypertension during the acute phase of STEMI, poor coronary collateral blood flow, Q waves on the ECG, use of corticosteroids or nonsteroidal antiinflammatory drugs (NSAIDs), and use of fibrinolytic therapy more than 14 hours after symptom onset.[15] Cardiac rupture typically occurs within 5 days of MT in 50% of patients and within 2 weeks of MI in 90% of patients.[49] Successful early reperfusion of the infarct-related artery and the presence of coronary collateral circulation are the most important determinants with regard to preventing free wall rupture.[15]

With acute cardiac rupture, bleeding into the pericardial sac results in cardiac tamponade, cardiogenic shock, pulseless electrical activity (PEA), and sudden death. Patients with a less rapid onset may complain of nausea, pain consistent with pericarditis, JVD, pulsus paradoxus, diminished heart sounds, a pericardial rub, and hypotension. ECG findings may reveal a junctional or idioventricular rhythm, low-voltage complexes, and tall T waves in the chest leads. Many patients have transient bradycardia just before rupture.[49] Pericardiocentesis is necessary to relieve the tamponade. Fluid replacement and the use of vasopressors to maintain blood pressure are temporizing measures that may be used until an emergency surgical repair can be attempted.

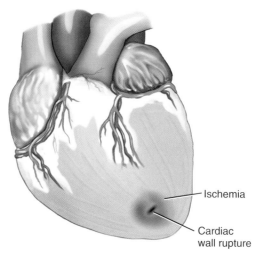

Figure 5-36 Cardiac wall rupture.

Hypotension

Adequate tissue perfusion requires an intact cardiovascular system. This includes an adequate fluid volume (the blood), a container to regulate the distribution of the fluid (the blood vessels), and a pump (the heart) with sufficient force to move the fluid throughout the container. A problem with any of these components can affect perfusion.

Hypotension occurs as a result of a problem with one of the parts of the cardiovascular triad. Shock is inadequate tissue perfusion that results from the failure of the cardiovascular system to deliver enough oxygen and nutrients to sustain vital organ function. The underlying cause must be recognized and treated promptly, or cell and organ dysfunction and death may result. Signs and symptoms differ according to underlying cause and compensatory mechanisms.

Keeping It Simple

Cardiovascular Triad
- Conduction system (rate)
- Myocardium (pump)
- Tank or vascular system (volume)

A problem with the conduction system can result in a rate problem; however, a "rate problem" is not synonymous with a "conduction problem." An adequate rate may be present, although a conduction defect exists. A rate that is too slow may be associated with a sinus bradycardia, second- and third-degree AV blocks or pacemaker failure. Sinus tachycardia, atrial flutter or AFib with a rapid ventricular response, SVT and VT are examples of rhythms that may produce a rapid ventricular rate. In general, if the patient is hypotensive (and symptomatic) and the heart rate is too slow, speed it up (i.e., use the bradycardia algorithm). If the patient is hypotensive (and symptomatic) and the heart rate is too fast, slow it down (i.e., determine the width of the QRS complex, and then use the appropriate tachycardia algorithm).

Hypotension may also occur as a result of a volume problem. Possible causes of a volume deficit are shown in Box 5-9. If a volume deficit exists, generally the first priority is fluid replacement to increase volume. It is reasonable to begin with a fluid challenge (250- to 500-mL IV boluses) and to then reassess the patient after each bolus. In some situations, a blood transfusion may be warranted. Consider vasopressors, if indicated, to improve vascular tone if there is no response to fluid challenges.

Pump failure as a result of acute MI may result in decreased cardiac output and there is produce signs and symptoms of tissue hypoperfusion or pulmonary congestion (Box 5-10). Pump problems may be primary or secondary. Causes of primary pump problems include MI, papillary muscle dysfunction, myocarditis, cardiomyopathies, acute aortic insufficiency, prosthetic valve dysfunction, septal

---

BOX 5-9   **Possible Causes of a Volume Deficit**

- Empty tank (absolute hypovolemia = actual fluid deficit)
  - Adrenal insufficiency (aldosterone)
  - Gastrointestinal loss (e.g., vomiting, diarrhea)
  - Hemorrhage
  - Insensible losses (e.g., perspiration, breathing)
  - Phlebotomy
  - Reduced fluid intake as a result of pain, nausea, or vomiting
  - Renal losses (e.g., polyuria)
- Change in tank size (relative hypovolemia = vasodilation from any cause or redistribution of fluid to third spaces)
  - Adrenal insufficiency (cortisol)
  - Anaphylaxis
  - Central nervous system injury
  - Drugs that alter vascular tone
  - Sepsis
  - Spinal injury
  - Third-space loss

BOX 5-10   **Signs And Symptoms of Tissue Hypoperfusion or Pulmonary Congestion**

Signs and Symptoms of Hypoperfusion
- Fatigue
- Hypotension
- Skin findings (e.g., pallor, sweating)
- Weak pulse
- Weakness

Signs and Symptoms of Pulmonary Congestion
- Cyanosis
- Dyspnea
- Frothy sputum
- Jugular venous distention
- Labored breathing
- Tachypnea

---

rupture, and drug overdose or poisoning. Secondary causes of pump failure include cardiac tamponade, pulmonary embolism, drugs that alter function, and superior vena cava syndrome. As oxygen, glucose, and adenosine triphosphate (ATP) are depleted, essentially all patients in shock will eventually develop a secondary pump problem.

Ventricular Failure

Left Ventricular Failure[54]

When the left ventricle fails, blood backs up behind it, causing a chain reaction (Figure 5-37). Blood builds up in the lungs because the left ventricle is unable to eject all of the blood within its walls. The left atrium swells with blood because it cannot empty the blood within its walls into the left ventricle. Stretching of the atrial muscle fibers may result in atrial dysrhythmias. The pulmonary veins cannot empty the blood from the pulmonary arteries into the left atrium because it already is full. Pressure within the pulmonary vessels increases, forcing fluid from the pulmonary capillaries across the alveolar walls into the alveoli of the lungs; this results in pulmonary edema. The congestion heard in the lungs is the reason heart failure often is called *congestive heart failure*. The buildup of fluid widens the gap between the alveolar-capillary membrane, impairing the diffusion of oxygen and carbon dioxide.

Cardiogenic shock is a form of severe left ventricular failure. It may occur as a complication of shock of any cause and can also occur if myocardial contractility is decreased as a result of prolonged cardiac surgery, ventricular aneurysm, cardiac arrest, or rupture of the ventricular wall. Other causes of cardiogenic shock include cardiac dysrhythmias, rupture of the ventricular septum, myocarditis, cardiomyopathy, myocardial trauma, heart failure, hypothermia, severe electrolyte or acid–base imbalances, and severe congenital heart disease.

Patients with cardiogenic shock who have had a recent MI are more likely to be older, have had a STEMI, have a history of a previous MI or heart failure, and have had an anterior infarction at the time shock develops. Although cardiogenic shock is associated more often with STEMI than NSTEMI,

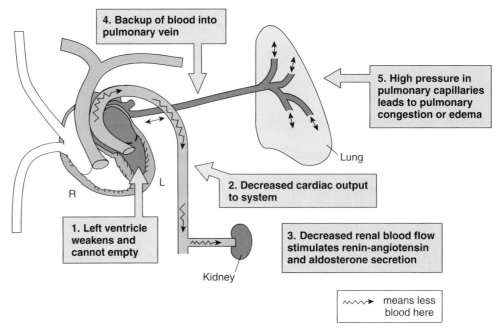

Figure 5-37 Left ventricular failure.

a 1999 study found that approximately 20% of all cardiogenic shock complicating MI was associated with NSTEMI.[55] Cardiogenic shock occurs in up to 5% of patients with NSTEMI and mortality rates are greater than 60%.[56,57]

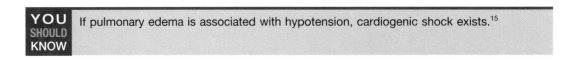

YOU SHOULD KNOW If pulmonary edema is associated with hypotension, cardiogenic shock exists.[15]

In compensated cardiogenic shock, the patient's mental status initially may be normal. As perfusion to the brain decreases, the patient becomes restless, agitated, and confused. Breath sounds reveal crackles in most patients. However, patients with RVI or those who are hypovolemic may have less evidence of pulmonary congestion. JVD, indicating right ventricular failure (RVF), may be present. If the patient is hypovolemic, JVD will be absent. Peripheral pulses often are weak and rapid. However, pulses may be weak and slow if an AV block is present. The patient's skin is usually pale or mottled. The extremities often feel cool and moist. Initially the patient's systolic blood pressure may be normal, but pulse pressure is usually narrowed. If cardiogenic shock is associated with cardiac tamponade, heart sounds may be muffled.

In decompensated cardiogenic shock, the patient usually has an altered mental status or may be unresponsive. Breathing is often rapid and shallow. Breath sounds usually reveal increasing pulmonary congestion and crackles. Peripheral pulses may be absent. Central pulses are often weak and rapid. The patient's skin is usually pale, mottled, or cyanotic. The extremities feel cold and sweaty. As ventricular function worsens and cardiac output falls, the systolic blood pressure progressively decreases.

The treatment of cardiogenic shock is generally based on increasing contractility without significant increases in heart rate, altering preload and afterload, and controlling dysrhythmias if they are present and contributing to shock. Apply a pulse oximeter and administer supplemental oxygen as indicated. Place the patient on a cardiac monitor and establish IV access. Obtain a 12-lead ECG and maintain normal body temperature. Cardiogenic shock and heart failure are not contraindications to fibrinolysis. Primary PCI is considered a reasonable treatment option for patients who develop shock within 36 hours of symptom onset and who are suitable candidates for revascularization that can be performed within 18 hours of the onset of shock.[32] Intra-aortic balloon counterpulsation may also be considered.

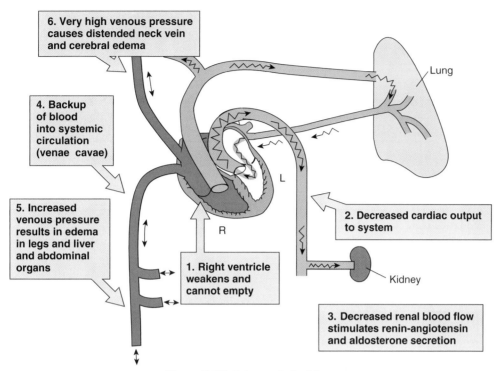

6. Very high venous pressure causes distended neck vein and cerebral edema

4. Backup of blood into systemic circulation (venae cavae)

5. Increased venous pressure results in edema in legs and liver and abdominal organs

1. Right ventricle weakens and cannot empty

2. Decreased cardiac output to system

3. Decreased renal blood flow stimulates renin-angiotensin and aldosterone secretion

Lung

Kidney

L

R

Figure 5-38 Right ventricular failure.

Right Ventricular Failure[54]

To eject the blood within its walls, the right ventricle must work harder to overcome the high pressure and congestion within the pulmonary vessels. When it cannot keep up with the increased workload, the right ventricle fails (Figure 5-38). Blood backs up behind the right ventricle, increasing the pressure in the right atrium. If the right atrium is unable to eject the blood within its walls, blood backs up into the superior and inferior venae cavae. Veins become congested with blood because the superior and inferior venae cavae cannot drain into an already full right atrium. Because venous return is delayed, organs become congested with blood. For example, the liver enlarges (i.e., hepatomegaly) and becomes tender because of increased pressure in the hepatic veins. As venous congestion worsens, increased pressure within the veins forces serous fluid through capillary walls and into body tissues, producing edema. Peripheral edema is most easily seen in dependent areas of the body, such as the feet and ankles. Serous fluid may build up in the abdomen (i.e., ascites), pleural cavity (i.e., pleural effusion), or pericardial cavity (i.e., pericardial effusion). As RVF worsens, generalized edema of the entire body (i.e., anasarca) may be seen.

Initial Management of Ventricular Failure

Treatment of ventricular failure focuses on correcting hypoxia, reducing preload, reducing afterload, and improving myocardial contractility. Place the patient in a position of comfort. Limit the patient's physical activity. If pulmonary congestion is present and the patient's blood pressure will tolerate it, place him or her in a sitting position with the feet dangling. This will help decrease venous return and decrease the work of breathing.

Apply a pulse oximeter and administer oxygen as needed to maintain the patient's oxygen saturation at 94% or higher. If oxygen is indicated and breathing is adequate, give oxygen by mask if the patient will tolerate it. Some patients will feel they are suffocating if a mask in used. You may need to reassure the patient that the oxygen mask is necessary and will help with their breathing. If you are unable to convince the patient to accept the mask, you may have to resort to using blow-by oxygen or a nasal cannula. If the patient is unresponsive or his or her breathing is inadequate, administer oxygen using positive pressure ventilation.

Obtain a portable radiograph, place the patient on a cardiac monitor, and obtain a 12-lead ECG. Heart failure may occur as a result of a dysrhythmia. Alternatively, hypoxia and acidosis predispose patients with heart failure to dysrhythmias. Dysrhythmias may range from tachycardias to bradycardias.

Establish IV access. To help ensure that the patient in heart failure does not receive too much IV fluid, it is common clinical practice to use a heparin lock or a saline lock. If your facility or agency protocols require you to use an IV bag and tubing, infuse the fluid at a to-keep-open rate (i.e., 30 mL/hr).

> **ACLS Pearl**
>
> Check and recheck the volume of fluid in the IV bag while the patient with heart failure is in your care. Be certain to document the amount of fluid in the bag when you started the IV and the amount of fluid remaining in the bag when you transfer patient care.

Medications used for the treatment of heart failure may include the following:
- Antiarrhythmics to treat dysrhythmias
- Analgesics to treat pain, if present
- Diuretics (e.g., furosemide) to reduce preload (Table 5-9)
- Venodilators (e.g., NTG) to reduce preload
- Positive inotropic agents (e.g., dopamine, dobutamine) to increase myocardial contractility (Table 5-10)
- Angiotensin-converting enzyme inhibitors, angiotensin receptor blockers, or beta-blockers to reduce afterload

> **ACLS Pearl**
>
> The term *inotrope* refers to a drug's effect on myocardial contractility. A drug that is a positive inotrope increases the heart's force of contraction. Digitalis, dopamine, dobutamine, and epinephrine are examples of drugs that are positive inotropes. Negative inotropes decrease the heart's force of contraction. Calcium channel blockers and beta-blockers are examples of negative inotropes.

> **ACLS Pearl**
>
> The patient who is experiencing pump failure may require:
> - Treatment of a coexisting rate or volume problem
> - Correction of underlying problems (i.e., hypoglycemia, hypoxia, drug overdose, poisoning)
> - Support for the failing pump
>   - Inotropic agents to increase contractility
>   - Vasodilators to decrease afterload
>   - Vasodilators and diuretics to decrease preload
>   - Mechanical assistance (e.g., intra-aortic balloon pump)
>   - Surgery (e.g., CABG, valve repair or replacement, heart transplant)

TABLE 5-9 Diuretics

Medication	Mechanism of Action	Dosing	Comments
furosemide (Lasix) Class: Loop diuretic	• Inhibits the reabsorption of sodium and chloride in the ascending limb of the loop of Henle, resulting in an increase in the urinary excretion of sodium, chloride, and water → profound diuresis • Furosemide increases excretion of potassium, hydrogen, calcium, magnesium, bicarbonate, ammonium, and phosphate • Venodilation—increases venous capacitance, decreases preload (venous return)	Initial dose is 0.5 to 1-mg/kg IV bolus at a rate no faster than 20 mg/min Use less than 0.5 mg/kg for new onset acute pulmonary edema without hypovolemia. Use 1 mg/kg for acute or chronic volume overload, renal insufficiency.[15]	Ototoxicity and resulting transient deafness can occur with rapid administration. Do not exceed the recommended rate of administration. Can cause excessive fluid loss and dehydration, resulting in hypovolemia and electrolyte imbalance.

TABLE 5-10	Drugs Used to Improve Cardiac Output and Blood Pressure		
Medication	**Mechanism of Action**	**Dosing**	**Comments**
dobutamine (Dobutrex) Class: Direct-acting sympathomimetic, cardiac stimulant, adrenergic agonist agent	Stimulates alpha, beta$_1$, and beta$_2$ receptors Potent inotropic effect (i.e., increased myocardial contractility, increased stroke volume, increased cardiac output) • Less chronotropic effect (heart rate) • Minimal alpha effect (vasoconstriction)	Given by continuous IV infusion. Usual dose is 2 to 20 mcg/kg/min IV, but patient response varies.	Onset of action 1 to 2 min. Correct hypovolemia before treatment with dobutamine. Tachycardia may occur with high doses, although this occurs less commonly than with dopamine. Continuously monitor ECG and blood pressure.
norepinephrine (Levophed) Class: Direct-acting adrenergic agent	Norepinephrine functions as a peripheral vasoconstrictor (alpha-adrenergic action) and as an inotropic stimulator of the heart and dilator of coronary arteries (beta-adrenergic action); alpha activity dominant	0.5 to 1 mcg/min by continuous IV infusion titrated to improve blood pressure (up to 30 mcg/min); usual dose range is 8 to 12 mcg/min	Onset of action immediate. Should be administered via an infusion pump into a central vein or a large peripheral vein (e.g., antecubital vein) to reduce the risk of necrosis of the overlying skin from prolonged vasoconstriction. Monitor blood pressure every 2 to 3 min until stabilized, then every 5 min. Monitor the patient's ECG continuously.

Pericarditis

Acute pericarditis is an inflammatory process, often with fluid accumulation, involving the pericardium that results in a clinical syndrome with the triad of chest pain, pericardial friction rub, and ECG changes.[58] Although common causes include infection, renal failure, MI, malignancy, mediastinal radiation, systemic autoimmune disease, and trauma, the cause is viral or unknown in 90% of cases.[59] Pericarditis that occurs as a late complication of acute MI is known as *Dressler's syndrome*.

Most patients with acute pericarditis experience "sharp" or "stabbing" chest discomfort unlike the more typical "pressure" or "heaviness" that accompanies infarction. The pain of pericarditis can often be localized with one finger. By contrast, the discomfort associated with acute MI is typically over a larger area that cannot be localized with one finger. The pain of pericarditis tends to be affected by movement, breathing, and position. The pain is usually worse with inspiration, intensified when lying supine, and lessened by sitting forward. If the pain radiates, the patient may report that it is felt around the base of the neck or in the area between the shoulder blades, presumably as a result of irritation of the phrenic nerves, which pass next to the pericardium.[59] A pericardial friction rub, which is a high-pitched, scratchy sound that corresponds with cardiac motion within the pericardial sac, is a classic initial finding in patients with acute pericarditis. The friction rub results from pericardial inflammation and can occur within 2 to 7 days after an MI. A low-grade fever is common.

The ECG changes associated with acute pericarditis have been described as evolving in four phases: phase I, diffuse ST-segment elevation and PR-segment depression; phase II, normalization of the ST and PR segments; phase III, widespread T wave inversions; and phase IV, normalization of the T waves (Figure 5-39).[59]

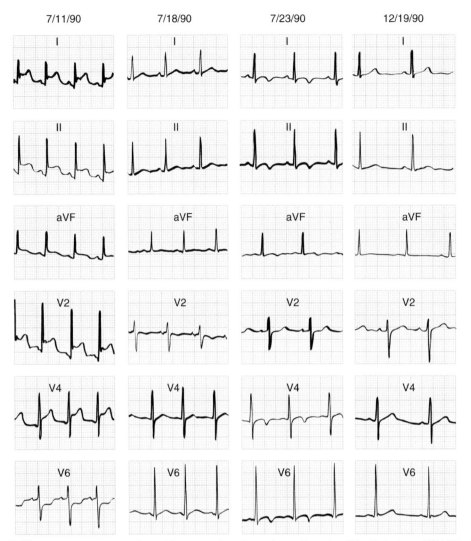

Figure 5-39 The classic electrocardiographic progression of a patient with pericarditis. First phase (7/11/90): Diffuse ST-segment elevation. Second phase (7/18/90): ST segment is back to isoelectric, but decreased T wave amplitude. Third phase (7/23/90): T wave inversion. Fourth phase (12/19/90): Complete resolution. Notice that the first three phases of the electrocardiogram (ECG) abnormalities of pericarditis in this patient are evident during the first 2 weeks of his illness. A follow-up ECG obtained 5 months later reveals a complete resolution of all the previous ECG abnormalities.

Nonsteroidal antiinflammatory drugs (NSAIDs) can be used for relief of pain but are contraindicated in the early period (less than 7 to 10 days) after MI (may predispose to cardiac rupture), and aspirin should be used instead.[58] Additional examples of complications of MI are shown in Figure 5-40 (see next page).

Embolic Complications

Most episodes of systemic emboli occur within the first 10 days after acute MI.[49] Abnormalities in left ventricular wall motion or left ventricular aneurysms are often the cause of systemic emboli, although AFib in the setting of ischemia may also contribute to systemic embolization.[49]

It is estimated that an acute stroke complicates 0.75% to 1.2% of MIs; mortality from post-STEMI stroke remains at more than 40%.[15] The major risk factors for embolic stroke include prior stroke, hypertension, old age, decreased ejection fraction or multiple ulcerated plaques, and AFib, which is by far the most important of these risk factors. Embolic stroke after STEMI occurs even in patients who have been treated with fibrinolysis.[15]

Pulmonary emboli commonly arise from thrombi in the leg veins. Although deep venous thrombosis and pulmonary embolism were once relatively frequent complications of MI, their incidence has declined because most patients now receive anticoagulant therapy.

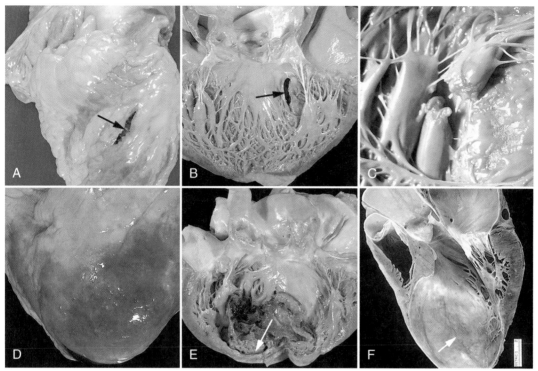

Figure 5-40 Complications of myocardial infarction (MI). A-C, Cardiac rupture. **A,** Anterior myocardial rupture in an acute infarct (*arrow*). **B,** Rupture of the ventricular septum (*arrow*). **C,** Complete rupture of a necrotic papillary muscle. **D,** Fibrinous pericarditis, showing a dark, roughened epicardial surface overlying an acute infarct. **E,** Early expansion of anteroapical infarct with wall thinning (*arrow*) and mural thrombus. **F,** Large apical left ventricular aneurysm (*arrow*).

STOP AND REVIEW

True/False

Indicate whether the statement is true or false.

_____ 1. Myocardial ischemia prolonged more than just a few minutes can result in myocardial injury.

_____ 2. Fibrinolytic therapy is an essential intervention in the treatment of all patients with unstable angina/non–ST-elevation myocardial infarction.

_____ 3. In the early acute phase, telling the difference between a patient with unstable angina and a patient having an acute myocardial infarction is often impossible because their clinical presentations and ECG findings may be identical.

_____ 4. A patient experiencing atypical chest pain has discomfort that is localized to the chest area but may have musculoskeletal, positional, or pleuritic features.

_____ 5. In prehospital or emergency department settings, glycoprotein IIb/IIIa inhibitors should be routinely used in the management of acute coronary syndromes with and without ST elevation.

_____ 6. Decisions regarding the care of a patient experiencing an acute coronary syndrome are primarily based on his or her assessment findings and symptoms, oxygen saturation, and presence of cardiac risk factors.

_____ 7. Angiotensin-converting enzyme inhibitors act on $beta_1$ and $beta_2$ receptors to slow sinus rate, depress AV conduction, and reduce blood pressure.

Multiple Choice

Identify the choice that best completes the statement or answers the question.

_____ 8. Which of the following correctly reflects the ECG hallmarks of ischemia?
a. Pathologic Q waves, ST-segment elevation
b. ST-segment depression, T wave inversion
c. Pathologic Q waves, ST-segment depression
d. ST-segment elevation, T wave inversion

_____ 9. Beta-blockers:
a. Reduce myocardial contractility
b. Increase myocardial oxygen demand
c. Increase atrioventricular node conduction velocity
d. Increase the rate of discharge of the sinoatrial node

_____ 10. The recommended initial dose of aspirin is:
a. 35 to 75 mg
b. 75 to 162 mg
c. 162 to 325 mg
d. 325 to 500 mg

____ 11. Dopamine:
a. Suppresses ventricular ectopy
b. Is used to increase heart rate and blood pressure
c. Should be given until the QRS lengthens to more than 50% of its original width
d. Is useful in relieving chest discomfort associated with acute coronary syndromes

____ 12. The highest incidence of ventricular fibrillation occurs about __ hours after ST-elevation MI symptom onset.
a. 4
b. 12
c. 24
d. 48

____ 13. Examples of electrical complications of an acute myocardial infarction include:
a. Acute stroke and pulmonary embolism
b. Ventricular aneurysm and pericarditis
c. Sinus bradycardia and bundle branch blocks
d. Papillary muscle disorders and left ventricular failure

____ 14. The medication of choice for relief of persistent chest discomfort associated with an ST-elevation myocardial infarction that is unresponsive to nitrates is:
a. Aspirin
b. Morphine
c. Midazolam (Versed)
d. Diltiazem (Cardizem)

____ 15. Acute pericarditis:
a. occurs most often because of chest trauma
b. is usually intensified when sitting forward and lessened by lying supine.
c. typically results in a clinical syndrome of chest pain, pericardial friction rub, and ECG changes
d. is usually associated with discomfort over a widespread area that cannot be localized with one finger

Questions 16 to 26 pertain to the following scenario:

A 62-year-old man is complaining of chest discomfort. The patient states his discomfort is located in the center of his chest and radiates to his left arm. He was reading the newspaper when his discomfort began about 1½ hours ago. On a 0 to 10 scale, the patient rates his discomfort a "9." He has no significant past medical history, takes no medications regularly, and states he has "never had anything like this before." His father died of a heart attack at the age of 66. The patient is an investment banker and states he is under considerable daily stress. The following questions refer to the initial assessment and management of this patient.

____ 16. Initial management of this patient should include primary and secondary surveys, oxygen (if indicated), IV, monitor, and:
a. Aspirin and a 12-lead ECG
b. Preparations for transcutaneous pacing
c. Preparations for immediate defibrillation
d. A 500-mL fluid challenge of normal saline

____ 17. The patient's vital signs are as follows: Blood pressure 146/74, pulse 128 (regular), ventilations 18, oxygen saturation 97% on oxygen at 4 liters/min. Breath sounds are clear bila0terally. The patient's skin is warm and moist. The cardiac monitor shows a sinus tachycardia. This rhythm:
   a. Requires immediate treatment with synchronized cardioversion
   b. Requires immediate treatment with vagal maneuvers and adenosine
   c. Is common and no reason for concern in a patient experiencing an acute coronary syndrome
   d. Is most likely associated with the discomfort and acute coronary syndrome the patient is experiencing

____ 18. An IV has been established. The cardiac monitor now reveals sinus tachycardia with occasional uniform premature ventricular complexes. Which of the following statements is true regarding obtaining a 12-lead ECG in this situation?
   a. A 12-lead ECG is necessary only if the patient's symptoms persist for more than 30 minutes.
   b. A 12-lead ECG should be obtained within 10 minutes of patient contact (prehospital) or arrival in the emergency department.
   c. A 12-lead ECG is an unnecessary expense and should be reserved for those situations in which you are unsure if the patient is experiencing an acute coronary syndrome.
   d. A 12-lead ECG is essential to decision making in the emergency care of a patient with an acute coronary syndrome and should be obtained with 30 minutes of patient contact (prehospital) or arrival in the emergency department.

____ 19. Sublingual nitroglycerin (NTG) is ordered for this patient. What is the rationale for giving NTG in this situation?
   a. NTG is a potent narcotic analgesic.
   b. NTG increases myocardial oxygen consumption.
   c. NTG relaxes vascular smooth muscle, including dilation of the coronary arteries.
   d. NTG blocks the formation of thromboxane A_2, which causes platelets to clump and arteries to constrict.

____ 20. What precautions should be taken before giving NTG?
   a. Make sure the patient's heart rate is at least 70 beats/min.
   b. Make sure there is no evidence of a right ventricular infarction.
   c. Make sure the patient's systolic blood pressure is more than 140 mm Hg.
   d. Make sure the patient has not used a diuretic or antihypertensive medication in the past 24 hours.

____ 21. NTG sublingual tablets or spray may be given:
   a. Every 5 minutes until discomfort is relieved
   b. At 3- to 5-minute intervals to a maximum of 3 doses
   c. Only once. If no relief of discomfort after one dose, give morphine
   d. At 15-minute intervals to a maximum of two doses. If no relief of discomfort after 2 doses, give midazolam (Versed) or meperidine (Demerol).

____ 22. A 12-lead ECG has been obtained. Which of the following components of the ECG should be carefully examined to determine the most appropriate treatment course for this patient?
a. P waves and PR intervals
b. ST segments, Q waves, and T waves
c. P waves and QRS complexes
d. ST segments and PR intervals

____ 23. When viewing the ECG of a patient experiencing an acute coronary syndrome, the presence of ST-segment elevation in the leads facing the affected area suggests myocardial __ .
a. Ischemia
b. Injury
c. Infarction
d. Necrosis

____ 24. The patient's 12-lead ECG reveals 3-mm ST-segment elevation in leads V_1, V_2, V_3, and V_4. What portion of the heart do these leads "see?"
a. The septum and anterior surface of the left ventricle
b. The right ventricle and the lateral surface of the left ventricle
c. The anterior and inferior surfaces of the left ventricle
d. The posterior and lateral surfaces of the left ventricle

____ 25. The patient rates his chest discomfort a "9" despite sublingual NTG therapy. His blood pressure is 140/70, pulse 120, and ventilations 18. Assuming the patient's vital signs remain stable, which of the following statements is true about relieving this patient's chest discomfort?
a. Give morphine 10 mg slow IV push and repeat every 90 minutes until the patient determines his discomfort is tolerable.
b. Give morphine 5 mg IV and reassess the degree of the patient's discomfort every 30 minutes.
c. Give morphine 8 mg IV, repeat every 30 minutes until the patient is pain free, and obtain a 12-lead ECG after each dose.
d. Give morphine 2 mg IV, reassess vital signs and level of discomfort after each dose, and give additional doses 5- to 15-minute intervals until the patient is pain free.

____ 26. The patient has been diagnosed with an anteroseptal myocardial infarction. Which of the following complications should be reasonably anticipated with this type of infarction?
a. Atrial fibrillation and stroke
b. Heart failure and cardiogenic shock
c. Bradycardias and pulmonary embolism
d. Tension pneumothorax and bundle branch blocks

Completion
Complete each statement.

27. _____ is a decreased supply of oxygenated blood to a body part or organ.

28. In an acute coronary syndrome, the zone of injury produces ST-segment _____ in the leads facing the affected area due to abnormal repolarization.

29. _____ therapy is one reperfusion option for patients with ST elevation MI.

30. A positive inotropic effect refers to a(n) _____ in _____
    _____.

31. _____ _____ is an anticoagulant that indirectly inhibits thrombin, acting
    at multiple sites in the normal coagulation system.

Matching
Match each description below with its corresponding answer.

a. The time from onset of symptoms of STEMI to start of reperfusion therapy
b. A combination of medications (such as fibrinolytics and/or glycoprotein IIb/IIIa inhibitors) and PCI
c. ECG changes seen in leads opposite the affected area are called __ changes.
d. Examples of beta-blockers
e. This type of angina is the result of intense spasm of a segment of a coronary artery
f. A procedure in which a catheter is used to open a coronary artery blocked or narrowed by coronary artery disease
g. Contraindicated in the early period (less than 7 to 10 days) after MI because they may predispose to cardiac rupture
h. Memory aid used to recall the medications typically given in the management of acute coronary syndromes
i. An actual fluid deficit is also called a(n) __ hypovolemia.
j. A classic initial finding in patients with acute pericarditis
k. Vasopressor that stimulates dopaminergic, beta, and alpha-adrenergic receptor sites
l. Examples of calcium channel blockers
m. Prevent new clots from forming, but do not dissolve previously formed clots
n. Blood tests used to help verify the presence of a myocardial infarction
o. Example of an antiplatelet agent
p. Potent peripheral vasoconstrictor
q. PCI performed after an unsuccessful reperfusion attempt with fibrinolytics
r. Treatment for sustained monomorphic and polymorphic VT that is not associated with hemodynamic compromise
s. Treatment for sustained monomorphic ventricular tachycardia associated with hemodynamic compromise
t. PCI performed alone as the primary treatment after diagnostic angiography
u. The most common electrical complication in the first few hours following MI

_____ 32. Percutaneous coronary intervention (PCI)

_____ 33. Dopamine

_____ 34. MONA

_____ 35. Anticoagulants

_____ 36. Norepinephrine

_____ 37. Facilitated PCI

_____ 38. Absolute

_____ 39. Rescue PCI

_____ 40. Atenolol (Tenormin), metoprolol (Lopressor)

_____ 41.   Reciprocal

_____ 42.   Pericardial friction rub

_____ 43.   Antiarrhythmics

_____ 44.   Cardiac biomarkers

_____ 45.   Prinzmetal's

_____ 46.   Primary PCI

_____ 47.   Diltiazem (Cardizem), verapamil (Calan, Isoptin, Verelan)

_____ 48.   Dysrhythmias

_____ 49.   Total ischemic time

_____ 50.   Clopidogrel (Plavix)

_____ 51.   Synchronized cardioversion

_____ 52.   Nonsteroidal antiinflammatory drugs (NSAIDs)

Short Answer

53. The 12-lead ECG plays a central role in the management of a patient with an acute coronary syndrome. When the patient's initial 12-lead is obtained, the ECG should be carefully reviewed and then the patient should be categorized into one of three groups, based on the 12-lead findings. What are the three groups?
    1.
    2.
    3.

54. Describe the characteristics of unstable angina.

55. How does myocardial injury differ from myocardial infarction?

56. What is meant by the phrase, "anginal equivalent" symptoms?

57. When are two ECG leads considered contiguous?

58. In a standard 12-lead ECG, how many leads look at tissue supplied by the right coronary artery?

59. List four examples of anginal equivalents.
    1.
    2.
    3.
    4.

REFERENCES

1. Lloyd-Jones D, Adams RJ, Brown TM, et al: Heart disease and stroke statistics—2010 update. A report from the American Heart Association Statistics Committee and Stroke Statistics Subcommittee, *Circulation* 121:e1–e170, 2010.
2. Sapin PM, Muller JE: Triggers of acute coronary syndromes. In: Cannon C, editor: *Management of Acute Coronary Syndromes*, 2nd ed, Totowa, NJ, 2003, Humana Press, pp 61–94.
3. Shah PK: Mechanisms of plaque vulnerability and rupture, *J Am Coll Cardiol* 19:41(4 Suppl S):15S–22S, 2003.
4. Becker R, Armani A: Linking biochemistry, vascular biology, and clinical events in acute coronary syndromes. In: Cannon C, editor: *Management of acute coronary syndromes*, 2nd ed, Totowa, NJ, 2003, Humana Press, pp 19–60.
5. Karve AM, Bossone E, Mehta RH: Acute ST-segment elevation myocardial infarction: critical care perspective, *Crit Care Clin* 23:685–707, 2007.
6. McCord J, Jneid H, Hollander JE, et al: Management of cocaine-associated chest pain and myocardial infarction: a scientific statement from the American Heart Association Acute Cardiac Care Committee of the Council on Clinical Cardiology, *Circulation* 117(14):1897–1907, 2008.
7. Hollander JE, Hoffman RS: Cocaine-induced myocardial infarction: an analysis and review of the literature, *J Emerg Med* 10:169–177, 1992.
8. Hollander JE, Hoffman RS, Burstein JL, et al: Cocaine-associated myocardial infarction. Mortality and complications. Cocaine-Associated Myocardial Infarction Study Group, *Arch Intern Med* 155:1081–1086, 1995.
9. Kontos MC, Jesse RL, Tatum JL, Ornato JP: Coronary angiographic findings in patients with cocaine-associated chest pain, *J Emerg Med* 24:9–13, 2003.
10. Anderson JL, Adams CD, Antman EM, et al: ACC/AHA 2007 guidelines for the management of patients with unstable angina/non–ST-elevation myocardial infarction: a report of the American College of Cardiology/American Heart Association Task Force on Practice Guidelines (Writing Committee to Revise the 2002 Guidelines for the Management of Patients With Unstable Angina/Non–ST-Elevation Myocardial Infarction): developed in collaboration with the American College of Emergency Physicians, American College of

Physicians, Society for Academic Emergency Medicine, Society for Cardiovascular Angiography and Interventions, and Society of Thoracic Surgeons, *J Am Coll Cardiol* 50:e1–e157, 2007.

11. Kawano H, Motoyama T, Yasue H, et al: Endothelial function fluctuates with diurnal variation in the frequency of ischemic episodes in patients with variant angina, *J Am Coll Cardiol* 40:266–270, 2002.

12. Phalen T, Aehlert B: The 12-Lead ECG. In *Acute coronary syndromes*, ed 3, St. Louis, 2012, Elsevier, pp 59–126.

13. Thygesen K, Alpert JS, White HD: Joint ESC/ACCF/AHA/WHF Task Force for the Redefinition of Myocardial Infarction. Universal definition of myocardial infarction, *J Am Coll Cardiol* 50:2173–2195, 2007.

14. Bolooki HM, Bajzer CT: Acute myocardial infarction. In *Cleveland Clinic: current clinical medicine*, Philadelphia, 2009, Elsevier, pp 58–65.

15. Antman EM, Anbe DT, Armstrong PW, et al: ACC/AHA guidelines for the management of patients with ST-elevation myocardial infarction: a report of the American College of Cardiology/American Heart Association Task Force on Practice Guidelines (Committee to Revise the 1999 Guidelines for the Management of Patients With Acute Myocardial Infarction). 2004. Available at www.acc.org/clinical/guidelines/stemi/index.pdf, *J Am Coll Cardiol* 44(3):E1–E211, 2004. Accessed August 29, 2011.

16. Gnecchi-Ruscone T, Piccaluga E, Guzzetti S, et al: Morning and Monday: critical periods for the onset of acute myocardial infarction. The GISSI 2 Study experience, *Eur Heart J* 15(7):882–887, 1994.

17. ISIS-2 (Second International Study of Infarct Survival) Collaborative Group: Morning peak in the incidence of myocardial infarction: experience in the ISIS-2 trial, *Eur Heart J* 13(5):594–598, 1992.

18. Tofler GH, Muller JE, Stone PH, et al: Modifiers of timing and possible triggers of acute myocardial infarction in the Thrombolysis in Myocardial Infarction Phase II (TIMI II) Study Group, *J Am Coll Cardiol* 20(5):1049–1055, 1992.

19. Behar S, Halabi M, Reicher-Reiss H, et al: Circadian variation and possible external triggers of onset of myocardial infarction. SPRINT Study Group, *Am J Med* 94(4):395–400, 1993.

20. Willich SN, Löwel H, Lewis M, et al: Weekly variation of acute myocardial infarction. Increased Monday risk in the working population, *Circulation* 90(1):87–93, 1994.

21. Sayer JW, Wilkinson P, Ranjadayalan K, et al: Attenuation or absence of circadian and seasonal rhythms of acute myocardial infarction, *Heart* 77(4):325–329, 1997.

22. Marchant B, Ranjadayalan K, Stevenson R, et al: Circadian and seasonal factors in the pathogenesis of acute myocardial infarction: the influence of environmental temperature, *Br Heart J* 69(5):385–387, 1993.

23. Tofler GH, Stone PH, Maclure M, et al: Analysis of possible triggers of acute myocardial infarction (the MILIS study), *Am J Cardiol* 66(1):22–27, 1990.

24. Culić V, Eterović D, Mirić D: Meta-analysis of possible external triggers of acute myocardial infarction, *Int J Cardiol* 99(1):1–8, 2005.

25. Harskamp RE: Acute respiratory tract infections: a potential trigger for the acute coronary syndrome, *Ann Med* 40(2):121–128, 2008.

26. Hammoudeh AJ, Alhaddad IA: Triggers and the onset of acute myocardial infarction, *Cardiol Rev* 17(6):270–274, 2009.

27. Servoss SJ: Triggers of acute coronary syndromes. *Prog Cardiovasc Dis* 44(5):369–380, 2002.

28. Antman EM, Braunwald E: ST-elevation myocardial infarction: pathology, pathophysiology, and clinical features. In Libby P, Bonow RO, Mann DL, et al, editors: *Braunwald's heart disease: a textbook of cardiovascular medicine*, ed 8, Philadelphia, 2007, Saunders, pp 1207–1232.

29. McSweeney JC, O'Sullivan P, Cleves MA, et al: Racial differences in women's prodromal and acute symptoms of myocardial infarction, *Am J Crit Care* 19(1):63–73, 2010.

30. Rautaharju PM, Surawicz B, Gettes LS: AHA/ACCF/HRS recommendations for the standardization and interpretation of the electrocardiogram: part IV: the ST segment, T and U waves, and the QT interval: a scientific statement from the American Heart Association Electrocardiography and Arrhythmias Committee, Council on Clinical Cardiology; the American College of Cardiology Foundation; and the Heart Rhythm Society, *J Am Coll Cardiol* 53:982–991, 2009.

31. Wagner GS, Macfarlane P, Wellens H, et al: AHA/ACCF/HRS recommendations for the standardization and interpretation of the electrocardiogram: part VI: acute ischemia/infarction: a scientific statement from the American Heart Association Electrocardiography and Arrhythmias Committee, Council on Clinical Cardiology; the American College of Cardiology Foundation; and the Heart Rhythm Society, *J Am Coll Cardiol* 53:1003–1011, 2009.

32. O'Connor RE, Brady W, Brooks SC, et al: Part 10: acute coronary syndromes: 2010 American Heart Association guidelines for cardiopulmonary resuscitation and emergency cardiovascular care, *Circulation* 122(Suppl 3):S787–S817, 2010.

33. Aehlert B: *ECGs Made Easy*, ed 4, St. Louis, 2011, Mosby.

34. Nair R, Glancy DL: ECG discrimination between right and left circumflex coronary arterial occlusion in patients with acute inferior myocardial infarction: value of old criteria and use of lead aVR, *Chest* 122(1):134–139, 2002.

35. Chia BL, Yip JW, Tan HC, Lim YT: Usefulness of ST elevation II/III ratio and ST deviation in lead I for identifying the culprit artery in inferior wall acute myocardial infarction, *Am J Cardiol* 86(3):341–343, 2000.

36. Anderson JL: ST segment elevation acute myocardial infarction and complications of myocardial infarction. In Goldman L, Ausiello D, editors: *Cecil medicine*, ed 23, Philadelphia, 2007, Saunders.

37. Hollander JE, Levitt MA, Young GP, et al: Effect of recent cocaine use on the specificity of cardiac markers for diagnosis of acute myocardial infarction, *Am Heart J* 135(pt 1):245–252, 1998.

38. Drew BJ, Califf RM, Funk M, et al: Practice standards for electrocardiographic monitoring in hospital settings: an American Heart Association scientific statement from the Councils on Cardiovascular Nursing, Clinical Cardiology, and Cardiovascular Disease in the Young: endorsed by the International Society of Computerized Electrocardiology and the American Association of Critical-Care Nurses [published correction appears in Circulation, 2005;111(3):378], *Circulation* 110(17):2721–2746, 2004.

39. Meine TJ, Roe MT, Chen AY, et al: Association of intravenous morphine use and outcomes in acute coronary syndromes: results from the CRUSADE quality improvement initiative, *Am Heart J* 149:1043–1049, 2005.

40. Chen ZM, Pan HC, Chen YP, et al: Early intravenous then oral metoprolol in 45,852 patients with acute myocardial infarction: randomized placebo-controlled trial, *Lancet* 366:1622–1632, 2005.

41. O'Connor RE, Bossaert L, Arntz H-R, et al; on behalf of the Acute Coronary Syndrome Chapter Collaborators. Part 9: acute coronary syndromes: 2010 international consensus on cardiopulmonary resuscitation and emergency cardiovascular care science with treatment recommendations, *Circulation* 122(Suppl 2):S422–S465, 2010.

42. Innes GD, Zed PJ: Basic pharmacology and advances in emergency medicine, *Emerg Med Clin N Am* 23:433–465, 2005.

43. Antman EM, Hand M, Armstrong PW, et al; 2004 Writing Committee Members, Anbe DT, Kushner FG, Ornato JP, et al: 2007 Focused update of the ACC/AHA 2004 guidelines for the management of patients with ST-elevation myocardial infarction: a report of the American College of Cardiology/American Heart Association Task Force on Practice Guidelines: developed in collaboration with the Canadian Cardiovascular Society endorsed by the American Academy of Family Physicians: 2007 Writing Group to Review New Evidence and Update the ACC/AHA 2004 Guidelines for the Management of Patients With ST-Elevation Myocardial Infarction, Writing on behalf of the 2004 Writing Committee, *Circulation* 117(2):296–329, 2008 Jan 15. Epub 2007 Dec 10.

44. Kushner FG, Hand M, Smith SC Jr, et al: 2009 focused updates: ACC/AHA guidelines for the management of patients with ST-elevation myocardial infarction (updating the 2004 guideline and 2007 focused update) and ACC/AHA/SCAI guidelines on percutaneous coronary intervention (updating the 2005 guideline and 2007 focused update): a report of the American College of Cardiology Foundation/American Heart Association Task Force on Practice Guidelines, *J Am Coll Cardiol* 54:2205–2241, 2009.

45. O'Donoghue M, Boden WE, Braunwald E, et al: Early invasive vs conservative treatment strategies in women and men with unstable angina and non-ST-segment elevation myocardial infarction: a meta-analysis, *JAMA* 300(1):71–80, 2008.

46. Faxon DP: Development of systems of care for ST-elevation myocardial infarction patients: current state of ST-elevation myocardial infarction care, *Circulation* 116(2):e29–e32. Epub 2007 May 30, 2007.

47. Desai ND, Fremes SE: Radial artery conduit for coronary revascularization: as good as an internal thoracic artery? *Curr Opin Cardiol* 22(6):534–540, 2007.

48. Jorapur V, Cano-Gomez A, Conde CA: Should saphenous vein grafts be the conduits of last resort for coronary artery bypass surgery? *Cardiol Rev* 17(5):235–242, 2009.

49. Brener SJ, Tschopp D: Complications of acute myocardial infarction. In *Cleveland Clinic: current clinical medicine*, Philadelphia, 2009, Elsevier, pp 103–111.

50. Glower DD, Lowe JE: Left ventricular aneurysm. In Cohn LH, Edmunds LH Jr, editors: *Cardiac surgery in the adult*, New York, 2003, McGraw-Hill, pp 771–788.

51. Ba'albaki HA, Clements SD Jr: Left ventricular aneurysm: a review, *Clin Cardiol* 12:5–13, 1989.

52. Urden LD, Stacy KM, Lough ME: Cardiovascular disorders. In *Critical care nursing: diagnosis and management*, 6th ed, St. Louis, 2009, Mosby, pp 426–494.

53. Voci P, Bilotta F, Caretta Q, et al: Papillary muscle perfusion pattern. A hypothesis for ischemic papillary muscle dysfunction, *Circulation* 91:1714–1718, 1995.

54. Aehlert B: *Paramedic practice today*, St. Louis, 2010, Mosby.

55. Hochman JS, Sleeper LA, Godfrey E, et al: Should we emergently revascularize occluded coronaries for cardiogenic shock: an international randomized trial of emergency PTCA/CABG-trial design. The SHOCK Trial Study Group, *Am Heart J* 137:313–321, 1999.

56. The PURSUIT Trial Investigators: Inhibition of platelet glycoprotein IIb/IIIa with eptifibatide in patients with acute coronary syndromes. Platelet Glycoprotein IIb/IIIa in Unstable Angina: Receptor Suppression Using Integrilin Therapy, *N Engl J Med* 339:436–443, 1998.

57. Holmes DR Jr, Berger PB, Hochman JS, et al: Cardiogenic shock in patients with acute ischemic syndromes with and without ST segment elevation, *Circulation* 100:2067–2073, 1999.

58. Jacob R, Grimm RA: Pericardial disease. In *Cleveland Clinic: current clinical medicine*, Philadelphia, 2009, Elsevier, pp 171–179.

59. Little WC, Freeman GL: Pericardial disease, *Circulation* 113:1622–1632, 2006.

Acute Stroke

Upon completion of this chapter, you will be able to:

1. Describe the two major types of stroke.
2. Describe the initial emergency care for acute ischemic stroke.

INTRODUCTION

A **stroke** is a sudden change in neurologic function caused by a change in cerebral blood flow. A stroke is also called a *brain attack*. The public is familiar with the phrase *heart attack*. Because a stroke happens in the brain rather than in the heart, the phrase *brain attack* may convey the events involved in a stroke more clearly to the public than the word *stroke*. The term *brain attack* and its application to stroke are credited to Vladimir C. Hachinski, M.D., and John Norris, M.D., neurologists from Canada. The National Stroke Association (NSA) began using the term in 1990. The term **cerebrovascular accident**, a term that was used for many years as a synonym for stroke, has lost favor because strokes are not really accidents.[1]

In this chapter, stroke types, assessment findings and symptoms, and initial emergency care for acute ischemic stroke are discussed.

STROKE FACTS

- Of the 795,000 strokes that occur in the United States each year, about 610,000 of these are first attacks, and 185,000 are recurrent attacks.
- Stroke is the third leading cause of death in the United States, after heart disease and cancer.
- Stroke is a leading cause of long-term disability in the United States.
- Stroke kills more than twice as many American women every year as breast cancer.

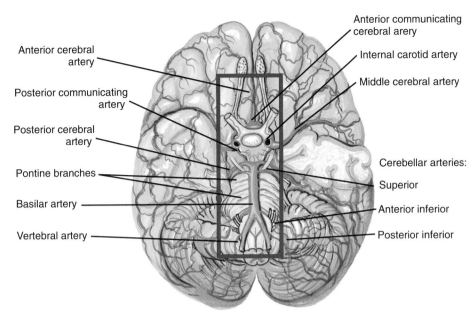

Figure 6-1 Arterial blood supply to the brain.

Deaths from stroke can be reduced or delayed by preventing and controlling risk factors. Nonmodifiable risk factors for stroke include older age, family history of stroke or cardiovascular disease, male gender, and ethnicity (higher rates are seen in African Americans compared with whites). Modifiable risk factors include alcohol consumption, asymptomatic carotid bruit/stenosis, cardiac disease, cigarette smoking, diabetes mellitus, dyslipidemia, hypercoagulopathy, hypertension, illicit drug use, increased fibrinogen, obesity, oral contraceptive use, prior history of stroke, and transient ischemic attacks. Other factors may affect the risk of stroke. Because stroke deaths tend to occur more often during extremely hot or cold weather, season and climate may increase the risk of stroke. People of lower income and educational levels may also be at increased risk for stroke.

Classification of Stroke by Anatomic Location

Eighty percent of blood flow to the brain is supplied by the carotid arteries. Twenty percent is supplied through the vertebrobasilar system (Figure 6-1). Strokes involving the carotid arteries are called *anterior circulation strokes* or *carotid territory strokes*. They usually involve the cerebral hemispheres. Strokes affecting the vertebrobasilar arteries are called *posterior circulation strokes* or *vertebrobasilar territory strokes*. They usually affect the brain stem or cerebellum. Approximately 75% to 80% of ischemic strokes occur in the carotid (or anterior) circulation and 20% to 25% occur in the vertebrobasilar (or posterior) circulation.[3] Signs and symptoms of stroke are shown in Table 6-1.

ISCHEMIC AND HEMORRHAGIC STROKE

[Objective 1]
There are two major types of stroke: ischemic and hemorrhagic. An ischemic stroke occurs when a blood vessel supplying the brain is blocked. It can be life-threatening, but rarely leads to death within the first hour. A hemorrhagic stroke occurs when a cerebral artery bursts. It can be fatal at onset.

Ischemic Stroke

Of the approximately 795,000 strokes that occur each year, about 87% are ischemic, 10% are intracerebral hemorrhage, and 3% are subarachnoid hemorrhage.[2,4] About 8% to 12% of ischemic strokes result in death within 30 days.[3]

There are two types of ischemic strokes: thrombotic and embolic. It is estimated that about 45% of ischemic strokes are caused by a small (~25%) or large artery (~20%) thrombus, about 20% are embolic in origin (most often from atrial fibrillation),[5] and about 30% have an unknown cause.[6]

Table 6-1	Signs and Symptoms of Stroke	
Affected Artery	**Structures Supplied by Affected Vessel**	**Signs and Symptoms of Blockage**
Anterior cerebral	Supplies medial surfaces and upper portions of frontal and parietal lobes	Confusion Contralateral motor or sensory loss in leg greater than arm Loss of coordination Personality changes, emotional lability Urinary incontinence Weakness, numbness on affected side
Middle cerebral (most commonly blocked vessel in stroke)	Supplies a portion of the frontal lobe, lateral surface of the temporal and parietal lobes, including the primary motor and sensory areas of the face, throat, hand, and arm and in the dominant hemisphere, the areas for speech	Altered level of responsiveness Contralateral motor loss in lower face Contralateral motor or sensory loss (arm greater than leg) Contralateral visual field deficits Language deficit (dominant hemisphere) Spatial-perceptual deficit (nondominant hemisphere)
Posterior cerebral	Supplies medial and inferior temporal lobes, medial occipital lobe, thalamus, posterior hypothalamus, visual receptive area	Contralateral sensory impairment or loss Cortical blindness from ischemia Ipsilateral visual field deficits
Internal carotid	Supplies cerebral hemispheres and diencephalon	Altered level of responsiveness Bruits over the carotid artery Headaches Ipsilateral blindness Profound aphasia Ptosis Weakness, paralysis, numbness, sensory changes, and visual deficits (blurring) on the affected side
Vertebral or basilar	Supplies brainstem and cerebellum	*Incomplete blockage* Dysarthria Dysphagia Headache "Locked-in" syndrome—no movement except eyelids; sensation and consciousness preserved Nausea, vertigo, tinnitus Numbness Transient ischemic attacks Unilateral and bilateral weakness of extremities Visual deficits on affected side (diplopia, color blindness, lack of depth perception) *Complete blockage* Coma Extension (decerebrate) posturing Respiratory and circulatory abnormalities

A thrombotic stroke is the most common cause of stroke (Figure 6-2). In a thrombotic stroke, atherosclerosis of large vessels in the brain causes progressive narrowing and platelet clumping. Platelet clumping results in the development of blood clots within the brain artery itself (i.e., cerebral thrombosis). When the blood clots are of sufficient size to block blood flow through the artery, the area that was previously supplied by that artery becomes ischemic. Ischemia occurs because the tissue supplied by the blocked artery does not receive oxygen and the essential nutrients needed for normal brain function. The patient's signs and symptoms depend on the location of the artery affected and the areas of brain ischemia.

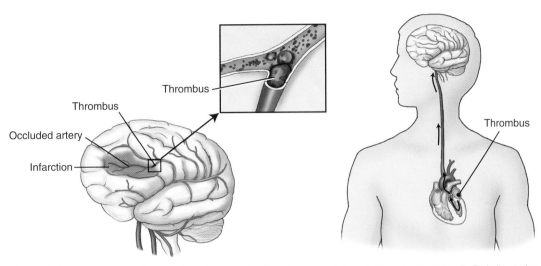

Figure 6-2 An ischemic stroke may occur because of a thrombus or embolus. **A,** Thrombotic stroke. **B,** Embolic stroke.

> **ACLS Pearl**
> About 5% of patients with acute ischemic stroke present with a seizure, and up to 30% have a headache.[7]

In an embolic stroke, material from an area outside the brain (e.g., heart, aorta, other major artery) becomes dislodged and travels through the bloodstream to the brain (i.e., cerebral embolism). Embolic material may consist of fragments of valves, tumors, or plaques; air; fat; amniotic fluid; a foreign body; or a blood clot. An embolus tends to become lodged where arteries branch because blood flow is most turbulent in these areas. Fragments of the embolus may become lodged in smaller vessels. As with thrombotic strokes, the patient's signs and symptoms depend on the location of the artery affected and the areas of brain ischemia.

> **ACLS Pearl**
> Similar to acute cardiac events, the time of onset of an ischemic stroke has also been shown to have a dominant peak between 6 am to noon. Even when accounting for stroke patients awakening with symptoms, when the time of onset may not be known, more than 50% of strokes in one study[8] and 38% in another[9] were thought to have had their onset between 6 am and noon.[10]

Evolution of an Ischemic Stroke

Complete blockage of an artery may lead to death of an area of cells in the brain because blood flow is obstructed (ischemic infarction). The evolution of the thrombosis may take place in a few minutes, hours, or even days. Large blood vessels, such as the carotid, middle cerebral, and basilar arteries, can take longer to become blocked than smaller vessels.

In an ischemic stroke, there are two main areas of injury (Figure 6-3). The first area is the zone of ischemia. Because of the blockage in the artery, there is little blood flow through this area. As a result, brain tissue previously supplied by the blocked vessel is deprived of oxygen, glucose, and other essential nutrients. Unless blood flow is quickly restored, nerve cells and other supporting nervous system cells will be irreversibly damaged or die (i.e., infarct) within a few minutes of the blockage.

Brain damage may occur because of the infarction as well as an excessive buildup of fluid in the brain (cerebral edema). As brain tissue dies, fluid begins to build up, resulting in swelling. Because the skull is a rigid container, as swelling increases, nearby brain tissue (nerve cells, nerve tracts, and cerebral arteries) is compressed, and intracranial pressure (ICP) increases. A sustained increase in pressure causes continued ischemia, irreparable damage to brain cells, and potentially death. Cerebral edema usually peaks 2 to 5 days after the onset of the stroke. The fluid buildup then stabilizes and may begin to decrease.

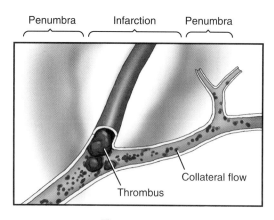
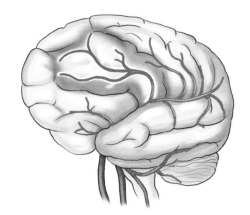

Figure 6-3 Ischemic stroke. Zone of ischemia and the ischemic penumbra.

The second area of injury is called the **ischemic penumbra** or the **transitional zone**. The penumbra is a rim of brain tissue that surrounds the zone of ischemia. It is supplied with blood by collateral arteries that connect with branches of the blocked vessel. The size of the penumbra depends on the number and patency of the collateral arteries. Blood flow to brain tissue in this area is decreased to between 20% and 50% of normal, but not absent. Brain tissue in the penumbra is "stunned" but not yet irreversibly damaged. Because the collateral blood supply is not enough to maintain the brain's demand for oxygen and glucose indefinitely, brain cells in the penumbra may live or die depending on how quickly blood flow is restored during the early hours of a stroke. Many acute stroke therapies are targeted toward restoring flow or function to the ischemic penumbra.[11]

A patient may experience warning signs of impending stroke. A transient ischemic attack (TIA) is one of the most important warning signs. A **transient ischemic attack** has been traditionally defined as a neurologic deficit caused by focal brain ischemia that completely resolves within 24 hours. Most TIAs last only about 5 to 20 minutes.[3] This definition has been changed to "a brief episode of neurologic dysfunction caused by focal brain or retinal ischemia, with clinical symptoms typically lasting less than one hour, and without evidence of acute infarction."[12] This definition is tissue based rather than time based because some patients with traditionally defined transient ischemic attacks have, in fact, had a stroke.[12] Some studies have shown positive magnetic resonance imaging (MRI) findings of stroke in up to two thirds of patients with a clinical transient ischemic attack diagnosis. The longer the duration of symptoms, the more likely that the MRI result will be positive.[12] A TIA should be treated with the same urgency as a completed stroke.

> **ACLS Pearl**
> When obtaining the patient's medical history, be sure to ask about previous TIAs and their frequency.

Reperfusion Therapy

The time from the onset of stroke symptoms to treatment is a key factor to the success of any therapy. The earlier the treatment for stroke is given, the more favorable the results are likely to be. Blood flow needs to be restored to the affected area as quickly as possible. In acute stroke management, the phrase **time is brain** reflects the need for rapid assessment and intervention because delays in diagnosis and treatment may leave the patient neurologically impaired and disabled.[13]

Intravenous administration of a recombinant form of tissue plasminogen activator (rtPA) has proved to be an effective cerebral reperfusion therapy. Since 1996, the window of opportunity for the use of intravenous rtPA for the treatment of ischemic stroke patients has been within 3 hours of symptom onset. This has required that patients be at a hospital within 60 minutes of symptom onset to be evaluated and receive treatment. Unfortunately, delay in seeking treatment is a common reason for ineligibility for rtPA. Patients not directly seeking medical attention and waiting to see if their symptoms would improve; delays in transfer to a hospital capable of treating the patient; and indeterminate time of symptom onset are among the reasons for treatment delays, precluding the use of rtPA.[14,15] The designation of a longer time window for treatment is one of the potential approaches that have been proposed to increase patient treatment opportunities.

 YOU SHOULD KNOW Although rtPA may be used for eligible patients with myocardial infarction (MI) and acute ischemic stroke, the dosing regimen of rtPA for MI and stroke patients differs. The dose used for acute ischemic stroke is less than the dose recommended for use in MI (or pulmonary embolism) treatment.

Hemorrhagic Stroke

A hemorrhagic stroke is caused by either rupture of an artery with bleeding into the spaces surrounding the brain (i.e., subarachnoid hemorrhage) or bleeding into the brain tissue (i.e., intracerebral hemorrhage) (Figure 6-4). Hemorrhagic strokes can occur in patients of any age. When they occur in young patients, they generally are caused by the rupture of an aneurysm or an arteriovenous malformation. Rarely do these patients have a history of hypertension.

Subarachnoid Hemorrhage

Subarachnoid hemorrhage (SAH) accounts for about 3% of all strokes.[4] A ruptured cerebral aneurysm is the most common cause of SAH. Patients often report a sudden onset "thunderclap" headache or describe the feeling as "the worst headache of my life." Assessment findings and symptoms may quickly progress to forceful vomiting (often without nausea), neurologic deficits, and visual disturbances (e.g., blurry or double vision), unconsciousness, and seizures. The patient also may show signs and symptoms of rising intracranial pressure, such as unilateral pupil dilation, nausea, vomiting, and vital sign changes.

Initial mortality is high and rebleeding is common. Mortality from rebleeding is also high. Rebleeding most commonly occurs during the first day, usually within 12 hours of the initial hemorrhage.

Intracerebral hemorrhage

Intracerebral hemorrhage (ICH) accounts for about 10% of all strokes.[4] Most intracerebral hemorrhages are associated with chronic hypertension, but other common causes and risk factors include bleeding disorders, African-American ethnicity, advanced age, vascular malformations, excessive use/abuse of alcohol, and liver dysfunction.[16] This type of stroke may require neurosurgery.

 YOU SHOULD KNOW Stroke care consists of two phases.[16] Phase 1 (emergency or hyperacute phase) encompasses the first 3 to 24 hours after stroke onset and includes prehospital and emergency department care. During this phase, attention is focused on identifying stroke symptoms and location of the infarction, evaluating the patient's risk for acute and long-term complications, and identifying treatment options. Phase 2 (acute care) encompasses the period 24 to 72 hours after stroke onset. This phase focuses on confirming the cause of stroke and preventing medical complications, preparing the patient and family for discharge, and establishing long-term secondary prevention measures.

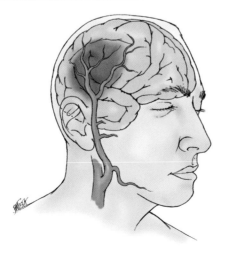

Figure 6-4 Hemorrhagic stroke.

STROKE CHAIN OF SURVIVAL

[Objective 2]

Like the Chain of Survival used to describe the sequence of events needed to survive sudden cardiac death, the Chain of Recovery is a metaphor for the series of events that must occur during the emergency care of the possible stroke patient to optimize his or her chances of full recovery. The critical links in the chain include:[17]

1. Identification of stroke signs and symptoms by the patient or bystanders
2. Immediate Emergency Medical System (EMS) activation and appropriate dispatch with prearrival instructions
3. Rapid EMS response, assessment, evacuation, and appropriate prehospital care
4. Forewarning of the receiving stroke center for resource preparation and mobilization
5. Rapid definitive diagnosis by experienced specialists at a stroke center

The Chain of Recovery has been modified in American Heart Association publications and is called the "Stroke Chain of Survival."[18,19] The chain consists of eight links, which are also referred to as the "Ds of stroke care": detection, dispatch, delivery, door, data, decision, drug, and disposition.[20]

Detection

The first link in the chain is *detection* of the onset of stroke signs and symptoms. Recognition of stroke signs and symptoms by the patient, family, or bystanders is critical. Patients and their families should be taught to consider the possibility of a stroke if any of the following signs and symptoms occur: sudden behavior changes or confusion; altered mental status; difficulty speaking (e.g., an inability to say what is meant, slurred speech); difficulty walking or maintaining balance; sudden weakness or numbness of the face, arm, or leg (particularly on one side of the body); facial droop; sudden visual changes in one or both eyes; difficulty swallowing; or a sudden severe headache with no known cause.

Dispatch

The second link in the chain is *dispatch* through activation of the EMS system, priority EMS dispatch, and prompt EMS response. Stroke victims and their families must be taught to activate the EMS system immediately upon recognition of stroke signs and symptoms. It is estimated that 29% to 65% of patients with signs or symptoms of acute stroke access their initial medical care using local EMS personnel.[14]

Delivery

Delivery (prompt transport of the patient to an appropriate receiving facility while providing appropriate prehospital assessment and care as well as prearrival notification) is the third link in the chain. Prehospital professionals should quickly perform a primary survey and stabilize the patient's airway, breathing, and circulation as necessary.

Obtain an accurate history and determine the patient's normal baseline mental status. Ask the patient (ideally), patient's family, or bystanders when the patient was last known to be symptom-free (i.e., last known well time). Determining and documenting the time of symptom onset is critical and the single most important determinant of treatment options during the hyperacute phase of stroke care (Box 6-1).[16] Perform a neurologic evaluation using the Cincinnati Prehospital Stroke Scale (CPSS) (Box 6-2) or with another validated evaluation tool. The CPSS is taught as the three Ds of "**d**rift (arm), **d**roop (facial weakness), and **d**ysarthria (slurred speech)," as well as using the acronym "FAST" for **f**acial droop, **a**rm drift, **s**peech (dysarthria and aphasia), and **t**ime of onset .[13,21]

If the patient's assessment findings and symptoms suggest an acute stroke, **immediately** *begin transport as soon as the patient's condition is assessed as stable*[16] (i.e., load and go) to the closest appropriate facility capable of treating acute stroke and notify the receiving facility that the patient is en route. Perform a focused or detailed physical examination during transport as dictated by the patient's condition.

Monitor the patient's breathing effort and be prepared to assist ventilations. Apply a pulse oximeter and a cardiac monitor. Give oxygen if the patient is hypoxemic (SpO_2 below 94%) or if the patient's oxygen saturation is unknown.[20] Obtain a 12-lead electrocardiogram (ECG) to establish a baseline.

BOX 6-1	Determining the Time of Symptom Onset

"For the purposes of treatment, the onset is assumed as the time that the patient was last known to be symptom-free. Because ischemic stroke is often painless, most patients are not awakened by its occurrence. Thus, for a patient with symptoms of stroke on awakening, the time of onset is assumed to be the time the patient was last known to be symptom-free before retiring. If a patient had mild impairments but then had worsening over the subsequent hours, the time the first symptom began is assumed to be the time of onset. In contrast, if a patient has symptoms that completely resolved (TIA) and then has a second event, the time of onset of the new symptoms is used."[22]

BOX 6-2	Cincinnati Prehospital Stroke Scale[23]

Facial droop/weakness: Ask patient to "Show me your teeth" or "Smile for me"
- Normal: Both sides of face move equally well
- Abnormal: One side of face does not move as well as the other

Motor weakness (arm drift): With eyes closed, ask patient to extend arms out in front of him or her 90 degrees (if sitting) or 45 degrees (if supine). Drift is scored if the arm falls before 10 seconds.
- Normal: Both arms move the same OR both arms do not move at all
- Abnormal: One arm either does not move OR one arm drifts down compared to the other

Aphasia (speech): Ask the patient to say "A rolling stone gathers no moss," "You can't teach an old dog new tricks," "The sky is blue in Cincinnati," or a similar phrase
- Normal: Phrase is repeated clearly and correctly with no slurring
- Abnormal: Patient uses inappropriate words, words are slurred, or the patient is unable to speak

Check the patient's serum glucose level; this helps to differentiate stroke from other common causes of stroke symptoms (e.g., hypoglycemia). Establish IV access with a saline lock or an IV line containing normal saline or lactated Ringer's solution and run it at a keep-open rate (i.e., 30 mL/hr) or per physician instructions. Avoid glucose-containing fluids unless the patient is hypoglycemic. Do not delay transport to perform these procedures. Unless contraindicated (e.g., hypotension), the patient should be transported with the head of the stretcher elevated 30 degrees. This position may help with oxygenation and may reduce the risk of aspiration.

Assess and support the patient's vital signs. Vital signs should be monitored at least every 15 minutes and more frequently if any vital sign is abnormal. In general, hypertension should not be treated in the prehospital setting. Hypotension should be treated in accordance with the underlying cause of the hypotension.

ACLS Pearl

Be familiar with the categorization/designation of hospitals in your area. Transport of the acute stroke patient to a receiving center where screening procedures such as computed tomography, angiography, endovascular techniques, and intra-arterial fibrinolytic therapy are available (such as a designated stroke center) is essential. The center should be notified of the patient's impending arrival.

Use a Prehospital Stroke Alert Checklist to screen patients for stroke signs and symptoms, time of onset, and contraindications to fibrinolytic therapy or other therapies that may become available. Any information obtained should be relayed to the receiving facility. Collect and document all medications. Medications that are particularly important include aspirin, warfarin (Coumadin), insulin, and antihypertensives.

Encourage family members or bystanders to accompany the patient to the hospital so they can provide historical information to the treating team and provide support to the patient. Although the family's support is always important, it is particularly important for the acute ischemic stroke patient who presents within the time frame for rtPA administration and whose language or decision-making capability is compromised. If the patient's family cannot go to the hospital, obtain a telephone number where they can be contacted and be certain to document this information for subsequent retrieval by other members of the health care team.

Because strokes are dynamic processes, reassess the patient often during transport. Document any changes in the patient's presentation from your initial assessment findings and relay this information to the appropriate receiving facility staff on arrival at the receiving facility.

Door

The fourth link in the chain is *door* (immediate emergency department triage). Hospital emergency departments that accept stroke patients from EMS professionals should have the necessary personnel and procedures in place (e.g., a stroke team) to rapidly assess and treat stroke patients. The National Institute of Neurological Disorders and Stroke (NINDS) has established recommended target times for hospitals that receive acute stroke patients: (1) Emergency department physician evaluation within 10 minutes of arrival; (2) stroke team notification within 15 minutes of arrival; (3) brain computed tomography (CT) scan within 25 minutes of arrival and interpretation within 45 minutes of arrival; (4) if indicated, door-to-drug/intervention time of less than 60 minutes from arrival in the emergency department for at least 80% of patients; (5) door to neurosurgical availability (on-site or by transport) of 2 hours or less; and (6) door to admission to monitored bed of 3 hours or less.[24] Recognizing that the door-to-drug time may need to be shortened to successfully begin fibrinolytic therapy within 3 hours of stroke onset in some cases, specific patients who meet eligibility criteria may be treated between a 3- and 4.5-hour window after the onset of stroke symptoms (discussed later in this chapter).[16] The American Heart Association's goals for management of patients with suspected stroke are shown in Figure 6-5.

Proper triage of stroke patients requires that emergency nurses be familiar with both typical and unusual stroke presentations.[16] Within minutes of the patient's arrival, reassess the patient's airway, breathing, and circulation (ABCs) and ensure that the patient has a secure airway and adequate breathing. Apply a pulse oximeter and check the patient's oxygen saturation level. Oxygen should be given to those patients who are hypoxemic (i.e., an SpO_2 of less than 94%) or if the patient's oxygen saturation level is unknown.[20] All patients with suspected acute stroke should receive continuous ECG monitoring to detect myocardial ischemia and cardiac dysrhythmias (e.g., atrial fibrillation). Cardiac monitoring is recommended for 24 to 48 hours in stroke patients who do not receive fibrinolytic therapy and for up to 72 hours or more for patients who do receive fibrinolytics.[16]

Diagnostic laboratory tests including serum glucose, complete blood count (including platelet count), electrolytes, cardiac biomarkers, renal function, prothrombin and partial thromboplastin times, should be drawn immediately and before IV fluids are started.[14] Three IV lines should be established if it is anticipated that the patient will received fibrinolytic therapy. One site is used for IV fluid administration, another for fibrinolytic administration, and the third for giving IV medications.[14] Avoid hypotonic solutions because they can contribute to worsening cerebral edema and increased intracranial pressure.[25,26] Check the patient's blood sugar and give dextrose if the patient is hypoglycemic. Administration of insulin is recommended if the patient's serum glucose level is more than 185 mg/dL in a patient with acute stroke.[20]

Verify the time of symptom onset. When was the last time the patient was known to be without symptoms? Was anyone with the patient when his or her symptoms started? What was the patient doing when the symptoms began? Did the patient complain of a headache? Did he or she have a seizure? Has there been a change in his or her level of responsiveness? Is there a history of any recent trauma? Review the patient's past medical history and determine the presence of stroke risk factors. Find out the medications the patient is currently taking (including anticoagulation therapy) and the patient's allergies to medications.

Perform a general neurologic screening assessment and alert the stroke team (if not already done). Scales are used in order to give quantifiable information to other members of the stroke team. Use the Glasgow Coma Scale (GCS) to determine the patient's level of responsiveness (Table 6-2). The GCS measures impairment but is of limited use in a patient who is intubated, a patient with orbital trauma, or a patient with previous neurologic impairment. Use the National Institutes of Health Stroke Scale (NIHSS) to localize the stroke lesion, determine the stroke's severity, and assessing neurologic outcome and degree of recovery (Table 6-3). The NIHSS is an 11-item, 42-point scale that assesses the patient's level of alertness and comprehension as well as motor, sensory, visual, and language function; it usually

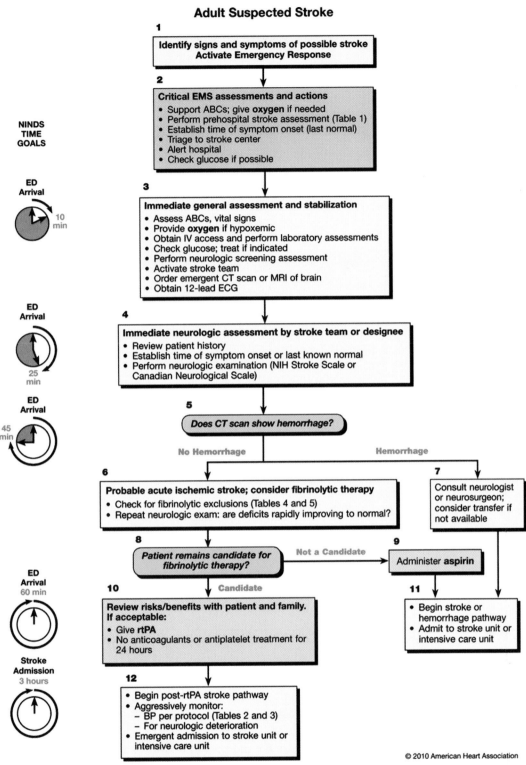

Figure 6-5 The American Heart Association's goals for management of patients with suspected stroke. ABCs, airway, breathing, circulation; BP, blood pressure; CT, computed tomography; ECG, electrocardiogram; ED, emergency department; MRI, magnetic resonance imaging; NIH, National Institutes of Health; NINDS, National Institute of Neurological Disorders and Stroke; rtPA, recombinant form of tissue plasminogen activator.

Table 6-2 Glasgow Coma Scale

Eye Opening	E-Score
Spontaneous	4
To speech	3
To pain	2
No response	1

Best Verbal Response	V-Score
Oriented	5
Confused	4
Inappropriate	3
Incomprehensible	2
No response	1

Best Motor Response	M-Score
Obeys commands	6
Localizes pain	5
Withdrawal	4
Abnormal flexion	3
Extension	2
No response	1
Score: E + V + M	15

BOX 6-3 Conditions that Mimic Stroke

- Bell's palsy
- Brain tumors
- Complicated migraine
- Concussion with head injury
- Conversion disorder
- Drug overdose
- Eclampsia
- Encephalopathies, encephalitis, meningitis
- Hypoglycemia
- Hyponatremia
- Seizures
- Subdural hematoma

is performed by stroke specialists. Initial treatment should not be delayed by using this scale. The NIHSS is performed before and after fibrinolytic administration and again at hospital discharge. Use of this scale allows a standardized way to assess outcome and compare outcomes with other centers.

 YOU SHOULD KNOW Assessment of the acute stroke patient may be enhanced by using the Miami Emergency Neurological Deficit (MEND) examination, which incorporates both the NIHSS and CPSS. Prehospital professionals are encouraged to use the CPSS when assessing "D" in the primary survey and then using the MEND examination when en route with the patient (but *not* on scene). The MEND examination is routinely used for neurologic assessment by hospital nursing personnel for patients with focal deficits.

When performing a physical exam, consider the presence of conditions that mimic stroke (Box 6-3). Obtain vital signs at least every 30 minutes while the patient is in the emergency department and more frequently if any vital sign is abnormal. Assess the patient's blood pressure (BP) in both upper extremities. BP elevation is common during the acute phase of stroke and may be a compensatory mechanism for reduced blood flow in the ischemic penumbra. A systolic BP greater than 185 mm Hg or a diastolic BP greater than 110 mm Hg is a contraindication to IV administration of rtPA. The American Heart Association Stroke Council recommends withholding antihypertensive agents unless the systolic BP is greater than 220 mm Hg or the diastolic BP is greater than 120 mm Hg in an acute ischemic stroke patient who is not treated with fibrinolytics.[14] If the lowering of BP is indicated, it should be instituted cautiously to avoid hypotension. Any treatment given should be based on multiple BP measurements taken at least 5 minutes apart.

Table 6-3 National Institutes of Health Stroke Scale

Item #	Category	Description	Score
1A	Level of consciousness (patients who score 2 or 3 on this item should be assessed using the Glasgow Coma Scale)	Alert Not alert (arousable—minor stimulation) Not alert (arousable—painful stimulation Unresponsive	0 1 2 3
1B	Orientation questions (two)–Ask patient month and age	Answers both correctly Answers one correctly Answers neither correctly	0 1 2
1C	Response to commands (two)–Ask patient to open/close eyes; make fist, release fist	Performs both tasks correctly Performs one task correctly Performs neither correctly	0 1 2
2	Best gaze–Look at position of eyes at rest, then ask patient to look to the left or right	Normal horizontal movements Partial gaze palsy Complete gaze palsy	0 1 2
3	Visual fields–Test by asking patient to count fingers in all four quadrants	No visual field defect Partial hemianopia Complete hemianopia Bilateral hemianopia	0 1 2 3
4	Facial movement–Ask patient to grimace or smile, puff out cheeks, pucker, and squeeze eyes shut	Normal Minor facial weakness/paralysis Partial facial weakness/paralysis Complete unilateral palsy	0 1 2 3
5	Motor function–Raise arm palm down to 90 degrees (sitting) or 45 degrees (supine) and score drift/movement a. Left arm b. Right arm	No drift–holds for full 10 seconds Drift before 5 seconds Falls before 10 seconds No effort against gravity No movement Not tested (amputation, joint fusion)	0 1 2 3 4 UN
6	Motor function–Raise leg to 30 degrees and score drift/movement a. Left leg b. Right leg	No drift–holds for full 5 seconds Drift before 5 seconds Falls before 5 seconds No effort against gravity No movement Not tested (amputation, joint fusion)	0 1 2 3 4 UN
7	Limb ataxia–Finger-to-nose and heel-to-shin tests	No ataxia Ataxia in one limb Ataxia in two limbs	0 1 2
8	Sensory–Pinprick to face, arm, trunk, leg–compare side to side	No sensory loss Mild sensory loss Severe sensory loss	0 1 2
9	Language–Name groups of objects, read short sentences, describe a picture	Normal Mild aphasia Severe aphasia Mute or global aphasia	0 1 2 3
10	Articulation (speech clarity)–Ask patient to read words or repeat a phrase	Normal Mild dysarthria Severe dysarthria	0 1 2
11	Extinction and inattention (neglect)–Ask patient to describe features on right and left sides of a picture	Absent/no neglect Partial neglect (mild; 1 sensory modality) Complete neglect (severe; 2 sensory modalities)	0 1 2
		Total:	

Note: The full NIH Stroke Scale is available at www.ninds.nih.gov/doctors/NIH_Stroke_Scale.pdf.

A noncontrast brain computed tomography (CT) scan or brain MRI scan should be obtained for all patients with suspected acute ischemic stroke. Additional diagnostic studies should be obtained in selected cases such as pregnancy testing, blood alcohol level, urine or blood toxicology screen (for patients with possible substance abuse), liver function tests and ammonia level (for patients with an unexplained altered level of consciousness),[26] lumbar puncture (for suspected meningitis or if subarachnoid hemorrhage is suspected and CT is negative for blood), electroencephalogram (for suspected seizures), and arterial blood gas tests (for suspected hypoxia).[14] A 12-lead ECG should be obtained to evaluate for preexisting cardiac disease and concurrent myocardial injury.[13] A chest radiograph should be obtained because aspiration is a concern in stroke patients with dysphagia or if lung disease is suspected, and for patients with respiratory distress or hypoxia.[13,14,26]

Data

Collection of *data* (emergency department evaluation, prompt laboratory studies, and computed tomography) is the fifth link in the chain. Data from the patient's history and physical examination, laboratory studies, and imaging studies are used to help determine his or her treatment plan.

Decision

The sixth link is making a *decision* about potential therapies. It is made on the basis of the data gathered and the type (i.e., hemorrhagic vs. nonhemorrhagic), location (e.g., carotid/vertebrobasilar), and severity of the stroke.

Drug

Drug (administration of appropriate drugs or other therapy) is the seventh link. If the patient meets the inclusion criteria, fibrinolytic therapy may be ordered for the treatment of acute ischemic stroke. Characteristics of patients with ischemic stroke who could be treated with rtPA are shown in Box 6-4.

BOX 6-4 **Characteristics of Patients with Ischemic Stroke Who Could Be Treated with rtPA**[14]

Diagnosis of ischemic stroke causing measurable neurological deficit
The neurological signs should not be clearing spontaneously.
The neurological signs should not be minor and isolated.
Caution should be exercised in treating a patient with major deficits.
The symptoms of stroke should not be suggestive of subarachnoid hemorrhage.
Onset of symptoms less than 3 hours before beginning treatment
No head trauma or prior stroke in previous 3 months
No myocardial infarction in the previous 3 months
No gastrointestinal or urinary tract hemorrhage in previous 21 days
No major surgery in the previous 14 days
No arterial puncture at a noncompressible site in the previous 7 days
No history of previous intracranial hemorrhage
Blood pressure not elevated (systolic less than 185 mm Hg and diastolic less than 110 mm Hg)
No evidence of active bleeding or acute trauma (fracture) on examination
Not taking an oral anticoagulant or, if anticoagulant being taken, international normalized ratio (INR) 1.7 or less
If receiving heparin in previous 48 hours, activated partial thromboplastin time (aPTT) must be in normal range.
Platelet count 100,000 mm^3 or more
Blood glucose concentration 50 mg/dL or more (2.7 mmol/L)
No seizure with postictal residual neurological impairments
CT does not show a multilobar infarction (hypodensity more than one third of cerebral hemisphere).
The patient or family members understand the potential risks and benefits of treatment

rtPA, recombinant form of tissue plasminogen activator.

Currently, an estimated 1.8% to 2.1% of acute ischemic stroke patients receive IV rtPA.[13,27] Possible reasons for the low frequency of use of IV rtPA include lack of a well-developed local care system to implement treatment, delayed emergency department arrival times after stroke onset, lack of EMS delivery system use, poor physician motivation, and poor patient awareness.[13]

A science advisory issued by the American Heart Association/American Stroke Association[28] reports that although the degree of clinical benefit is smaller than it is for patients who are treated within 3 hours, studies demonstrated clinical improvement when IV rtPA was administered to a carefully selected group of patients who presented within a 3- to 4.5-hour window after the onset of acute stroke symptoms. Patients excluded from the extended window for rtPA administration included individuals who were older than 80 years, those taking oral anticoagulants with an international normalized ratio of less than 1.7, those with an NIHSS score higher than 25, and those with a history of stroke and diabetes. The American Heart Association states that administration of IV rtPA to patients with acute ischemic stroke who meet specific eligibility criteria is recommended if rtPA is administered by physicians in the setting of a clearly defined protocol, a knowledgeable team, and institutional commitment.[20] As of this writing, the use of rtPA for selected acute ischemic stroke patients presenting within 3 to 4.5 hours of symptom onset has not yet been approved by the U.S. Food and Drug Administration.

If the decision is made to use fibrinolytic therapy (rtPA), close monitoring of the patient is critical. The rtPA dose is 0.9 mg/kg, not to exceed 90 mg. Ten percent of the dose is given as an initial IV bolus followed by the remaining 90% of the dose infused during the next hour. The patient should be admitted to an intensive care or stroke unit for close monitoring. Neurologic assessments and BP monitoring should be checked at least every 15 minutes during the infusion, then every 30 minutes for 6 hours, and then every hour until 24 hours after the infusion. The physician should be notified and the rtPA infusion stopped if a decrease in the patient's level of responsiveness or worsening neurologic deficit occurs during infusion. Do not give antiplatelet or anticoagulant therapies for 24 hours and do not perform invasive procedures, intramuscular injections, or arterial punctures on noncompressible sites for 24 hours. Obtain a brain CT scan 24 hours postinfusion or sooner if neurologic deterioration occurs.

Direct administration of intra-arterial (IA) fibrinolytic agents into the clot while passing the catheter through the clot and mechanically disrupting it has been pursued as an alternative strategy to treat selected patients who have a large stroke of less than 6 hours duration as a result of occlusion of the middle cerebral artery, for those who have a life-threatening vertebrobasilar stroke in the posterior circulation, and for those in whom IV rtPA is contraindicated (e.g., those who have undergone a recent surgery).[22,29] Because IA therapy requires access to emergent cerebral angiography, experienced stroke physicians, and neurointerventionalists, it should be performed only at an experienced center.

The use of IV rtPA followed by IA rtPA is called *bridging therapy* and is sometimes used to treat acute stroke in areas that do not have neurointerventional teams available. For example, with the use of telemedicine, which is also called telestroke, the patient may receive IV rtPA at the transferring hospital followed by IA rtPA when he or she reaches a hospital with a neurointerventional team qualified to administer IA therapy.

Disposition

The final link in the chain is *disposition*. It is recommended that the stroke patient be admitted to a stroke unit or an intensive care unit for ongoing care and close observation within 3 hours of arrival, especially after administration of IV rtPA.[20] This phase of stroke care focuses on prevention of hypoxia; performing frequent evaluations of neurologic status; blood pressure monitoring and management; controlling temperature and glucose levels; establishing the cause of the stroke; providing nutritional support; preventing complications (e.g., aspiration pneumonia, urinary tract infections, deep venous thrombosis); and evaluating secondary prevention strategies.[16, 20]

STOP AND REVIEW

True/False
Indicate whether the statement is true or false.

_____ 1. Breast cancer affects more American women every year than stroke.

_____ 2. One possible cause of a hemorrhagic stroke is the rupture of an artery with bleeding into the brain tissue. This type of bleeding is called a subarachnoid hemorrhage.

_____ 3. The National Institutes of Health Stroke Scale is limited to evaluation of eye opening, verbal response, and motor response.

_____ 4. A noncontrast brain CT or brain MRI should be obtained in all patients with suspected acute ischemic stroke.

Multiple Choice
Identify the choice that best completes the statement or answers the question.

_____ 5. Paramedics are at the home of a 62-year-old man presenting with signs and symptoms suggesting a stroke. Which of the following is the most important question that should be asked of this patient, bystanders, or both?
a. "When did you last see a physician?"
b. "When did your symptoms begin?"
c. "What hospital would you prefer to be taken to?"
d. "Do you have a history of hypertension?"

_____ 6. What is the most common cause of a stroke?
a. Cerebral hemorrhage
b. A thrombus
c. Dissecting cerebral aneurysm
d. Cerebral vasospasm

_____ 7. The most commonly blocked vessel in a stroke is the:
a. Vertebral artery
b. Middle cerebral artery
c. Posterior cerebral artery
d. Anterior cerebral artery

_____ 8. Current stroke protocols recommend that a possible stroke patient presenting to the emergency department should be seen by a physician within __ of his or her arrival and a CT scan should be completed within __.
a. 5 minutes, 15 minutes
b. 10 minutes, 25 minutes
c. 30 minutes, 45 minutes
d. 45 minutes, 60 minutes

_____ 9. Which of the following dysrhythmias is most likely to precipitate a stroke?
a. Sinus bradycardia
b. Junctional rhythm
c. Atrial fibrillation
d. Ventricular escape rhythm

_____ 10. Currently, the "window of opportunity" to use IV rtPA to treat most ischemic stroke patients is within __ of the onset of symptoms.
a. 1 hour
b. 3 hours
c. 6 hours
d. 12 hours

_____ 11. The three areas measured with the Glasgow Coma Scale are:
a. Eye opening, verbal response, and motor response
b. Vital signs, eye opening, and pupil reaction
c. Level of consciousness, vital signs, and breathing pattern
d. Open wounds, peripheral pulses, and motor response

_____ 12. Current stroke guidelines recommend that antihypertensive agents should be withheld in acute ischemic stroke patients who are not potential candidates for acute reperfusion therapy unless the systolic blood pressure is greater than __ mm Hg or the diastolic blood pressure is greater than __ mm Hg.
a. 165, 100
b. 185, 110
c. 200, 100
d. 220, 120

_____ 13. A patient is experiencing signs and symptoms consistent with a possible stroke. Which of the following is a contraindication to fibrinolytic therapy for this patient?
a. The patient's symptoms began 30 minutes ago.
b. The patient is 43 years old.
c. The patient has a history of a myocardial infarction in 1996.
d. The patient had a laparoscopic cholecystectomy 2 weeks ago.

_____ 14. A 52-year-old woman presents with a sudden onset of numbness and weakness in her right arm and leg. Family members state her signs and symptoms began while the patient was preparing breakfast 1 hour ago. Examination reveals unequal grips with marked weakness on the patient's right side. Her blood pressure is 174/86, pulse 88, respirations 16. Her oxygen saturation on room air is 90%. As you give oxygen and start an IV, you note improvement in the patient's symptoms. After 25 minutes, her grips become equal and there is no weakness on the patient's right side. You suspect:
a. Ischemic stroke
b. Transient ischemic attack
c. Hemorrhagic stroke
d. Hypoglycemia

Short Answer

15. Briefly explain the difference between the two types of stroke.

16. What are the two main areas of injury in an ischemic stroke?

1.
2.

17. Why should the serum glucose level be determined during the initial management of a possible stroke patient?

18. The Cincinnati Prehospital Stroke Scale effectively identifies patients with stroke. List the three major physical findings evaluated with this scale.

1.
2.
3.

REFERENCES

1. Zivin JA: Approach to cerebrovascular diseases. In Lee Goldman, Dennis Ausiello, editors: *Cecil Medicine*, 23rd ed, Philadelphia, 2007, Saunders Book Co.
2. Lloyd-Jones D, Adams RJ, Brown TM, et al: Heart disease and stroke statistics—2010 update. A report from the American Heart Association Statistics Committee and Stroke Statistics Subcommittee, *Circulation* 121:e1–e170, 2010.
3. Biller J, Love BB, Schneck MJ: Vascular diseases of the nervous system: ischemic cerebrovascular disease. In Bradley Walter G, editor: *Neurology in clinical practice*, 5th ed, Philadelphia, 2008, Butterworth-Heinemann, pp 1165–1220.
4. Rosamond W, Flegal K, Furie K, et al: Heart disease and stroke statistics: 2008 update: a report from the American Heart Association Statistics Committee and Stroke Statistics Subcommittee, *Circulation* 117:e25–e146, 2008.
5. Albers GW, Amarenco P, Easton JD, et al: Antithrombotic and thrombolytic therapy for ischemic stroke: the Seventh ACCP Conference on Antithrombotic and Thrombolytic Therapy, *Chest* 126(Suppl):483S–512S, 2004.
6. Hickey JV, Hock NH: Stroke and other cerebrovascular diseases. In Hickey JV, editor: *The clinical practice of neurological and neurosurgical nursing*, 5th ed, Philadelphia, 2003, Lippincott, Williams, & Wilkins, pp 559–587.
7. Lewandowski CA, Libman R: Acute presentation of stroke, *J Stroke Cerebrovasc Dis* 8:117–126, 1999.
8. Argentino C, Toni D, Rasura M, et al: Circadian variation in the frequency of ischemic stroke, *Stroke* 21(3):387–389, 1990.
9. Marler JR, Price TR, Clark GL, et al: Morning increase in onset of ischemic stroke, *Stroke* 20(4):473–476, 1989.
10. Sapin PM, Muller JE: Triggers of acute coronary syndromes. In: Cannon C, editor: *Management of acute coronary syndromes*, 2nd ed, Totowa, NJ, 2003, Humana Press, 61–94.
11. Khaja AM: Acute ischemic stroke management: administration of thrombolytics, neuroprotectants, and general principles of medical management, *Neurol Clin* 26(4):943–961, viii, 2008.
12. Albers GW, Caplan LR, Coull BM: Transient ischemic attack: proposal for a new definition, *N Engl J Med* 347:1713–1716, 2002.
13. Gorelick AR, Gorelick PB, Sloan EP: Emergency department evaluation and management of stroke: acute assessment, stroke teams and care pathways, *Neurol Clin* 26(4):923–942, viii, 2008.
14. Adams HP Jr, del Zoppo G, Alberts MJ, et al: Guidelines for the early management of adults with ischemic stroke: a guideline from the American Heart Association/American Stroke Association Stroke Council, Clinical Cardiology Council, Cardiovascular Radiology and Intervention Council, and the Atherosclerotic Peripheral Vascular Disease and Quality of Care Outcomes in Research Interdisciplinary Working Groups [published corrections appear in Stroke, 2007;38:e38 and Stroke. 2007;38:e96], *Stroke* 38:1655–1711, 2007.
15. Barber PA, Zhang J, Demchuk AM, et al: Why are stroke patients excluded from TPA therapy? An analysis of patient eligibility, *Neurology* 56(8):1015–1020, 2001.
16. Summers D, Leonard A, Wentworth D, et al; American Heart Association Council on Cardiovascular Nursing and the Stroke Council. Comprehensive overview of nursing and interdisciplinary care of the acute ischemic stroke patient: a scientific statement from the American Heart Association, *Stroke* 40(8):2911–2944, Epub 2009 May 28, 2009.

17. Pepe PE: Overview: prehospital emergency medical care systems. The initial links in the chain of recovery for brain attack—access, prehospital care, notification, and transport. In Marler JR, Winters Jones P, Emr M, editors: Proceedings of a National Symposium on Rapid Identification and Treatment of Acute Stroke, Bethesda, MD, 1997, The National Institute of Neurological Disorders and Stroke, National Institutes of Health, pp 17–28.

18. Hazinski MF: Demystifying recognition and management of stroke, *Curr Emerg Cardiac Care* 7:8, 1996.

19. Cummins RO, editor: *Textbook of advanced cardiac life support*, Dallas, 1997, American Heart Association.

20. Jauch EC, Cucchiara B, Adeoye O, et al: Part 11: adult stroke: 2010 American Heart Association guidelines for cardiopulmonary resuscitation and emergency cardiovascular care, *Circulation* 122(Suppl 3):S818–S828, 2010.

21. Harbison J, Houssain O, Jenkinson D, et al: Diagnostic accuracy of stroke referrals from primary care, emergency room physicians, and ambulance staff using the face, arm, speech test, *Stroke* 34:71–76, 2003.

22. Adams HP Jr, Adams RJ, Brott T, et al; Stroke Council of the American Stroke Association: Guidelines for the early management of patients with ischemic stroke: A scientific statement from the Stroke Council of the American Stroke Association, *Stroke* 34(4):1056–1083, 2003.

23. Kothari RU, Pancioli A, Liu T, Brott T, Broderick J: Cincinnati Prehospital Stroke Scale: Reproducibility and validity, *Ann Emerg Med*, 33(4), 373–378, 1999.

24. Bock BF: Response system for patients presenting with acute stroke. In: Marler JR, Jones PM, Emr M, editors: *Proceeding of a national symposium on rapid identification and treatment of acute stroke: 1997*, Bethesda (MD), 1997, National Institute of Neurological Disorders and Stroke, National Institutes of Health, pp 55–62.

25. White OB, Norris JW, Hachinski VC, Lewis A: Death in early stroke: causes and mechanisms, *Stroke* 10(6):743, 1979.

26. Finley Caulfield A, Wijman CA: Management of acute ischemic stroke, *Neurol Clin* 26(2):345–371, vii, 2008.

27. Kleindorfer D, Lindsell CJ, Brass L, et al: National US estimates of recombinant tissue plasminogen activator use. ICD-9 codes substantially underestimate, *Stroke* 39:924–928, 2008.

28. Del Zoppo GJ, Saver JL, Jauch EC, Adams HP Jr; American Heart Association Stroke Council: Expansion of the time window for treatment of acute ischemic stroke with intravenous tissue plasminogen activator: a science advisory from the American Heart Association/American Stroke Association, *Stroke* 40(8):2945–2948, Epub 2009 May 28, 2009.

29. Agarwal P, Kumar S, Hariharan S, et al: Hyperdense middle cerebral artery sign: can it be used to select intraarterial versus intravenous thrombolysis in acute ischemic stroke? *Cerebrovasc Dis* 17:182–190, 2004.

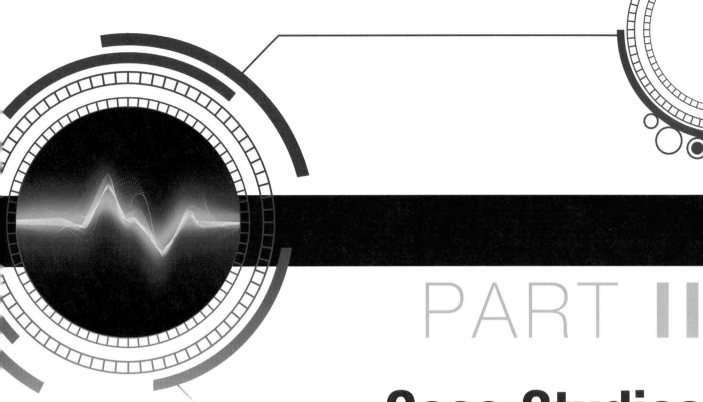

PART II

Case Studies

Case Studies

The first section of this book provided the "why," "when," and "how" for the case studies that follow. It has been proved that in order to learn how to do something, you must actually do it. The opportunity to "do" the skills taught in an advanced cardiac life support (ACLS) course and make decisions regarding patient care is provided in 10 "core" case studies in the ACLS student course. The ten "core" cases presented during an ACLS course include the following:

1. Respiratory arrest
2. Pulseless ventricular tachycardia (VT)/ventricular fibrillation (VF) treated with an automated external defibrillator (AED)
3. Pulseless VT/VF
4. Asystole
5. Pulseless electrical activity (PEA)
6. Acute coronary syndromes (ACSs)
7. Symptomatic bradycardia
8. Unstable tachycardia
9. Stable tachycardia
10. Acute ischemic stroke

During an ACLS course, discussion pertaining to each of the core ACLS cases may occur between the course instructor and the entire class, between several instructors and small groups of course participants, or between groups of students who alternate playing the role of the patient, rescuers, and coach with oversight by an instructor.

Each of the "core" ACLS cases is presented on the following pages. The case studies presented here are not intended to cover every possible dysrhythmia or patient condition that may be presented in an actual ACLS course. Rather, they are provided as examples to help you integrate the information presented in the preparatory section of this book.

Each ACLS case is presented using scenario-based skill sheets. A sample scenario sheet is shown below. Read the entire sheet, paying particular attention to the "Necessary Tasks" section, which reflects what you are expected to do. After you have read the sheet, ask another person to assist you by assuming the role of "coach." Information that should be read aloud to you appears in italics. As you practice, assume that you are the person responsible for directing the actions of a team providing emergency care for the patient. Assume that each team member will correctly carry out your instructions; however, they will not do anything without your direction. Perform a patient assessment as you would in an actual situation, including communicating with your patient. The coach should assume the role of the patient, family members, bystanders, or others as necessary. As you progress through the case study, state everything you are assessing. Ask the coach questions about the patient's vital signs, history, and response to the treatments performed as needed. If you have trouble deciding what to do, the coach can help you by reading what Emergency Action Step is next or by telling you what Necessary Tasks should be performed. The coach should acknowledge your interventions and ask you for additional information if clarification is needed. After completing each scenario, briefly review with the coach what went right and what needed improvement. Remember, practice makes perfect.

ACLS Pearl

The case studies presented here simulate situations that you may encounter as an ACLS provider. Although case studies provide opportunities for problem solving and help "put it all together," they are imperfect simulations of reality. It is impossible to predict all possible actions for a given situation, or patient responses to a particular intervention. As you practice with each of the case studies presented here, please understand that there may be alternative actions that are perfectly acceptable, yet not presented in the case study.

Sample Scenario Sheet

Emergency Action Steps	Necessary Tasks
Scene Survey	Ensures scene safety. Takes or communicates standard precautions. *Coach: The scene is safe.*

Initial Assessment

General Impression	Verbalizes general impression of patient (appearance, breathing, circulation) *Coach: The patient is not moving. There is no obvious movement of his chest. His skin looks pale.*

Primary Survey

Responsiveness/Airway	Assesses airway … *Coach:*
Breathing	Assesses breathing … *Coach:*
Circulation	Assesses pulses, skin (e.g., color, temperature and moisture), estimates heart rate *Coach:*
Defibrillation/Disability	Based on information obtained, determines need for a defibrillator *Coach:*

Secondary Survey

Vital Signs/History	Obtains baseline vital signs, history *Coach:*
Airway, Breathing, Circulation	Assesses need for advanced airway, gives O_2, establishes vascular access … *Coach:*
Differential Diagnosis, Evaluates Interventions	Determines treatment plan, begins appropriate care, evaluates patient response, facilitates family presence when applicable *Coach:*

Post-resuscitation Support/Reassessment

Begins Postresuscitation Support/ Performs Reassessment	Repeats initial assessment *Coach:* Repeats vital signs *Coach:* Evaluates response to care *Coach:*

CASE 1: RESPIRATORY ARREST

Objective	Given a patient situation, describe and demonstrate the initial emergency care for a patient who has experienced a respiratory arrest.
Skills to Master	Primary and secondary surveys
	Recognition of a patient with respiratory compromise/arrest
	Head tilt–chin lift, jaw thrust without head tilt
	Insertion of an oral or nasal airway
	Pocket face mask or bag-mask ventilation
	Upper airway suctioning
	Attachment and use of electrocardiogram (ECG) monitoring leads
	Use of a pulse oximeter and capnometer
	IV access
Rhythms to Master	Sinus bradycardia
	Sinus rhythm
	Sinus arrhythmia
Medications to Master	O_2
Related Text Chapters	Chapter 1: The ABCDs of Emergency Cardiovascular Care
	Chapter 2: Airway Management: Oxygenation and Ventilation
Essential Actions	• Ensure scene safety, use personal protective equipment
	• Perform a primary and secondary survey
	• Consider possible causes of the event
	• Transfer patient for definitive care
Unacceptable Actions	• Failure to use personal protective equipment
	• Failure to recognize signs of deterioration to respiratory failure or arrest and the need for more aggressive intervention
	• Giving O_2 by a means other than positive pressure ventilation
	• Failure to ventilate the patient at appropriate rate
	• Failure to monitor the cardiac rhythm in any patient who displays abnormal ventilatory rate or effort, abnormal heart rate, perfusion, blood pressure, or acute altered mental status
	• Failure to confirm advanced airway placement
	• Failure to properly secure an advanced airway
	• Failure to recognize right primary bronchus intubation or esophageal intubation
	• Interruption of ventilations for more than 30 seconds at any time
	• Failure to oxygenate the patient between intubation attempts

Case 1: Scenario Sheet

Scenario: Your patient is a 42-year-old woman who was pulled out of a backyard swimming pool. It is a warm July day. The time is 1523. You have four other advanced life support (ALS) personnel available to assist you. Emergency equipment is immediately available.

Emergency Action Steps	**Necessary Tasks**
Scene Survey	I am putting on personal protective equipment. Is the scene safe to enter?
	Coach: The scene is safe.

Initial Assessment

General Impression	As I approach the patient and form a general impression (assessing the patient's appearance, work of breathing, and circulation), what do I see?
	Coach: You see a woman supine on a stretcher. Her eyes are closed and her hair and clothing are wet. You see no signs of breathing. Her skin looks pale.

Primary Survey

Responsiveness/Airway

I will quickly approach the patient and assess her level of responsiveness. Does she respond when I call her name?

Coach: There is no response.

Does she respond when I pinch her hand?

Coach: The patient is unresponsive.

I will open the patient's airway using a jaw thrust without head tilt maneuver. Do I see anything in the patient's mouth such as blood, broken teeth or loose dentures, gastric contents, or a foreign object?

Coach: You see a small amount of pink fluid in the patient's mouth.

I will ask an assistant to clear the patient's upper airway with suctioning.

Coach: The airway is now clear. What should be done now?

Breathing

Is the patient breathing?

Coach: The patient is not breathing.

I will ask the airway team member to size and insert an oral airway and begin positive pressure ventilation with a bag-mask device connected to 100% O_2 while I continue the primary survey. I want the airway team member to maintain proper head position and a good seal with the mask against the patient's face. I want a second team member to assume responsibility for compressing the bag with just enough force to produce gentle chest rise.

Coach: An oral airway has been inserted and the patient is being ventilated with a bag-mask. You see gentle chest rise with bagging. At what rate should this patient be ventilated?

The patient should be ventilated at a rate of 10 to 12/min (i.e., one ventilation every 5 to 6 seconds). Each ventilation should be given over 1 second. I will ask an assistant to assess baseline breath sounds while the patient is being ventilated and then prepare the intubation equipment.

Circulation

I will ask the defibrillation team member to attach a pulse oximeter and the ECG monitoring leads while I feel for a carotid pulse for up to 10 seconds. Do I feel a pulse?

Coach: A pulse is present. Current resuscitation guidelines generally begin with a C-A-B sequence. You have chosen the traditional A-B-C approach. Why?

Hypoxia is the most unfavorable consequence of submersion. CPR for drowning victims requires modification of the C-A-B sequence and involves the use of the traditional A-B-C approach because of the hypoxic nature of the arrest.[1] While I am feeling the patient's pulse, I will assess her skin condition. What is her skin temperature, color, and condition?

Coach: The patient's skin is cool, pale, and wet. What should be done now?

Defibrillation/Disability

I will assess the need for a defibrillator. Because the patient has a slow pulse, defibrillation is not necessary right now. I will ask a team member to obtain the patient's baseline vital signs while I begin the secondary survey.

Secondary Survey

Vital Signs/History

What are the patient's vital signs?

Coach: The patient remains unresponsive and apneic. Breath sounds are clear and equal bilaterally with bag-mask ventilation. The patient's heart rate is 44 beats/min. Her blood pressure is 86/54 mm Hg. The patient has been placed on the cardiac monitor (Figure 7-1). What is the rhythm on the monitor?

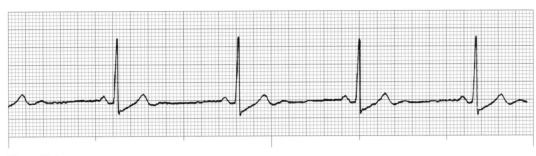

Figure 7-1

The rhythm is a sinus bradycardia. Is there someone available who may know what happened to this patient?

Coach: (See SAMPLE history obtained from the patient's husband).

Sample History

Signs/symptoms	Submersion incident
Allergies	None
Medications	Unknown
Past medical history	Depression
Last oral intake	Unknown
Events prior	The patient was retrieved from the swimming pool by her husband. He estimates she was in the water for less than 10 minutes.

Airway, Breathing, Circulation

I want my most experienced assistant to intubate the patient. I want the IV team member to start an IV with normal saline. I would also like a team member to obtain a 12-lead ECG while I perform a focused physical examination.

Coach: (See physical examination findings). A tracheal tube has been inserted and the cuff inflated. An IV has been established with normal saline. Describe how you will confirm placement of the tracheal tube.

Physical Examination Findings

Head, ears, eyes, nose, and throat	Pink fluid initially present in mouth (cleared with suctioning)
Neck	Trachea midline, no jugular venous distention
Chest	Breath sounds clear and equal with bag-mask ventilation
Abdomen	No abnormalities noted
Pelvis	No abnormalities noted
Extremities	No abnormalities noted
Posterior body	Unremarkable

I will confirm placement of the tracheal tube starting with a 5-point auscultation of the chest. I will listen first over the epigastrium. What do I hear? Next, I will listen to the right and left sides of the chest in four areas. What do I hear?

Coach: There are no sounds heard over the epigastrium. Breath sounds are diminished on the left side of the chest with bag-mask ventilation. They are clearly heard on the right. What would you like to do now?

On the basis of these findings, I suspect a right primary bronchus intubation. I will ask the airway team member to deflate the cuff, pull back slightly on the tracheal tube, reinflate the cuff, and reassess the patient's breath sounds.

Coach: Breath sounds with bag-mask ventilation now reveal clear and equal breath sounds. What would you like to do now?

Differential Diagnosis, Evaluates Interventions

If capnography confirms the presence of CO_2, I will ask the airway team member to note the centimeter markings on the tracheal tube and then secure the tube in place.

Coach: Waveform capnography confirms the presence of CO_2. The tracheal tube has been secured. What should be done now?

Postresuscitation Support/Reassessment

Begins Postresuscitation Support/Performs Reassessment

I would like to repeat the primary survey and obtain another set of vital signs. Is the patient attempting to breathe spontaneously? What is the rate and quality of the patient's pulse? What is the patient's blood pressure?

Coach: The patient is attempting to breathe spontaneously at a rate of 6 to 8/ min. Her vital signs are now: Blood pressure 112/74, pulse strong and regular at 75 beats/min; ventilatory rate 10/min via bag-mask; SpO_2 97% with bagging. What is the rhythm on the cardiac monitor (Figure 7-2)? What would you like to do next?

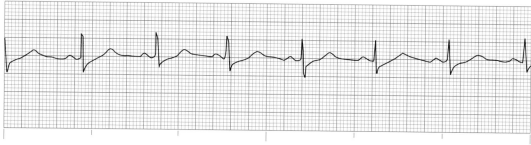

Figure 7-2

The monitor shows a sinus rhythm. Although the patient is beginning to breathe on her own, I want the airway team member to continue assisting her ventilations until the rate and quality of the patient's spontaneous breathing effort improves. I will evaluate the patient's 12-lead ECG results and transfer the patient for continued monitoring and care.

CASE 2: PULSELESS VT/VF WITH AN AED

Objective

Given a patient situation, describe and demonstrate the initial emergency care for a patient in cardiac arrest due to pulseless VT/VF and with an AED immediately available.

Skills to Master

Primary and secondary surveys
Recognition of a patient in cardiac arrest
Head tilt–chin lift, jaw thrust without head tilt
Insertion of an oral or nasal airway
CPR
Pocket face mask or bag-mask ventilation
Upper airway suctioning
Operation of an AED
Vascular access
IV/intraosseous (IO) medication administration

Rhythms to Master	None (rhythm analysis performed by AED)
Medications to Master	O_2
	Epinephrine
	Vasopressin
	Amiodarone
	Lidocaine
Related Text Chapters	Chapter 1: The ABCDs of Emergency Cardiac Care
	Chapter 2: Airway Management: Oxygenation and Ventilation
	Chapter 3: Rhythms and Management
	Chapter 4: Electrical Therapy
Essential Actions	• Ensure scene safety, use personal protective equipment
	• Perform a primary and secondary survey
	• Begin CPR
	• Demonstrate safe operation of the defibrillator, including ensuring the O_2 is not flowing over the patient's chest during each shock if electrical therapy is indicated
	• Give O_2 using positive pressure ventilation
	• Establish vascular access
	• Know the actions, indications, dosages, adverse effects, and contraindications for the medications used in the treatment of pulseless VT/VF
	• Follow each medication given in a cardiac arrest with a 20 mL fluid flush and elevation of the affected extremity
	• Consider possible reversible causes of the arrest
	• Facilitate family presence during resuscitative efforts according to agency/institution protocol
Unacceptable Actions	• Failure to use personal protective equipment
	• Failure to begin CPR
	• Performing CPR incorrectly (e.g., incorrect hand position, depth of compressions, compression rate, ventilation rate)
	• Unsafe operation of AED (e.g., failure to clear self or others before shocking)
	• Giving O_2 by a means other than positive pressure ventilation
	• Failure to establish vascular access
	• Failure to give medications appropriate for the dysrhythmia
	• Failure to consider the possible reversible causes of the arrest
	• Medication errors
	• Performing any technique resulting in potential harm to the patient

Case 2: Scenario Sheet

Scenario: Your patient is a 52-year-old woman who was found unresponsive on her kitchen floor by a neighbor. The time is 1442. You have four other ALS personnel available to assist you. Emergency equipment is immediately available.

Emergency Action Steps	**Necessary Tasks**
Scene Survey	I am putting on personal protective equipment. Is the scene safe to enter?
	Coach: The scene is safe.

Initial Assessment

General Impression	As I approach the patient and form a general impression (assessing the patient's appearance, work of breathing, and circulation), what do I see?
	Coach: A woman is supine on a stretcher. Her eyes are closed. You do not see any signs of breathing. Her skin is pale and her lips are blue. What would you like to do now?

Primary Survey

Responsiveness/Breathing

I will approach the patient and assess her level of responsiveness. Is she aware of my approach?

Coach: The patient is unresponsive. How would you like to proceed?

I will quickly check for breathing.

Coach: The patient is not breathing. How would you like to proceed?

Circulation

I will feel for a carotid pulse for up to 10 seconds and assess the patient's skin temperature, color, and moisture at the same time. Is a pulse present?

Coach: There is no pulse. Her skin is cool, pale, and dry. What should be done now?

I will ask the CPR team member to begin chest compressions.

Coach: At what rate should compressions be performed? How far should the patient's chest be compressed?

Compressions should be performed at a rate of at least 100/min. An adult's chest should be compressed at least 2 inches (5 cm).

Coach: Compressions are being performed as requested. How would you like to proceed?

Airway

Although there are no visible signs of trauma, I will open the patient's airway using a jaw thrust without head tilt because I understand that the patient was found on the floor and I cannot rule out a trauma as a result of a possible fall injury. Do I see anything in the patient's mouth such as blood, broken teeth or loose dentures, gastric contents, or a foreign object?

Coach: The patient's airway is clear. What should be done now?

Breathing

I will ask the airway team member to quickly size and insert an oral airway. I will ask the airway team member and an assistant to perform two-person ventilation with a bag-mask device connected to 100% O_2. I want the patient ventilated with just enough force to produce gentle chest rise. I will ask another assistant to assess the patient's baseline breath sounds while the patient is being ventilated.

Coach: An oral airway has been inserted. The patient is being ventilated with a bag-mask. You see gentle chest rise with bagging. What would you like to do next?

Defibrillation/Disability

I want the chest compressor and airway team member to automatically rotate positions after every five cycles (about 2 minutes) of CPR so they do not become fatigued. Without interrupting CPR, I will ask the defibrillation team member to power on the AED and then to apply the AED pads to the patient's bare chest.

Coach: The power to the AED is on. The AED pads are in place on the patient's chest. How do you want to proceed?

I will ask my team to briefly interrupt chest compressions and ask the defibrillation team member to press the "Analyze" button on the AED.

Coach: The AED advises a shock.

As soon as the defibrillation team member indicates that he is ready to shock, I want all team members to clear the patient. I want the chest compressor to switch positions with the airway team member. As the airway team member clears the patient and assumes the compressor role, I will ask her to ensure that O_2 is not flowing over the patient's chest as we prepare to defibrillate the patient.

Coach: Everyone cleared the patient and she has been defibrillated.

I want my team to resume CPR immediately, beginning with chest compressions. After five cycles of CPR (about 2 minutes), the defibrillation team member will reanalyze the patient's rhythm.

Coach: The AED states, "No shock advised."

I will check for a pulse and repeat the primary survey. Is the patient responsive? Is she breathing? Does she have a pulse?

Coach: A strong carotid pulse is present. The patient is waking up and breathing on her own about 12 times/min. What should be done now?

Secondary Survey
Vital Signs/History

I will ask an assistant to obtain a complete set of vital signs. Is there someone available who can provide additional information about this patient?

Coach: The patient's heart rate is strong and regular at a rate of 80 beats/min. Ventilations are occurring at a rate of 12/min. The patient's blood pressure is 98/60. (See SAMPLE history obtained from neighbor and physical examination findings). What would you like to do next?

Sample History

Signs/symptoms	Found unresponsive by neighbor
Allergies	Unknown
Medications	Azithromycin (Zithromax), alendronate (Fosamax)
Past medical history	"Intestinal problems"
Last oral intake	Unknown
Events prior	Found unresponsive on the kitchen floor by a neighbor who had last spoken to patient about 25 minutes prior

Physical Examination Findings

Head, ears, eyes, nose, and throat	Cyanosis of lips
Neck	Trachea midline, no jugular venous distention
Chest	Breath sounds clear and equal with positive pressure ventilation
Abdomen	No abnormalities noted
Pelvis	No abnormalities noted
Extremities	No abnormalities noted
Posterior body	No abnormalities noted

Post–cardiac Arrest Support/Reassessment

Begins Post–cardiac Arrest Support/Performs Reassessment

I want the airway team member to apply a pulse oximeter and capnometer to assess the patient's oxygenation and ventilatory efforts. I will ask the airway team member to apply an oxygen delivery device (if the patient's breathing is adequate) or continue to assist the patient's breathing with a bag-mask device connected to O_2 (if the patient's breathing is inadequate) as indicated. I will order a cardiology consult and continue to monitor the patient's vital signs and ECG every 5 minutes as I prepare to transfer the patient for continued care.

CASE 3: PULSELESS VT/VF

Objective	Given a patient situation, describe and demonstrate the initial emergency care for a patient in cardiac arrest due to pulseless VT/VF.
Skills to Master	Primary and secondary surveys
	Recognition of a patient in cardiac arrest
	Head tilt–chin lift, jaw thrust without head tilt
	Insertion of an oral or nasal airway
	Pocket face mask or bag-mask ventilation
	Upper airway suctioning
	CPR
	Attachment and use of ECG monitoring leads
	Operation of a manual defibrillator
	Vascular access
	IV/IO medication administration
Rhythms to Master	VT
	VF
Medications to Master	O_2
	Epinephrine
	Vasopressin
	Amiodarone
	Lidocaine
Related Text Chapters	Chapter 1: The ABCDs of Emergency Cardiac Care
	Chapter 2: Airway Management: Oxygenation and Ventilation
	Chapter 3: Rhythms and Management
	Chapter 4: Electrical Therapy
Essential Actions	• Ensure scene safety, use personal protective equipment
	• Perform a primary and secondary survey
	• Begin CPR
	• Demonstrate safe operation of the defibrillator, including ensuring the O_2 is not flowing over the patient's chest during each shock if electrical therapy is indicated
	• Give O_2 using positive pressure ventilation
	• Establish vascular access
	• Know the actions, indications, dosages, adverse effects, and contraindications for the medications used in the treatment of pulseless VT/VF
	• Follow each medication given in a cardiac arrest with a 20 mL IV fluid flush and elevation of the affected extremity for 10 to 20 seconds
	• Consider possible reversible causes of the arrest
	• Facilitate family presence during resuscitative efforts according to agency/institution protocol
Unacceptable Actions	• Failure to use personal protective equipment
	• Failure to begin CPR
	• Performing CPR incorrectly (e.g., incorrect hand position, depth of compressions, compression rate, ventilation rate)
	• Failure to correctly identify the ECG rhythm
	• Unsafe operation of defibrillator (e.g., failure to clear self or others before shocking)
	• Giving O_2 by a means other than positive pressure ventilation
	• Failure to establish vascular access
	• Failure to give medications appropriate for the dysrhythmia
	• Failure to consider the possible reversible causes of the arrest
	• Failure to recognize rhythm change
	• Medication errors
	• Performing any technique resulting in potential harm to the patient

Case 3: Scenario Sheet

Scenario: Your patient is 35-year-old man found unresponsive by his wife. It has been about 15 minutes since the patient collapsed. The time is 1740. You have five other ALS personnel available to assist you. Emergency equipment, including a biphasic manual defibrillator, is immediately available.

Emergency Action Steps	Necessary Tasks
Scene Survey	I am putting on personal protective equipment. Is the scene safe to enter? *Coach: The scene is safe.*

Initial Assessment

General Impression	As I approach the patient and form a general impression, what do I see? *Coach: The patient is supine on a stretcher. His eyes are closed. The patient does not appear to be breathing and his skin looks pale.*

Primary Survey

Responsiveness/ Breathing	I will quickly approach the patient and assess his level of responsiveness. *Coach: The patient is unresponsive.* I will quickly check for breathing. *Coach: The patient is not breathing. How would you like to proceed?*
Circulation	I feel for a carotid pulse for up to 10 seconds. Do I feel a carotid pulse? What is the condition of the patient's skin? *Coach: There is no pulse. The patient's skin is cool, pale, and dry. What should be done now?* I will ask the CPR team member to begin chest compressions and ask for the defibrillator immediately. Without interrupting CPR, I want the defibrillation team member to attach combination pads to the patient's bare chest. *Coach: Compressions are being performed as requested. How would you like to proceed?*
Airway	I will open the patient's airway using a head tilt–chin lift maneuver because I understand that the patient was assisted to the floor when he collapsed, and no head or neck trauma is suspected. Is there anything visible in the patient's mouth such as blood, broken teeth or loose dentures, gastric contents, or a foreign object? *Coach: The patient's airway is clear. What should be done now?*
Breathing	I will ask the airway team member to size and insert an oral airway. I want the airway team member and an assistant to begin positive pressure ventilation with a bag-mask connected to 100% O_2. I want the airway team member to maintain proper head position and a good seal with the mask against the patient's face. I want a second team member to assume responsibility for compressing the bag with just enough force to produce gentle chest rise. I will ask another assistant to assess baseline breath sounds while the patient is being ventilated. *Coach: An oral airway has been inserted. Two-person bag-mask ventilation is being performed. You see gentle chest rise with bagging. Breath sounds are clear and equal with positive pressure ventilation. Combination pads are in place on the patient's chest as requested. What should be done now?*

Defibrillation/Disability | I will ask for the defibrillator immediately. I want the CPR team member and the airway team member to automatically rotate positions after every five cycles (about 2 minutes) of CPR. I want the patient's ECG rhythm checked every 2 minutes as the team members change positions.

Coach: A biphasic defibrillator is within arm's reach. You see this rhythm on the cardiac monitor (Figure 7-3). What is the rhythm on the monitor? How do you want to proceed?

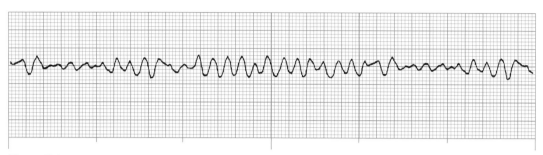

Figure 7-3

The rhythm is ventricular fibrillation. I will ask the airway team member to ensure that O_2 is not flowing over the patient's chest as the defibrillation team member prepares to shock the patient. I want the IV team member to prepare the initial medications that will be used and start an IV after the first shock is delivered.

Coach: What initial medications do you want the IV team member to prepare?

I want the IV team member to prepare epinephrine, vasopressin, and amiodarone.

Coach: What energy setting will you use for your initial shock?

I am using a biphasic defibrillator. The manufacturer of the machine I am using recommends 200 J for the initial shock.

As the machine charges, I want all team members (with the exception of the chest compressor) to immediately clear the patient. I want the chest compressor to continue CPR while the machine is charging. When the defibrillator is charged, I want the chest compressor to immediately clear the patient. After making sure that the chest compressor is clear, I will ask the defibrillation team member to defibrillate the patient with 200 J.

Coach: Shock delivered. What would you like to do next?

Secondary Survey

Vital Signs/History | I want my team to resume CPR immediately, beginning with chest compressions. After five cycles of CPR (about 2 minutes), I will recheck the patient's rhythm.

Airway, Breathing, Circulation | Without interrupting CPR, I want the IV team member to start an IV of normal saline and then give the patient 1 mg of epinephrine using a 1:10,000 solution IV push. I want the medication flushed with 20 mL of normal saline and then raise the arm into which the medication was administered for about 20 seconds.

Coach: An IV has been started with normal saline in the patient's left antecubital vein. Epinephrine has been given IV as ordered.

Differential Diagnosis, Evaluates Interventions | I am considering possible causes of the arrest. Is there someone available who may know what happened before the patient collapsed?

Coach: (See SAMPLE history obtained from the patient's wife and coworkers and physical examination findings).

Sample History

Signs/symptoms	Collapsed about 15 minutes ago
Allergies	Codeine, penicillin
Medications	Divalproex sodium (Depakote)
Past medical history	Epilepsy, substance abuse
Last oral intake	Unknown
Events prior	Sudden collapse

Physical Examination Findings

Head, ears, eyes, nose, and throat	No abnormalities noted
Neck	Trachea midline, no jugular venous distention
Chest	Breath sounds clear and equal with positive pressure ventilation
Abdomen	No abnormalities noted
Pelvis	No abnormalities noted
Extremities	No abnormalities noted
Posterior body	No abnormalities noted

The cardiac monitor still shows ventricular fibrillation. While CPR continues, I want the IV team member to administer IV amiodarone.

Coach: The IV team member requests clarification regarding your amiodarone order. What dosage that should be administered at this time?

In cardiac arrest, the loading dose of amiodarone is 300 mg IV. I want 300 mg of amiodarone given IV at this time.

Coach: Amiodarone has been given as instructed. The patient's cardiac rhythm remains unchanged and CPR is ongoing. What would you like to do now?

I will prepare to defibrillate with 300 J, as recommended by the manufacturer of the defibrillator I am using. As with the first shock delivered, I will ensure that all team members, with the exception of the chest compressor, are clear of the patient. The defibrillator is now charged and I will ask the chest compressor to clear the patient and then ask the defibrillation team member to defibrillate the patient with 300 J.

Coach: The shock has been delivered. A team member calls your attention to a rhythm change on the cardiac monitor. What is the rhythm on the monitor (Figure 7-4)?

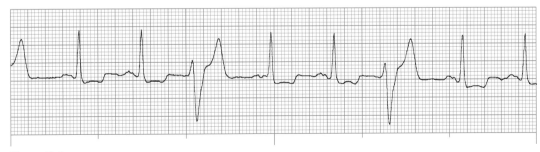

Figure 7-4

The monitor shows a sinus rhythm with uniform premature ventricular complexes.

Coach: What would you like to do next?

Because there is an organized rhythm on the monitor, I will ask the CPR team member to stop CPR and check for a pulse.[2]

Coach: A strong carotid pulse is present. What should be done now?

Post–cardiac Arrest Support/Reassessment

Begins Post–cardiac Arrest Support/Performs Reassessment	I will ask an assistant to obtain a complete set of vital signs while I will repeat the primary survey. Is the patient responsive? Is he breathing?
	Coach: The patient is unresponsive but breathing shallowly at a rate of approximately 4 breaths/min. A strong pulse is present at a rate of about 80 beats/min. His blood pressure is 88/62 mm Hg. His color is improving. What should be done now?
	I will recheck the patient's vital signs and ECG every 5 minutes. I want a team member to apply a pulse oximeter and capnometer, obtain a 12-lead ECG, and order a cardiology consult. Until the patient's spontaneous breathing is adequate, I want the airway team member to continue assisting the patient's breathing with the bag-mask until arrangements can be made for mechanical ventilation. I want the IV team member to prepare an IV infusion of amiodarone while I arrange for the patient's transfer for further care.

CASE 4: ASYSTOLE

Objective	Given a patient situation, describe and demonstrate the initial emergency care for a patient in asystole.
Skills to Master	Primary and secondary surveys
	Recognition of a patient in cardiac arrest
	Head tilt–chin lift, jaw thrust without head tilt
	Insertion of an oral or nasal airway
	CPR
	Pocket face mask or bag-mask ventilation
	Upper airway suctioning
	Attachment and use of ECG monitoring leads
	Use of a pulse oximeter and capnometer
	IV/IO access
	IV/IO medication administration
Rhythms to Master	Asystole
Medications to Master	O_2
	Epinephrine
	Vasopressin
Related Text Chapters	Chapter 1: The ABCDs of Emergency Cardiac Care
	Chapter 2: Airway Management: Oxygenation and Ventilation
	Chapter 3: Rhythms and Management
Essential Actions	• Ensure scene safety, use personal protective equipment
	• Perform a primary and secondary survey
	• Recognize asystole
	• Check for signs of obvious death, do not attempt resuscitation order
	• Begin CPR
	• Give O_2 using positive pressure ventilation
	• Establish vascular access
	• Know the actions, indications, dosages, adverse effects, and contraindications for the medications used in the treatment of asystole
	• Follow each medication given in a cardiac arrest with a 20 mL fluid flush and elevation of the affected extremity for 10 to 20 seconds
	• Consider possible reversible causes of the arrest
	• Facilitate family presence during resuscitative efforts according to agency/institution protocol

Unacceptable Actions

- Failure to use personal protective equipment
- Failure to begin CPR
- Performing CPR incorrectly (e.g., incorrect hand position, depth of compressions, compression rate, ventilation rate)
- Failure to correctly identify the ECG rhythm
- Giving O_2 by a means other than positive pressure ventilation
- Failure to establish vascular access
- Defibrillating asystole
- Failure to give medications appropriate for the dysrhythmia
- Failure to consider the possible reversible causes of asystole
- Failure to recognize rhythm change
- Medication errors
- Performing any technique resulting in potential harm to the patient

Case 4: Scenario Sheet

Scenario: Your patient is a 24-year-old man who was found unresponsive in his home by his girlfriend. She told law enforcement personnel that he was fine about 15 minutes ago and then she heard a gunshot. The time is 1415. You have four other ALS personnel available to assist you. Emergency equipment is immediately available.

Emergency Action Steps	Necessary Tasks
Scene Survey	I am putting on personal protective equipment. Is the scene safe to enter?
	Coach: While law enforcement personnel remain at his residence, the patient has been transported to the emergency department of the closest trauma center. It is safe to enter the patient's room.

Initial Assessment

General Impression	As I approach the patient and form a general impression (assessing the patient's appearance, work of breathing, and circulation), what do I see?
	Coach: You see a young man supine on a stretcher. He is unaware of your approach. There is no obvious rise and fall of his chest. His skin is pale. You observe minimal bleeding from a chest wound on the patient's right sternum. What would you like to do now?

Primary Survey

Responsiveness/Breathing	I will quickly approach the patient and assess his level of responsiveness. Does he respond when I call his name?
	Coach: The patient is unresponsive.
	I will quickly check for breathing.
	Coach: The patient is not breathing. How would you like to proceed?
Circulation	I feel for a carotid pulse for up to 10 seconds. Do I feel a carotid pulse? What is the condition of the patient's skin?
	Coach: There is no pulse. The patient's skin is cool, pale, and dry. What should be done now?
	I will ask the CPR team member to begin chest compressions and ask for the defibrillator immediately. Without interrupting CPR, I want the defibrillation team member to attach combination pads to the patient's bare chest.
	Coach: Compressions are being performed as requested. How would you like to proceed?

Airway

I will open the patient's airway using a jaw thrust without head tilt maneuver because I understand that the patient was found on the floor and I cannot rule out trauma as a result of a possible fall injury. Is there anything visible in the patient's mouth such as blood, broken teeth, gastric contents, or a foreign object?

Coach: The patient's airway is clear. What should be done now?

Breathing

I will ask the airway team member to size and insert an oral airway. I want the airway team member and an assistant to perform two-person ventilation with a bag-mask connected to 100% O_2. Each ventilation should be given over 1 second. I will ask another assistant to assess baseline breath sounds while the patient is being ventilated.

Coach: An oral airway has been inserted. Two-person bag-mask ventilation is being performed. You see gentle chest rise with bagging. Breath sounds are clear and equal with positive pressure ventilation. Combination pads are in place on the patient's chest as requested. A biphasic defibrillator is within arm's reach. What should be done now?

Defibrillation/Disability

I will assess the rhythm on the cardiac monitor and decide if defibrillation is needed. I want the CPR team member and the airway team member to automatically rotate positions after every five cycles (about 2 minutes) of CPR. I want the patient's ECG rhythm checked every 2 minutes as the team members change positions.

Coach: You see this rhythm on the cardiac monitor (Figure 7-5). What is the rhythm? How do you want to proceed?

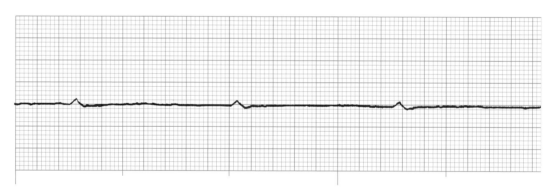

Figure 7-5

Secondary Survey
Vital Signs/History

The rhythm is P-wave asystole. I will perform a focused physical examination, looking for possible clues as to the cause of the arrest. Is the patient's girlfriend available to tell us what happened before the patient collapsed? What can she tell me about his medical history? Without interrupting CPR, I want the IV team member to start an IV and prepare epinephrine and vasopressin for administration.

Coach: (See SAMPLE history and physical examination findings). What do you want to do next?

Sample History

Signs/symptoms	Found unresponsive by girlfriend after she heard a gunshot; minimal bleeding from chest wound on right sternum
Allergies	None
Medications	None
Past medical history	None
Last oral intake	Lunch 2 hours ago
Events prior	Last seen 15 minutes ago; law-enforcement personnel report that the patient shot himself in the chest with a .45 caliber gun; an estimated 1 to 2 L of blood have been lost at the scene

Physical Examination Findings

Head, ears, eyes, nose, and throat	No abnormalities noted
Neck	Trachea midline, jugular veins flat
Chest	Gunshot wound present on the right of the sternum; breath sounds diminished on the left with positive pressure ventilation
Abdomen	No abnormalities noted
Pelvis	No abnormalities noted
Extremities	No abnormalities noted
Posterior body	Large exit wound lateral to left scapula

Airway, Breathing, Circulation

I will ask a qualified airway team member to insert an advanced airway. On the basis of the patient's mechanism of injury and the amount of blood loss at the scene, I want the IV team member to give an initial fluid bolus of 20 mL/kg and administer 1 mg of IV epinephrine (1 : 10,000 solution) to the patient and then raise the arm into which the drug was administered.

Coach: The airway team member has successfully inserted a Combitube. The IV team member has successfully placed an IV in the right antecubital vein.

I will confirm placement of the Combitube starting with a five-point auscultation of the chest. I am listening over the epigastrium and then to the right and left sides of the chest in four areas. What do I hear?

Coach: There are no sounds heard over the epigastrium. Breath sounds are diminished on the left and present on the right with positive pressure ventilation.

Does waveform capnography indicate that the Combitube is in the trachea?

Coach: Yes, waveform capnography confirms proper placement of the Combitube.

I will ask the airway team member to secure the Combitube in place.

Coach: The Combitube has been secured. The IV fluid bolus that you ordered is infusing and 1 mg of 1 : 10,000 epinephrine has been given. CPR is ongoing and the rhythm on the cardiac monitor is unchanged. Does placement of an advanced airway necessitate any changes in bag-mask ventilation?

Differential Diagnosis, Evaluates Interventions

I will instruct the airway team member to continue positive pressure ventilation at a rate of 8 to 10 breaths/min. I will instruct the CPR team member to continue chest compressions without pausing for ventilations. I want the IV team member to give 40 units of vasopressin IV push at this time.

Coach: After 40 minutes of high-quality CPR, the rhythm on the cardiac monitor is unchanged. Epinephrine has been given every 3 to 5 minutes and one dose of vasopressin was administered. What would you like to do now?

I would like to consult with a physician and the members of my team about termination of resuscitation efforts.

CASE 5: PULSELESS ELECTRICAL ACTIVITY

Objective	Given a patient situation, describe and demonstrate the initial emergency care for a patient in cardiac arrest due to pulseless electrical activity.
Skills to Master	Primary and secondary surveys Recognition of a patient in cardiac arrest Head tilt–chin lift, jaw thrust without head tilt Insertion of an oral or nasal airway CPR Pocket face mask or bag-mask ventilation Upper airway suctioning Attachment and use of ECG monitoring leads Upper airway suctioning Use of a pulse oximeter and capnometer IV/IO access IV/IO medication administration
Rhythms to Master	Junctional escape rhythm Idioventricular (ventricular escape) rhythm Sinus tachycardia Sinus bradycardia
Medications to Master	O_2 Epinephrine Vasopressin
Related Text Chapters	Chapter 1: The ABCDs of Emergency Cardiac Care Chapter 2: Airway Management: Oxygenation and Ventilation Chapter 3: Rhythms and Management
Essential Actions	• Ensure scene safety, use personal protective equipment • Perform a primary and secondary survey • Check for signs of obvious death, do not attempt resuscitation order • Begin CPR • Establish vascular access • Know the actions, indications, dosages, adverse effects, and contraindications for the medications used in the treatment of pulseless electrical activity • Follow each medication given in a cardiac arrest with a 20 mL IV fluid flush and elevation of the affected extremity • Consider possible reversible causes of the arrest • Facilitate family presence during resuscitative efforts according to agency/institution protocol
Unacceptable Actions	• Failure to use personal protective equipment • Failure to begin CPR • Performing CPR incorrectly (e.g., incorrect hand position, depth of compressions, compression rate, ventilation rate) • Failure to correctly identify the ECG rhythm • Giving O_2 by a means other than positive pressure ventilation • Failure to establish vascular access • Defibrillating PEA • Failure to give medications appropriate for the dysrhythmia

- Failure to consider the possible reversible causes of PEA
- Failure to recognize rhythm change
- Medication errors
- Performing any technique resulting in potential harm to the patient

Case 5: Scenario Sheet

Scenario: Your patient is a 53-year-old woman who was found unresponsive by her husband. The time is 1700. You have five other ALS personnel available to assist you. Emergency equipment is immediately available.

Emergency Action Steps	Necessary Tasks
Scene Survey	I am putting on personal protective equipment. Is the scene safe to enter? *Coach: The scene is safe.*

Initial Assessment

General Impression	As I approach the patient and form a general impression by assessing the patient's appearance, work of breathing, and circulation. What do I see? *Coach: You see a middle-aged woman lying supine on a stretcher. You estimate the patient weighs about 100 kg. Her eyes are closed and you do not observe any rise and fall of her chest.*

Primary Survey

Responsiveness/Breathing	I will quickly approach the patient and assess her level of responsiveness. Does she respond when I call her name? *Coach: The patient is unresponsive.* I will quickly check for breathing. *Coach: The patient is not breathing. How would you like to proceed?*
Circulation	I will feel for a carotid pulse for up to 10 seconds and assess the patient's skin condition at the same time. Is a pulse present? *Coach: There is no pulse. Her skin is cool, pale, and dry. What should be done now?* Because the patient is pulseless, I will ask the CPR team member to begin chest compressions and ask for the defibrillator immediately. Without interrupting CPR, I want the defibrillation team member to attach combination pads to the patient's bare chest. *Coach: Compressions are being performed and combination pads have been applied to the patient's chest as requested. How would you like to proceed?*
Airway	I will open the patient's airway using a head tilt–chin lift. Do I see anything in the patient's mouth such as blood, broken teeth or loose dentures, gastric contents, or a foreign object? *Coach: The patient's airway is clear. What should be done now?*
Breathing	I will ask the airway team member to size and insert an oral airway. I want the airway team member and an assistant to perform two-person ventilation with a bag-mask device connected to 100% O_2. The patient should be ventilated once every 5 to 6 seconds. I will ask another assistant to assess baseline breath sounds while the patient is being ventilated. *Coach: An oral airway has been inserted. Two-person bag-mask ventilation is being performed. You see gentle chest rise with bagging. Breath sounds are clear and equal with positive pressure ventilation. The defibrillator you requested is within arm's reach. What would you like to do next?*

Defibrillation/Disability

I want the CPR team member and airway team member to automatically rotate positions after every five cycles (about 2 minutes) of CPR so they do not become fatigued. I will assess the rhythm on the cardiac monitor. I want the patient's ECG rhythm checked every 2 minutes as the team members change positions.

Coach: You see this rhythm on the cardiac monitor (Figure 7-6). What is the rhythm? What do you want to do next?

Secondary Survey

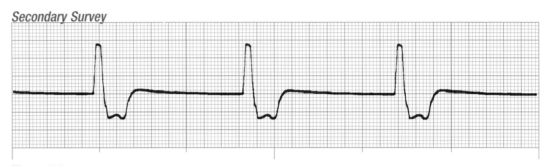

Figure 7-6

Vital Signs/History

The monitor shows an idioventricular rhythm. Although an organized rhythm is present on the monitor, the patient has no pulse, which means this is PEA. I will attempt to obtain a history from the patient's husband and perform a focused physical examination, looking for possible clues regarding the cause of the arrest.

Coach: (See SAMPLE history and physical examination findings). How would you like to proceed?

Sample History

Signs/symptoms	Unresponsive, apneic, pulseless
Allergies	Unknown
Medications	Unknown
Past medical history	Unknown
Last oral intake	Unknown
Events prior	According to the patient's husband, the patient told her daughter she was not feeling well and went to take a nap in the bedroom about 2 hours prior. The husband went to awaken his wife for dinner but could not arouse her. He reports that his wife has had no recent surgery or trauma. They returned from a 6-day stay in Mexico yesterday.

Physical Examination Findings

Head, ears, eyes, nose, and throat	Upper body blue
Neck	Trachea midline, no jugular venous distention
Chest	Breath sounds clear and equal with positive pressure ventilation; blue from the chest up
Abdomen	No abnormalities noted
Pelvis	No abnormalities noted
Extremities	No abnormalities noted
Posterior body	No abnormalities noted

Airway, Breathing, Circulation	I will ask my most experienced team member to intubate the patient. I want the IV team member to start an IV of normal saline without interrupting CPR and then administer 1 mg IV epinephrine (1:10,000 solution). I want each dose of epinephrine followed by flushing with 20 mL of normal saline IV and elevation of the patient's arm.

Coach: The airway team member states the tracheal tube is in place. The IV team member has successfully placed an IV in the left antecubital vein and epinephrine was administered as ordered. What should be done now?

Differential Diagnosis, Evaluates Interventions	I would like a cardiology consult right away. I want to confirm placement of the tracheal tube starting with a five-point auscultation of the patient's chest. I am listening over the epigastrium and then the right and left sides of the chest in four areas. What do I hear?

Coach: Breath sounds are clear and equal with bag-mask ventilation. A cardiology consult has been ordered.

I want to confirm placement with an esophageal detector device and waveform capnography. If proper tracheal tube position is confirmed, I will ask the airway team member to note the centimeter markings on the tracheal tube and then secure the tube in place.

Coach: The esophageal detector and waveform capnography confirm proper tube placement. The tracheal tube has been secured. What should be done now?

I will instruct the airway team member to continue positive pressure ventilation at a rate of 8 to 10 ventilations/min. I will instruct the CPR team member to continue chest compressions without pausing for ventilations. I will recheck the patient's cardiac rhythm.

Coach: High-quality CPR is continuing. The cardiac rhythm is unchanged and the patient still has no pulse.

I want the IV team member to give 1 mg of 1:10,000 epinephrine IV push now and every 3 to 5 minutes as long as the patient has no pulse. Flush each dose with 20 mL of normal saline and raise the patient's arm into which the drug was administered.

Coach: Epinephrine is being given IV as instructed. On the basis of the information available to you, what possible causes of this patient's cardiac arrest have you considered?

I suspect that two possible causes of the patient's PEA include hypoxia and a pulmonary embolism. I would like to order laboratory studies and a cardiology consult at this time.

Coach: You observe a change on the cardiac monitor (Figure 7-7). What is the rhythm? Does the change in the patient's cardiac rhythm necessitate any changes in the management of the patient at this time?

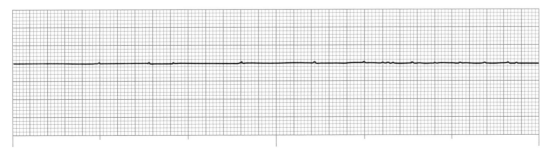

Figure 7-7

The monitor shows asystole and this does not necessitate any changes in patient management because PEA and asystole are managed similarly. I would like to reassess the quality of the CPR being performed and the assisted ventilations being delivered at this time. How much time has elapsed since we began resuscitation efforts? What is the total amount of epinephrine that has been given thus far?

Coach: High-quality CPR is ongoing. There is gentle chest rise with bagging and breath sounds are clear and equal with positive pressure ventilation. Forty-five minutes have now elapsed since resuscitation efforts began. So far, 8 milligrams of epinephrine have been given in 1-mg doses. The patient's ECG rhythm and condition remain unchanged. What should be done now?

I would like to consult with the cardiologist and members of my team about termination of resuscitation efforts.

CASE 6: ACUTE CORONARY SYNDROMES

Objective	Given a patient situation, describe and demonstrate the initial emergency care for a patient experiencing an acute coronary syndrome.
Skills to Master	Primary and secondary surveys
	Supplemental O_2 delivery devices
	Attachment and use of ECG monitoring leads
	IV access
	IV medication administration
	Knowledge of the ECG criteria for myocardial ischemia, injury, and infarction
Rhythms to Master	Sinus rhythm, sinus bradycardia, sinus tachycardia
	Atrial fibrillation, atrial flutter
	Atrioventricular (AV) blocks: first-degree, second-degree type I, second-degree type II, third-degree AV block
	Premature atrial complexes
	Premature ventricular complexes
	VF, VT
Medications to Master	O_2
	Nitroglycerin (NTG)
	Morphine sulfate
	Aspirin
	Fibrinolytics
	Beta-blockers
	Heparin
	Glycoprotein IIb/IIIa inhibitors
	Angiotensin-converting enzyme (ACE) inhibitors
Related Text Chapters	Chapter 1: The ABCDs of Emergency Cardiac Care
	Chapter 2: Airway Management: Oxygenation and Ventilation
	Chapter 3: Rhythms and Management
	Chapter 5: Acute Coronary Syndromes
Essential Actions	• Ensure scene safety, use personal protective equipment
	• Perform a primary and secondary survey
	• Give O_2, start an IV, obtain vital signs, attach a pulse oximeter and cardiac monitor, obtain a 12-lead ECG, order laboratory studies
	• Review the patient's initial 12-lead ECG for evidence of myocardial ischemia, injury, or infarction

- Know the actions, indications, dosages, adverse effects, and contraindications for the medications used in the treatment of acute coronary syndromes
- Use a reperfusion checklist to evaluate the patient's candidacy for reperfusion therapy

Unacceptable Actions
- Failure to use personal protective equipment
- Failure to monitor the cardiac rhythm in any patient who displays an abnormal ventilatory rate or effort, abnormal heart rate, perfusion, blood pressure, or acute altered mental status
- Failure to correctly identify the ECG rhythm
- Failure to start an IV
- Failure to give medications appropriate for patients with ischemic chest discomfort
- Medication errors
- Performing any technique resulting in potential harm to the patient

Case 6: Scenario Sheet

Scenario: Your patient is a 52-year-old man who is complaining of shortness of breath and substernal chest discomfort. The time is 0719. You have five other ALS personnel available to assist you. Emergency equipment is immediately available.

Emergency Action Steps	Necessary Tasks
Scene Survey	I am putting on personal protective equipment. Is the scene safe to enter? *Coach: The scene is safe.*

Initial Assessment

General Impression	As I approach the patient and form a general impression (assessing the patient's appearance, work of breathing, and circulation), what do I see? *Coach: You see a 52-year-old anxious-looking man sitting in a chair. His breathing does not appear to be labored. His skin is pink. How would you like to proceed?*

Primary Survey

Responsiveness/Airway	I will approach the patient and begin a primary survey. Is the patient aware of my approach? Does he respond when I speak his name? *Coach: The patient is aware of your approach. He quickly tells you that he is short of breath and has severe chest discomfort.*
Breathing	What is the rate and quality of the patient's breathing? *Coach: The patient's ventilatory rate is 22 and unlabored. The patient is able to speak in complete sentences without hesitation.*
Circulation	What is his pulse rate and quality? What is his skin condition? *Coach: Radial and carotid pulses are strong and regular. You estimate the heart rate to be about 60 beats/min. His skin is warm, pink, and moist.*
Defibrillation/Disability	I will make sure a defibrillator is within reach, although it is not needed at this time. *Coach: A biphasic defibrillator is available to you.*

Secondary Survey
Vital Signs/History

I want the defibrillation team member to attach a pulse oximeter and place the patient on a cardiac monitor.

Coach: The patient's SpO$_2$ is 88% on room air. The patient has been placed on the cardiac monitor.

Because the patient's SpO$_2$ is less than 94%, I want the airway team member to apply a nasal cannula at 4 L/min and reassess his oxygen saturation frequently to ensure that it remains above 94%. I want a team member to obtain the patient's baseline vital signs while I obtain a SAMPLE history from the patient and perform a focused physical examination. What are the patient's vital signs?

Coach: The patient's vital signs are: blood pressure 127/88 mm Hg, heart rate is 58, ventilations 22 breaths/min. Breath sounds are clear and equal. The patient's SpO$_2$ is now 98% with 4 L/min O$_2$ by nasal cannula. (See SAMPLE history and physical examination findings). How would you like to proceed?

Sample History

Signs/symptoms	Shortness of breath and substernal chest discomfort
OPQRST	Symptoms began at rest; patient describes his chest discomfort as "pressure" with radiation down his left arm and rates his discomfort at 10/10; the symptoms have been present for about 1 hour
Allergies	None
Medications	NTG, chlorzoxazone (Parafon Forte), imipramine (Tofranil), alprazolam (Xanax), hydrochlorothiazide (Hydrodiuril)
Past medical history	Depression, hypertension, angina pectoris; patient is 5'9" and weighs 190 pounds
Last oral intake	Dinner last evening
Events prior	The patient states that he was watching the morning news on television when his symptoms began; he denies nausea, vomiting, and dizziness

Physical Examination Findings

Head, ears, eyes, nose, and throat	No abnormalities noted
Neck	Trachea midline, no jugular venous distention
Chest	Breath sounds clear bilaterally
Abdomen	No abnormalities noted
Pelvis	No abnormalities noted
Extremities	No abnormalities noted
Posterior body	No abnormalities noted

Airway, Breathing, Circulation

I want the IV team member to confirm that there are no contraindications, and then give the patient 325 mg of baby aspirin and ask the patient to chew and swallow it. I want the IV team member to start an IV of normal saline and then I want to order a 12-lead ECG. How does the patient rate his discomfort now?

Coach: An IV has been started. Aspirin has been given. The patient rates his discomfort at 10/10. A 12-lead ECG has been obtained as ordered (Figure 7-8). Are there any significant findings on this 12-lead?

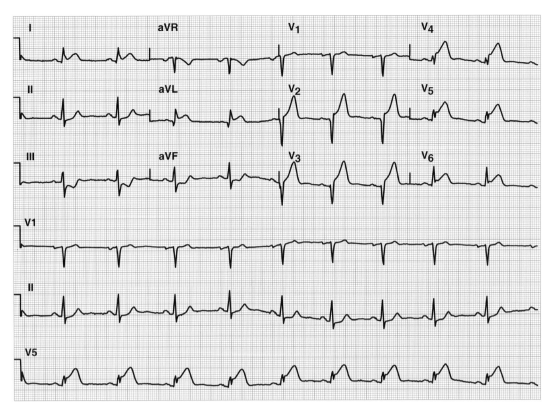

Figure 7-8

Differential Diagnosis, Evaluates Interventions

The 12-lead shows a sinus bradycardia at 58 beats/min. There is ST elevation in leads I, aVL, and V_2 through V_6. There is ST depression in leads II, III, and aVF. I want the IV team member to give a 300 mg loading dose of clopidogrel at this time. In addition, I want sublingual NTG given now and repeated every 5 minutes as needed to a maximum of three doses (assuming the patient's vital signs remain stable). I want the patient's blood pressure and level of discomfort reevaluated 5 minutes after each dose of NTG. I want another team member to order cardiac biomarkers and other laboratory work as well as a portable chest radiograph, and to begin a reperfusion therapy checklist right away.

Coach: The loading dose of clopidogrel was given as instructed. The patient rated his chest discomfort as 10/10 after the first dose of NTG. His BP remained stable and a second NTG dose was given. The patient's discomfort was subsequently noted as 8/10. A third dose of NTG was given (the patient's vital signs continued to remain stable), with no change in the patient's rating of his discomfort (i.e., 8/10). How would you like to proceed?

The patient's 12-lead ECG suggests an extensive anterior myocardial infarction (MI). A physician needs to review the 12-lead right away and to classify the patient as an ST elevation MI (STEMI). I would like the IV team member to give the patient 2 mg of morphine now. I want this repeated every 5 minutes as needed until the patient is pain free (assuming his vital signs remain stable). I want the patient's vital signs taken and recorded between doses.

Coach: What would you like to do next?

Postresuscitation Support/Reassessment

Begins Postresuscitation Support/Performs Reassessment	I want to repeat the primary survey and obtain another set of vital signs. How is the patient's discomfort? *Coach: The patient's blood pressure is now 131/91 mm Hg, his heart rate is 66 beats/min, and his ventilatory rate is 18 breaths/min. After two doses of IV morphine, he rates his discomfort as 0/10. What should be done now?* I want to make sure the reperfusion checklist is completed and schedule the patient for the cardiac catheterization laboratory.

CASE 7: SYMPTOMATIC BRADYCARDIA

Objective	Given a patient situation, describe and demonstrate the initial emergency care for a patient with a symptomatic bradycardia.
Skills to Master	Primary and secondary surveys Supplemental O_2 delivery devices Attachment and use of ECG monitoring leads IV access IV medication administration Operation of a transcutaneous pacemaker
Rhythms to Master	Sinus rhythm Sinus bradycardia Junctional rhythm Idioventricular (ventricular escape) rhythm AV blocks: first-degree, second-degree type I, second-degree type II, third-degree AV block
Medications to Master	O_2 Atropine Dopamine Epinephrine Isoproterenol
Related Text Chapters	Chapter 1: The ABCDs of Emergency Cardiac Care Chapter 2: Airway Management: Oxygenation and Ventilation Chapter 3: Rhythms and Management Chapter 4: Electrical Therapy Chapter 5: Acute Coronary Syndromes
Essential Actions	• Ensure scene safety, use personal protective equipment • Perform a primary and secondary survey • Give O_2, start an IV, obtain vital signs, attach a pulse oximeter and cardiac monitor, obtain a 12-lead ECG • Recognize first-degree, second-degree type I, second-degree type II, and third-degree AV blocks • Obtain a history and perform a physical examination, recognizing a symptomatic bradycardia • Give medications as indicated • Perform transcutaneous pacing as indicated • Consider reperfusion therapy if the patient's signs and symptoms are consistent with an acute coronary syndrome and there are no contraindications
Unacceptable Actions	• Failure to use personal protective equipment • Failure to monitor the cardiac rhythm in any patient who displays abnormal ventilatory rate or effort, abnormal heart rate, perfusion, blood pressure, or acute altered mental status • Failure to correctly identify the ECG rhythm • Failure to start an IV

- Failure to correctly operate a transcutaneous pacemaker (if pacing is indicated and ordered)
- Giving lidocaine for ventricular escape rhythms
- Treating an asymptomatic bradycardia with medications or pacing
- Medication errors
- Performing any technique resulting in potential harm to the patient

Case 7: Scenario Sheet

Scenario: Your patient is a 76-year-old woman who is complaining of dizziness. The time is 1121. You have five other ALS personnel available to assist you. Emergency equipment is immediately available.

Emergency Action Steps	Necessary Tasks
Scene Survey	I am putting on personal protective equipment. Is the scene safe to enter? *Coach: The scene is safe.*

Initial Assessment

General Impression	As I approach the patient and form a general impression (assessing the patient's appearance, work of breathing, and circulation), what do I see? *Coach: You see an ill-appearing woman lying on a stretcher. Her eyes are closed. You can see equal rise and fall of her chest. Her skin is pale. How would you like to proceed?*

Primary Survey

Responsiveness/Airway	I will approach the patient and begin a primary survey. Is the patient aware of my approach? Does she respond when I speak her name? *Coach: The patient opens her eyes as you approach and tells you that she is very dizzy.*
Breathing	What is the rate and quality of the patient's breathing? *Coach: The patient's ventilatory rate is 18 breaths/min and unlabored.*
Circulation	What is her pulse rate and quality? What is her skin condition? *Coach: The patient's carotid pulse is weak but regular. You estimate the rate to be about 30 beats/min. You are unable to palpate a radial pulse. Her skin is cool, pale, and dry.*
Defibrillation/Disability	I will make sure a defibrillator is within reach, although it is not needed at this time. *Coach: A biphasic defibrillator is available to you.*

Secondary Survey

Vital Signs/History	I want a team member to attach a pulse oximeter and place the patient on a cardiac monitor. I want another team member to obtain the patient's baseline vital signs while I obtain a SAMPLE history from the patient and perform a focused physical examination. What are the patient's vital signs? *Coach: The patient's vital signs are as follows: blood pressure 64/42 mm Hg, heart rate approximately 30 beats/min, and ventilatory rate is 18 breaths/min. Breath sounds are clear and equal. The patient's SpO$_2$ is 90% on room air. The patient has been placed on the cardiac monitor (Figure 7-9). (See SAMPLE history and physical examination findings). What is the rhythm on the monitor? How would you like to proceed?*

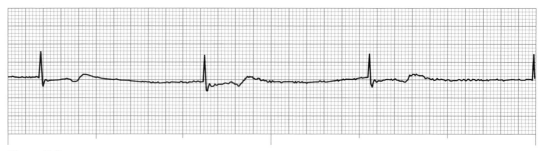

Figure 7-9

Sample History

Signs/ symptoms	Sudden onset of severe dizziness
Allergies	None
Medications	Furosemide (Lasix), aspirin, olanzapine (Zyprexa), pantoprazole (Protonix), paroxetine (Paxil)
Past medical history	Arthritis, osteoporosis, heart failure, schizophrenia, gastroesophageal reflux disease, depression
Last oral intake	Breakfast 3 hours ago
Events prior	Sudden onset of dizziness; symptoms started about 30 minutes ago while at rest

Physical Examination Findings

Head, ears, eyes, nose, and throat	No abnormalities noted
Neck	Trachea midline, no jugular venous distention
Chest	Breath sounds clear bilaterally
Abdomen	No abnormalities noted
Pelvis	No abnormalities noted
Extremities	No abnormalities noted
Posterior body	No abnormalities noted

Airway, Breathing, Circulation	The monitor shows a junctional bradycardia. I will ask the airway team member to place the patient on supplemental O₂ by nasal cannula at 4 L/min. I want the IV team member to start an IV of normal saline and I want to order a 12-lead ECG. I also want to make sure that my defibrillator has transcutaneous pacing capability.
	Coach: The patient has been placed on O₂ as instructed. An IV has been started. A 12-lead ECG has been ordered. The defibrillator available to you does have transcutaneous pacing capability.
Differential Diagnosis, Evaluates Interventions	I want to give the patient 0.5 mg of atropine IV now. In addition, I want to order cardiac biomarkers, additional laboratory studies, and a portable chest radiograph. I would like to order a cardiology consult as soon as possible and begin a reperfusion therapy checklist.
	Coach: Atropine has been given as ordered. Laboratory work and a chest radiograph have been ordered. A cardiology consult has been ordered. A reperfusion checklist has been started. What would you like to do next?

Postresuscitation Support/Reassessment

Begins Postresuscitation Support/Performs Reassessment	I want to repeat the primary survey and obtain another set of vital signs. Has there been any improvement in the patient's symptoms?

Coach: The patient's heart rate has increased to 48 beats/min (i.e., junctional rhythm). Her blood pressure is now 74/53 mm Hg, and her ventilatory rate is 16 breaths/min. What should be done now?

I want to give the patient another 0.5 mg of atropine IV and repeat the primary survey and vital signs.

Coach: A second dose of atropine has been given as ordered. The patient's blood pressure is now 110/66 mm Hg, her heart rate is 80 beats/min, and her ventilatory rate is 16 breaths/min. Her skin is now warm, pink, and dry. The patient states that she is feeling much better. What would you like to do next?

I will continue to monitor the patient's ECG and vital signs closely. I will review the results of the patient's 12-lead ECG and laboratory studies to try to determine the cause of the patient's bradycardia.

CASE 8: UNSTABLE TACHYCARDIA

Objective	Given a patient situation, describe and demonstrate the initial emergency care for an unstable patient with a narrow or wide-QRS tachycardia.
Skills to Master	Primary and secondary surveys Supplemental O_2 delivery devices Attachment and use of ECG monitoring leads IV access IV medication administration Synchronized cardioversion
Rhythms to Master	AV nodal reentrant tachycardia AV reentrant tachycardia Atrial tachycardia Junctional tachycardia Monomorphic ventricular tachycardia Polymorphic ventricular tachycardia Wide-complex tachycardia of unknown origin
Medications to Master	O_2 Adenosine Amiodarone Magnesium sulfate Procainamide Sotalol
Related Text Chapters	Chapter 1: The ABCDs of Emergency Cardiac Care Chapter 2: Airway Management: Oxygenation and Ventilation Chapter 3: Rhythms and Management Chapter 4: Electrical Therapy
Essential Actions	• Ensure scene safety, use personal protective equipment • Perform a primary and secondary survey • Quickly recognize if the patient is stable or unstable • Quickly identify the ECG rhythm, determining if the QRS is narrow or wide, regular or irregular • Recognize sinus tachycardia, AV nodal reentrant tachycardia, AV reentrant tachycardia, atrial tachycardia, junctional tachycardia, monomorphic ventricular tachycardia, polymorphic ventricular tachycardia, and wide-complex tachycardia of unknown origin • Obtain vital signs, start an IV, attach a pulse oximeter and cardiac monitor, give supplemental O_2 if indicated, obtain a 12-lead ECG • Obtain a history and perform a physical examination, recognizing a symptomatic tachycardia

- Know the actions, indications, dosages, adverse effects, and contraindications for the medications used in the treatment of a narrow-QRS or wide-QRS tachycardia
- Deliver the correct type of energy (synchronized cardioversion versus defibrillation) and the correct energy level for the tachycardia if electrical therapy is indicated
- Demonstrate safe operation of the defibrillator, including ensuring O_2 is not flowing over the patient's chest during each shock if electrical therapy is indicated
- Perform synchronized cardioversion as indicated
- Recognize the need to change from synchronized cardioversion to defibrillation if the rhythm changes to pulseless VT or VF

Unacceptable Actions
- Failure to use personal protective equipment
- Inability to quickly determine if the patient is stable or unstable
- Failure to monitor the cardiac rhythm in any patient who displays an abnormal ventilatory rate or effort, abnormal heart rate, perfusion, blood pressure, or acute altered mental status
- Failure to correctly identify the ECG rhythm
- Failure to start an IV
- Unsafe operation of defibrillator (failure to clear self or others before shocking)
- Medication errors
- Performing any technique resulting in potential harm to the patient

Case 8: Scenario Sheet

Scenario: Your patient is a 37-year-old man who states that he was awakened by heart palpitations. The time is 0023. You have five other ALS personnel available to assist you. Emergency equipment is immediately available.

Emergency Action Steps	Necessary Tasks
Scene Survey	I am putting on personal protective equipment. Is the scene safe to enter? *Coach: The scene is safe.*

Initial Assessment

General Impression	As I approach the patient and form a general impression (assessing the patient's appearance, work of breathing, and circulation), what do I see? *Coach: You see a man supine on a stretcher. He is awake and his skin looks very pale. You can see the rise and fall of his chest. How would you like to proceed?*

Primary Survey

Responsiveness/Airway	I will approach the patient and begin a primary survey. Does he respond when I speak his name? *Coach: The patient is aware of your approach and responds as you greet him.*
Breathing	What is the rate and quality of the patient's breathing? *Coach: The patient's breathing is unlabored at a rate of 16 breaths/min.*
Circulation	What is his pulse rate and quality? What is his skin condition? *Coach: You are unable to feel a radial pulse. A weak carotid pulse is present. You estimate the heart rate to be about 150 beats/min. The patient's skin is cool, pale, and moist.*
Defibrillation/Disability	I want to make sure that a defibrillator is within reach. *Coach: A biphasic defibrillator is available to you.*

Secondary Survey
Vital Signs/History

I want a team member to attach a pulse oximeter and place the patient on a cardiac monitor. I want a team member to obtain the patient's baseline vital signs while I obtain a SAMPLE history from the patient and perform a focused physical examination. What are the patient's vital signs?

Coach: The patient's vital signs are: blood pressure 50/24 mm Hg, heart rate is 150 beats/min, and ventilatory rate is 16 breaths/min. Breath sounds are clear and equal. The patient's SpO$_2$ is 88% on room air. The patient has been placed on the cardiac monitor (Figure 7-10). (See SAMPLE history and physical examination findings). What is the rhythm on the monitor? How would you like to proceed?

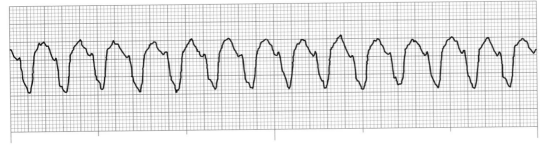

Figure 7-10

Sample History

Signs/symptoms	Heart palpitations
Allergies	Codeine, sulfa
Medications	Albuterol (Proventil), ipratropium (Atrovent)
Past medical history	Asthma
Last oral intake	Dinner at 1800
Events prior	Awakened from sleep by "heart palpitations"; symptoms present for 1.5 hours

Physical Examination Findings

Head, ears, eyes, nose, and throat	No abnormalities noted
Neck	Trachea midline, no jugular venous distention
Chest	Breath sounds clear and equal bilaterally
Abdomen	No abnormalities noted
Pelvis	No abnormalities noted
Extremities	No abnormalities noted
Posterior body	No abnormalities noted

Airway, Breathing, Circulation

The monitor shows monomorphic ventricular tachycardia (VT). The patient is unstable (e.g., severe hypotension). I want the airway team member to administer supplemental O$_2$ by nonrebreather mask for now and monitor the patient's oxygen saturation. I want the IV team member to start an IV of normal saline. I want to order a 12-lead ECG and cardiology consult as soon as possible. I will ask the defibrillation team member to apply combination pads to the patient's bare chest and prepare to shock the patient. While preparing to shock the patient, I will ask the IV team member to sedate the patient with midazolam (Versed).

Coach: An IV has been started. A 12-lead ECG has been ordered. Midazolam has been given as instructed. The cardiologist is en route. Are you going to perform synchronized cardioversion or will you defibrillate the patient?

Because the patient has a pulse and the rhythm is monomorphic VT, I want the defibrillation team member to perform synchronized cardioversion.

Coach: A biphasic manual defibrillator is available to you. What initial energy setting will you use?

Differential Diagnosis, Evaluates Interventions

I will begin synchronized cardioversion using 100 J, which is the energy setting recommended by the manufacturer. When the defibrillation team member is ready, he or she will make sure that oxygen is not flowing over the patient's chest and all team members (including himself or herself) are clear of the patient before delivering the shock.

Coach: A synchronized shock was delivered using 100 joules. You see the following rhythm on the monitor (Figure 7-11). What is the rhythm?

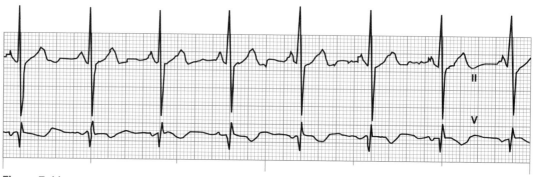

Figure 7-11

The monitor shows a sinus rhythm.

Coach: What would you like to do next?

Postresuscitation Support/Reassessment

Begins Postresuscitation Support/Performs Reassessment

I want to repeat the primary survey and obtain another set of vital signs.

Coach: Strong carotid and radial pulses are present. The patient's ventilatory rate is 14 breaths/min. Breath sounds are clear and equal. Blood pressure is 108/88 mm Hg, and his SpO$_2$ is 99%. The cardiologist is here.

I want the patient's vital signs monitored every 5 minutes for the next 30 minutes and will transfer patient care to the cardiologist.

CASE 9: STABLE TACHYCARDIA

Objective

Given a patient situation, describe and demonstrate the initial emergency care for a stable but symptomatic patient with a narrow or wide-QRS tachycardia.

Skills to Master

Primary and secondary surveys
Supplemental O$_2$ delivery devices
Attachment and use of ECG monitoring leads
IV access
IV medication administration

Rhythms to Master	Sinus tachycardia
	AV nodal reentrant tachycardia
	AV reentrant tachycardia
	Atrial tachycardia
	Junctional tachycardia
	Monomorphic ventricular tachycardia
	Polymorphic ventricular tachycardia
	Wide-complex tachycardia of unknown origin
Medications to Master	O_2
	Adenosine
	Amiodarone
	Beta-blockers
	Diltiazem
	Magnesium sulfate
	Procainamide
	Sotalol
	Verapamil
Related Text Chapters	Chapter 1: The ABCDs of Emergency Cardiac Care
	Chapter 2: Airway Management: Oxygenation and Ventilation
	Chapter 3: Rhythms and Management
	Chapter 4: Electrical Therapy

Essential Actions

- Ensure scene safety, use personal protective equipment
- Perform a primary and secondary survey
- Quickly recognize if the patient is stable or unstable
- Quickly identify the ECG rhythm, determining if the QRS is narrow or wide, regular or irregular
- Obtain vital signs, start an IV, attach a pulse oximeter and cardiac monitor, give supplemental O_2 if indicated, obtain a 12-lead ECG
- Recognize sinus tachycardia, AV nodal reentrant tachycardia, AV reentrant tachycardia, atrial tachycardia, junctional tachycardia, monomorphic ventricular tachycardia, polymorphic ventricular tachycardia, and wide-complex tachycardia of unknown origin
- Know what a vagal maneuver is, types, and when they are performed
- Know the actions, indications, dosages, adverse effects, and contraindications for the medications used in the treatment of a narrow-QRS or wide-QRS tachycardia

Unacceptable Actions

- Failure to use personal protective equipment
- Inability to quickly determine if the patient is stable or unstable
- Failure to monitor the cardiac rhythm in any patient who displays an abnormal ventilatory rate or effort, abnormal heart rate, perfusion, blood pressure, or acute altered mental status
- Failure to correctly identify the ECG rhythm
- Failure to start an IV
- Failure to give medications appropriate for the dysrhythmia
- Medication errors
- Performing any technique resulting in potential harm to the patient

Case 9: Scenario Sheet

Scenario: A 19-year-old man presents with a complaint of a "rapid heartbeat" and chest discomfort. You have four ALS personnel available to assist you. Emergency equipment is available.

Emergency Action Steps	Necessary Tasks

Scene Survey

I am putting on personal protective equipment. Is the scene safe to enter?
Coach: The scene is safe.

Initial Assessment

General Impression

As I approach the patient and form a general impression (assessing the patient's appearance, work of breathing, and circulation), what do I see?
Coach: You see a nervous-appearing young man sitting upright on a stretcher. His breathing is unlabored. His skin is pink. How would you like to proceed?

Primary Survey

Responsiveness/Airway

I will approach the patient and begin a primary survey. Is the patient aware of my approach? Does he respond when I speak his name?
Coach: As you approach, the patient speaks hurriedly, telling you that his heart is "racing and feels like it is going to pound out of my chest."

Breathing

What is the rate and quality of the patient's breathing?
Coach: The patient's ventilatory rate is 18 breaths/min and unlabored.

Circulation

What is his pulse rate and quality? What is his skin condition?
Coach: His radial and carotid pulses are strong but too fast to count accurately. You estimate the rate to be about 200 beats/min. His skin is warm, pink, and moist.

Defibrillation/Disability

I will assist the patient to a supine position and make sure a defibrillator is within reach.
Coach: A biphasic defibrillator is available to you.

Secondary Survey

Vital Signs/History

I want a team member to attach a pulse oximeter and place the patient on a cardiac monitor. I will ask the airway team member to administer supplemental O_2 if indicated. I want a team member to obtain the patient's baseline vital signs while I obtain a SAMPLE history and perform a focused physical examination. What are the patient's vital signs?
Coach: The patient's vital signs are: blood pressure 134/90 mm Hg, heart rate is 214 beats/min, and ventilatory rate is 18 breaths/min. Breath sounds are clear and equal. The patient's SpO_2 on room air is 99% and he has been placed on the cardiac monitor (Figure 7-12). (See SAMPLE history and physical examination findings). What is the rhythm shown on the monitor? How would you like to proceed?

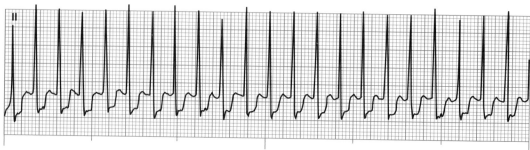

Figure 7-12

Sample History

Signs/ symptoms	Rapid heartbeat and chest discomfort
OPQRST	Symptoms began when the patient was at rest; he describes his chest discomfort as "pressure" and rates his discomfort at 1/10; his symptoms have been present for about 25 minutes
Allergies	None
Medications	None
Past medical history	None
Last oral intake	Caffeine-free soda 1 hour ago
Events prior	Patient was sitting in the college library when his symptoms began

Physical Examination Findings

Head, ears, eyes, nose, and throat	No abnormalities noted
Neck	Trachea midline, no jugular venous distention
Chest	Breath sounds clear bilaterally
Abdomen	No abnormalities noted
Pelvis	No abnormalities noted
Extremities	No abnormalities noted
Posterior body	No abnormalities noted

Airway, Breathing, Circulation	The monitor shows a narrow-QRS tachycardia with ST depression. I want the IV team member to start an IV of normal saline and I want to order a 12-lead ECG.
	Coach: An IV has been started in the right antecubital vein. A 12-lead has been ordered. What would you like to do now?
Differential Diagnosis, Evaluates Interventions	On the basis of the patient's history and physical findings, I believe the patient is stable at this time. I will ask the patient to perform a vagal maneuver (e.g., to bear down as if having a bowel movement).
	Coach: The patient has complied with your instructions, but no change is observed on the cardiac monitor.
	Because the rhythm is a narrow-QRS tachycardia, I will ask the IV team member to give 6 mg of adenosine via rapid IV bolus over 1 to 3 seconds, to follow with a 20-mL IV normal saline flush, and to then raise the patient's arm for 10 to 20 seconds.
	Coach: Adenosine has been given as ordered. What would you like to do next?

Postresuscitation Support/Reassessment

Begins Postresuscitation Support/Performs Reassessment	I would like to order a cardiology consult as soon as possible. I want to repeat the primary survey and obtain another set of vital signs. Has there been any change in the patient's rhythm or in the patient's condition?
	Coach: A cardiology consult has been requested. The cardiologist is en route and is expected to arrive in about 20 minutes. The monitor now shows the following rhythm (Figure 7-13). The patient's chest discomfort has resolved. His blood pressure is now 122/70, his heart rate is about 40 beats/min, and his ventilatory rate is 16 breaths/min. His skin is warm, pink, and dry. The patient states he "feels much better." What is the rhythm on the monitor? What should be done now?

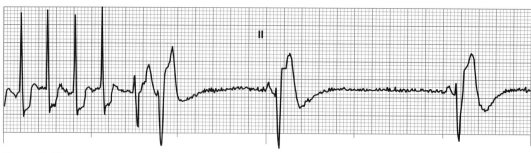

Figure 7-13

The monitor shows conversion from a narrow-QRS tachycardia–a sinus beat, a premature ventricular complex, and two sinus beats with ST elevation. Although the patient's heart rate is bradycardic at present, it is very likely that the rate will gradually increase over the next few minutes. I will continue to monitor the patient's ECG and vital signs closely while awaiting arrival of the cardiologist.

CASE 10: ACUTE ISCHEMIC STROKE

Objective	Given a patient situation, describe and demonstrate the initial emergency care for a patient experiencing an acute ischemic stroke.
Skills to Master	Primary and secondary surveys
	Supplemental O2 delivery devices
	Attachment and use of ECG monitoring leads
	Upper airway suctioning
	Serum glucose determination
	IV access
	IV medication administration
Rhythms to Master	Atrial fibrillation
	Sinus rhythm
Medications to Master	O_2
	Fibrinolytics
	Dextrose (if documented hypoglycemia)
Related Text Chapters	Chapter 1: The ABCDs of Emergency Cardiac Care
	Chapter 2: Airway Management: Oxygenation and Ventilation
	Chapter 3: Rhythms and Management
	Chapter 6: Acute Stroke

Essential Actions

- Ensure scene safety, use personal protective equipment
- Perform a primary and secondary survey
- Give O_2, start an IV, obtain vital signs, attach a pulse oximeter and cardiac monitor, check serum glucose, obtain 12-lead ECG, laboratory studies
- Give dextrose if documented hypoglycemia is present
- Obtain a focused history and perform a physical examination including vital signs, recognizing signs and symptoms of possible stroke
- Determine time of symptom onset
- Perform a general neurological screening assessment
- Order an urgent noncontrast CT scan
- Use a reperfusion checklist to determine the patient's eligibility for fibrinolytic therapy
- Consider fibrinolytics if the patient's presentation is consistent with acute ischemic stroke verified by CT scan and there are no contraindications

Unacceptable Actions

- Failure to use personal protective equipment
- Failure to monitor the cardiac rhythm in any patient who displays abnormal ventilatory rate or effort, abnormal heart rate, perfusion, blood pressure, or acute altered mental status
- Failure to establish IV access
- Failure to give medications appropriate for patients with acute ischemic stroke
- Medication errors
- Performing any technique resulting in potential harm to the patient

Case 10: Scenario Sheet

Scenario: A 73-year-old woman presents with a sudden onset of slurred speech. The patient's son is present. The time is 0906. You have four ALS personnel available to assist you. Emergency equipment is available.

Emergency Action Steps	Necessary Tasks

Scene Survey

I am putting on personal protective equipment. Is the scene safe to enter?
Coach: The scene is safe.

Initial Assessment

General Impression

As I approach the patient and form a general impression (assessing the patient's appearance, work of breathing, and circulation), what do I see?
Coach: You find the patient awake and supine on a stretcher. You see equal rise and fall of her chest. Her skin is pink and looks dry.

Primary Survey
Responsiveness

I will approach the patient and begin a primary survey. Is the patient aware of my approach? Does she respond when I speak her name?
Coach: The patient is aware of your approach and attempts to answer you, but her speech is garbled and unintelligible.

Airway/Breathing

I will look in the patient's mouth to make sure there is nothing present that may cause an airway obstruction or may explain the reason for the patient's garbled speech.
Coach: The patient's airway is clear.
What is the rate and quality of the patient's breathing?
Coach: Her breathing is quiet and unlabored at a rate of 18 breaths/min.

Circulation

What is her pulse rate and quality? What is her skin condition?
Coach: The patient's radial and carotid pulses are strong and regular at a rate of about 70 beats/min. The patient's skin is warm, pink, and dry.

Defibrillation/Disability

I want to make sure that a defibrillator is within reach, although it is not needed at this time.
Coach: A biphasic defibrillator is available to you.

Secondary Survey
Vital Signs/History

I want a team member to attach a pulse oximeter and place the patient on a cardiac monitor. I will ask the airway team member to administer O_2 if the patient's SpO_2 is less than 94%. I want the CPR team member to obtain the patient's baseline vital signs while I obtain a SAMPLE history from the patient and her son and perform a focused physical examination. I would like the patient's blood pressure assessed in both arms.

Coach: The patient's vital signs are as follows: blood pressure 217/93 in the left arm and 208/90 in the right arm, heart rate is strong and regular at 74 beats/min, and ventilatory rate is 18 breaths/min. Breath sounds are clear and equal. The patient's SpO$_2$ is 98% on room air. The patient has been placed on the cardiac monitor (Figure 7-14). (See SAMPLE history and physical examination findings). What is the rhythm shown on the monitor? How would you like to proceed?

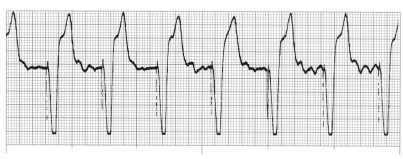

Figure 7-14

Sample History

Signs/ symptoms	Patient awoke at 0730 with slurred speech; it is apparent that the patient can understand you, although you cannot understand her
Allergies	None
Medications	Niaspan (Niacin), lisinopril with hydrochlorothiazide (Zestoretic), gabapentin (Neurontin)
Past medical history	Seizures, hypertension, pacemaker, high cholesterol
Last oral intake	Dinner about 1900 last evening
Events prior	The patient's son states that his mother has complained of heartburn and not feeling well for about 24 hours; she awoke this morning with slurred speech and said she was "feeling sick," with nausea, dizziness, and sweating.

Physical Examination Findings

Head, ears, eyes, nose, and throat	Pupils equal and reactive, but sluggish; right-sided facial droop present
Neck	Trachea midline, no jugular venous distention
Chest	Breath sounds clear bilaterally; pacemaker noted in left pectoral region
Abdomen	No abnormalities noted
Pelvis	No abnormalities noted
Extremities	Pulses, movement, and sensation equal bilaterally
Posterior body	No abnormalities noted

Airway, Breathing, Circulation	The monitor shows a ventricular paced rhythm. It looks like the patient's underlying rhythm is atrial flutter. I will ask the IV team member to start an IV of normal saline and check the patient's serum glucose level. I want to order a 12-lead ECG.

Coach: An IV has been started. A 12-lead ECG has been ordered. The patient's serum glucose level is 143 mg/dL. Why is it important to determine the serum glucose level of a patient with a suspected stroke?

Differential Diagnosis, Evaluates Interventions

A serum glucose level helps to differentiate a possible stroke from other common causes of stroke symptoms (e.g., hypoglycemia).

Coach: After obtaining the SAMPLE history, tell me three questions you should ask about a patient who presents with signs and symptoms of an acute stroke.

When was the last time the patient was known to be without symptoms? (i.e., the last known well time)

Was anyone with the patient with her symptoms started?

What was she doing when the symptoms began?

Did the patient complain of a headache?

Did she have a seizure?

Has there been a change in her level of responsiveness?

Is there a history of any recent trauma?

Coach: The patient's son states that his mother complained of heartburn and not feeling well for about 24 hours. She awoke at 0730 this morning with slurred speech (which is new for this patient) and said she was "feeling sick," with nausea, dizziness, and sweating. The patient does not have a headache, chest pain, or shortness of breath. Although the patient has a history of seizures, her last seizure was 4 months ago. There is no history of recent trauma. What would you like to do now?

On the basis of the patient's history and physical findings, I will alert the stroke team right away and order a 12-lead ECG, laboratory studies, and a portable chest radiograph. I will perform an initial neurologic evaluation using the Cincinnati Prehospital Stroke Scale.

Coach: What areas are assessed using this scale?

The Cincinnati Prehospital Stroke Scale assesses facial droop and weakness, arm drift, and speech. I will also attempt to establish the time of symptom onset.

Coach: Facial droop is present on the right. The patient is unable to repeat a phrase clearly. The upper extremities move equally. The patient has not been feeling well for 24 hours. She awoke at 0730 today with slurred speech.

I will begin completing a fibrinolytic therapy checklist to determine if the patient is a candidate for therapy and order a noncontrast computed tomography (CT) scan.

Coach: What is the time target for a possible stroke patient evaluation by a physician?

A patient who presents with a possible stroke should be seen by a physician within 10 minutes of arrival in the emergency department.

Coach: What are the time targets for obtaining and reading a CT scan?

A CT scan should be completed within 25 minutes of patient arrival and read by a physician within 45 minutes.

Coach: What would you like to do now?

Postresuscitation Support/Reassessment

Begins Postresuscitation Support/Performs Reassessment

I want to repeat the primary survey, obtain another set of vital signs, and transfer patient care to the stroke team.

Coach: The patient's airway remains clear and her breathing is adequate. Blood pressure is 210/95 mm Hg, ventilatory rate is 18 breaths/min, SpO$_2$ is 98%, and there is no change in the patient's heart rate. The patient's skin is warm and dry.

REFERENCES

1. Vanden Hoek TL, Morrison LJ, Shuster M, et al: Part 12: cardiac arrest in special situations: 2010 American Heart Association guidelines for cardiopulmonary resuscitation and emergency cardiovascular care, *Circulation* 122(Suppl 3):S829–S861, 2010.
2. Neumar RW, Otto CW, Link MS, et al. Part 8: adult advanced cardiovascular life support: 2010 American Heart Association Guidelines for Cardiopulmonary Resuscitation and Emergency Cardiovascular Care, *Circulation* 122(Suppl 3):S729–S767, 2010.

POSTTEST

Multiple Choice

Identify the choice that best completes the statement or answers the question.

_____ 1. From across the room, your general impression of a 78-year-old woman reveals that her eyes are closed, she is not moving, you can see no rise and fall of her chest or abdomen, and her skin color is pale. When you arrive at the patient's side, you confirm that she is unresponsive. Your best action in this situation will be to:
   a. Open her airway and give two breaths
   b. Apply the automated external defibrillator (AED)
   c. Check breathing and determine if she has a pulse
   d. Prepare the necessary equipment to insert an advanced airway

_____ 2. Which of the following statements about two-rescuer adult cardiopulmonary resuscitation (CPR) is correct?
   a. The compression to ventilation ratio is 15:2.
   b. Chest compressions should be performed at a rate of 80 to 100 per minute.
   c. The switch of compressor and ventilator roles should occur in 5 seconds or less when possible.
   d. Opening the airway and ventilating the victim are the initial actions performed when starting CPR in victims of cardiac arrest.

_____ 3. Assuming there are no contraindications, which of the following can be performed as an initial action in a stable but symptomatic patient with a narrow-QRS tachycardia?
   a. Vagal maneuvers
   b. Synchronized cardioversion
   c. Administration of diltiazem IV
   d. Administration of verapamil IV

_____ 4. Which of the following statements is true about the administration of epinephrine during cardiac arrest?
   a. One mg of epinephrine 1:1000 solution should be given in a slow IV push over 3 to 5 minutes.
   b. One mg of epinephrine 1:10,000 solution should be given rapid IV push every 3 to 5 minutes.
   c. Two to 2.5 mg of epinephrine 1:1000 solution should be given slow IV push over 3 to 5 minutes.
   d. Two to 2.5 mg of epinephrine 1:10,000 solution should be given rapid IV push every 3 to 5 minutes.

_____   5.   Which of the following statements is INCORRECT regarding safety precautions during defibrillation or synchronized cardioversion?
a. Use adult defibrillator paddles or pads for all patients.
b. When using handheld paddles, use gels or pastes that are specifically made for defibrillation.
c. When applying combination pads to a patient's bare chest, press from one edge of the pad across the entire surface to remove all air.
d. Remove supplemental oxygen sources from the area of the patient's bed before defibrillation and cardioversion attempts and place them at least 3.5 to 4 feet away from the patient's chest.

_____   6.   Which of the following situations does not require a reduction in the initial dose of IV adenosine?
a. Giving adenosine through a central IV line
b. Giving adenosine to a patient who is taking theophylline
c. Giving adenosine to a patient who has a transplanted heart
d. Giving adenosine to a patient who is taking carbamazepine (Tegretol)

_____   7.   A 60-year-old woman has suffered a cardiac arrest. A healthcare professional trained in tracheal intubation has intubated the patient. Which of the following findings would indicate inadvertent esophageal intubation?
a. Jugular vein distention
b. Subcutaneous emphysema
c. Gurgling sounds heard over the epigastrium
d. Breath sounds heard on only one side of the chest

_____   8.   In the management of a symptomatic bradycardia, if the maximum dose of atropine had been given and a pacemaker was not immediately available, your next course of action would include:
a. Dopamine infusion, 2 to 10 mcg/kg/min
b. Amiodarone 150 mg IV over 10 minutes
c. Epinephrine 1 mg IV bolus followed by a 20 mL saline flush
d. Lidocaine 1 to 1.5 mg/kg IV bolus followed by a 10 mL saline flush

_____   9.   At doses recommended for use in cardiac arrest, epinephrine and vasopressin:
a. Slow conduction through the AV node
b. Cause profound peripheral vasodilation
c. Cause significant peripheral vasoconstriction
d. Neutralize acid accumulated during cardiac arrest

_____   10.   A 62-year-old man is complaining of palpitations that came on suddenly after walking up a short flight of stairs. His symptoms have been present for about 20 minutes. He denies chest pain and is not short of breath. His skin is warm and dry, breath sounds are clear. BP 144/88, P 186, R 18. The cardiac monitor reveals sustained monomorphic ventricular tachycardia. An IV has been established. Which of the following medications is most appropriate in this situation?
a. Dopamine or sotalol
b. Furosemide or atropine
c. Nitroglycerin or morphine
d. Procainamide or amiodarone

____ 11. Which of the following statements regarding resuscitation efforts is INCORRECT?

a. Most resuscitation efforts result in a return of spontaneous circulation.

b. A resuscitation team member should be assigned to the family to answer questions, clarify information, and provide comfort.

c. Surveys have revealed that most relatives of patients requiring CPR would like to be offered the possibility of being in the resuscitation room.

d. If it is necessary to relay the news of a death to family members, the attitude of the news-giver is generally deemed more important by the family than the ability to answer questions.

____ 12. Complications associated with inferior wall myocardial infarction (MI) often include:

a. Cardiogenic shock

b. Ventricular rupture

c. Bradydysrhythmias

d. Tachydysrhythmias

____ 13. Which of the following could be administered tracheally if necessary during cardiac arrest?

a. Vasopressin, epinephrine, and lidocaine

b. Lidocaine, amiodarone, and procainamide

c. Procainamide, epinephrine, and adenosine

d. Amiodarone, dopamine, and procainamide

____ 14. A 56-year-old man has a permanent pacemaker in place. Should it be necessary to defibrillate this patient, adhesive pads or handheld defibrillator paddles should be placed:

a. One inch from the pacemaker generator

b. Directly over the pacemaker generator

c. Three inches or more from the pacemaker generator

d. At least 6 to 8 inches from the pacemaker generator

____ 15. The correct dose of epinephrine, when given by means of a tracheal tube during cardiac arrest, is:

a. 0.5 mg

b. 1 mg

c. 2 to 2.5 mg

d. 1 to 1.5 mg/kg

____ 16. In a patient presenting with an acute coronary syndrome (ACS), ST-segment depression of more than 0.5 mm in leads V_2 and V_3 and more than 1 mm in all other leads is suggestive of myocardial _____ when viewed in two or more anatomically contiguous leads.

a. Ischemia

b. Injury

c. Infarction

d. Necrosis

____ 17. During a cardiac arrest, at what rate should positive pressure ventilations be delivered after insertion of an advanced airway?

a. 4 to 6 breaths/min

b. 8 to 10 breaths/min

c. 10 to 12 breaths/min

d. 20 to 24 breaths/min

____ 18. A 62-year-old man is presenting with signs and symptoms suggesting a stroke. Realizing that the benefits of IV or intra-arterial fibrinolytics are time-dependent, which of the following is the most important question that you should ask this patient, family, and/or bystanders?
a. "When did your symptoms begin?"
b. "When did you last see a physician?"
c. "Do you have a history of hypertension?"
d. "What were you doing when your symptoms began?"

____ 19. Synchronized cardioversion:
a. Is used only for atrial dysrhythmias
b. Delivers a shock during ventricular depolarization
c. Delivers a shock between the peak and end of the T wave
d. Is used only for rhythms with a ventricular rate of less than 60 beats/min

____ 20. A 53-year-old woman is unresponsive. Her BP is 50/P, ventilations 10. The cardiac monitor initially showed a narrow-QRS tachycardia at 220 beats/min. Supplemental oxygen therapy was initiated and an IV established before the patient's collapse. You promptly delivered a synchronized shock. Reassessment reveals the patient is not breathing and has no pulse. The cardiac monitor now reveals ventricular fibrillation (VF). What course of action should you take at this time?
a. Defibrillate immediately.
b. Perform CPR for 2 minutes and then prepare to defibrillate.
c. Place an advanced airway and then begin transcutaneous pacing.
d. Press the "sync" control and deliver another synchronized shock.

____ 21. Magnesium sulfate is recommended in the management of:
a. Torsades de pointes
b. Asystolic cardiac arrest
c. Symptomatic bradycardia
d. Monomorphic ventricular tachycardia

____ 22. A 48-year-old man became unresponsive shortly after presenting to you with nausea and generalized chest discomfort. You observe gasping breathing and are unsure if you feel a pulse. You should now:
a. Call for help and begin chest compressions
b. Wait until breathing stops and then check again for a pulse
c. Begin chest compressions only if you are certain a pulse is absent
d. Observe the patient for 2 minutes, and then reassess his breathing and pulse

____ 23. An unstable patient with a regular narrow-QRS tachycardia requires electrical therapy. You have a biphasic defibrillator available to you. Which of the following correctly reflects the recommended energy that should be delivered in this situation?
a. Defibrillate with 120 J
b. Defibrillate with 360 J
c. Perform synchronized cardioversion with 50 J to 100 J for the initial shock
d. Perform synchronized cardioversion with 100 J to 200 J for the initial shock

____ 24. Select the INCORRECT statement regarding the use of cricoid pressure.
a. The use of cricoid pressure may impede advanced airway placement.
b. The use of cricoid pressure in adult cardiac arrest is not recommended.
c. Cricoid pressure is often applied incorrectly with too much or too little pressure.
d. Cricoid pressure eliminates the risk of aspiration during bag-mask ventilation or tracheal intubation.

_____ 25. Atypical symptoms or unusual presentations of ACSs are more common in:
a. Older adults, women, and diabetic individuals
b. Men, older adults, and individuals who have liver disease
c. Women, diabetic individuals, and individuals who have liver disease
d. Men, patients who have a history of coronary artery disease (CAD), and patients who have a history of hypertension

_____ 26. Which of the following statements is correct about the use of amiodarone in cardiac arrest?
a. Amiodarone is the drug of choice for cardiac arrest due to asystole.
b. Amiodarone should be given as soon as possible after an IV is established.
c. Amiodarone should be given immediately before the first shock if pulseless VT/VF is present.
d. Amiodarone can be considered if pulseless VT/VF continues despite two to three shocks, CPR, and administration of a vasopressor.

_____ 27. Which of the following statements is INCORRECT when considering potentially reversible causes of cardiac arrest?
a. Acute MI should be considered as a possible cause of pulseless VT/VF cardiac arrest.
b. A suspected tension pneumothorax should be treated with pericardiocentesis.
c. Fibrinolytic therapy may be considered if pulmonary embolism is presumed or known to be the cause of the arrest.
d. Cardiac arrest associated with severe blood volume loss may benefit from administration of crystalloid IV/IO infusion.

_____ 28. An 84-year-old man presents with an acute onset of altered mental status. The cardiac monitor shows a complete AV block with wide-QRS complexes at a rate of 30 beats/min. The patient's blood pressure is 58/30, ventilations 14. His skin is cool, moist, and pale. His SpO_2 on room air is 95%. An IV has been established. Based on the patient's signs and symptoms associated with this rhythm, you should:
a. Prepare for transcutaneous pacing.
b. Give atropine 1 mg IV every 3 to 5 minutes.
c. Give epinephrine 1 mg IV bolus and reassess.
d. Observe the patient and monitor for signs of deterioration.

_____ 29. The drug of choice for most forms of narrow-QRS tachycardia is:
a. Atropine
b. Adenosine
c. Amiodarone
d. Epinephrine

_____ 30. The three major physical findings evaluated with the Cincinnati Prehospital Stroke Scale are:
a. Eye movement, pupil reaction, and arm drift
b. Facial droop, arm drift, and speech abnormalities
c. Best verbal response, facial droop, and eye opening
d. Best motor response, pupil reaction, and speech abnormalities

_____ 31. Hypotension (i.e., a systolic blood pressure of less than 90 mm Hg) after the return of spontaneous circulation may necessitate the use of:
a. Fluid boluses and isoproterenol
b. Procainamide, epinephrine, or dopamine
c. Epinephrine, dopamine, or norepinephrine
d. Fluid boluses, procainamide, and isoproterenol

_____ 32. The 12-lead electrocardiogram (ECG) shown in Figure 8-1 is from a 50-year-old man complaining of chest discomfort.
Which of the following is true regarding this 12-lead ECG?
a. This 12-lead ECG reveals no significant findings.
b. ST elevation is present in leads V_2 through V_5. An anterior ST elevation myocardial infarction (STEMI) is suspected.
c. ST elevation is present in leads I, aVR, and V_6. A lateral STEMI is suspected.
d. ST depression is present in leads III and aVF. An inferior STEMI is suspected.

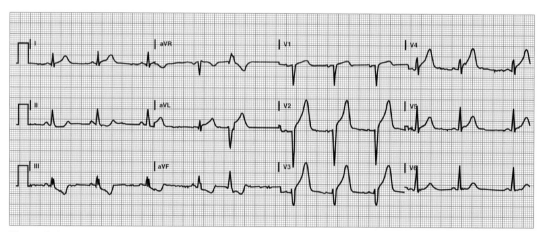

Figure 8-1

Questions 33 through 41 pertain to the following scenario:

A 55-year-old man is complaining of severe chest discomfort. He describes his discomfort as a "heavy pressure" in the middle of his chest that has been present for about 1 hour. He rates his discomfort 9/10. His blood pressure is 126/72 and ventilations 14. His SpO_2 on room air is 92%. The cardiac monitor shows a sinus rhythm at 75 beats/min.

_____ 33. Immediate management of this patient should include:
a. ABCs, oxygen, IV, and aspirin
b. ABCs, oxygen, IV, and atropine
c. ABCs, oxygen, IV, and adenosine
d. ABCs, oxygen, IV, and amiodarone

_____ 34. When the patient's 12-lead ECG is reviewed, the results should be used to classify the patient into one of three groups. Which of the following correctly reflects these categories?
a. ST elevation, normal ECG, Q waves
b. Q waves, ST depression, inconclusive ECG
c. ST depression, normal ECG, inconclusive ECG
d. ST elevation, ST depression, normal/nondiagnostic ECG

_____ 35. A 12-lead ECG has been obtained.

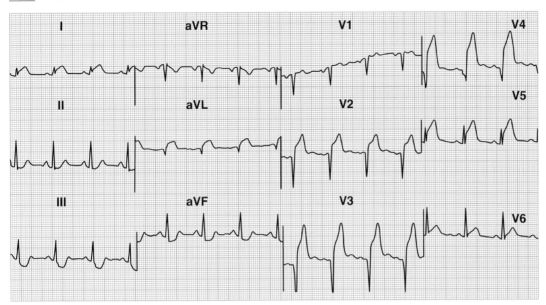

Figure 8-2

The patient's 12-lead ECG shows:
a. ST elevation in leads II, III, and aVF
b. ST depression in leads I, II, III, and aVL
c. ST depression in leads V_1, V_4, V_5, and V_6
d. ST elevation in leads I, aVL, V_2, V_3, V_4, and V_5

_____ 36. To be considered significant, ECG findings, such as ST elevation or depression, need to be viewed in two or more contiguous leads. Which of the following are contiguous leads?
a. V_1, V_4, and V_5
b. V_2, V_3, and V_4
c. I, II, III, and aVL
d. III, aVL, and aVF

_____ 37. In a patient presenting with an ACS, ST-segment elevation of more than _____ _____ _____ in men 40 years of age and older is suggestive of myocardial injury and warrants further evaluation.
a. 1 mm in leads V_1 and V_2 and 0.5 mm in all other leads
b. 2 mm in leads V_2 and V_3 and 1 mm in all other leads
c. 1 mm in leads V_1 through V_6 and 0.5 mm in all other leads
d. 2 mm in leads I, II, III, aVL, and aVF and 1 mm in all other leads

_____ 38. The patient's 12-lead ECG findings suggest a(n) _____ myocardial infarction.
a. Posterior
b. Anterolateral
c. Inferolateral
d. Non-ST elevation

_____ 39. Supplemental oxygen is being administered and an IV has been established. The patient's BP is 130/70, pulse 98, and ventilations 14. Assuming there are no contraindications for any of the following medications, which of the following would be appropriate for this patient at this time?
a. Aspirin and nitroglycerin
b. An IV beta-blocker and clopidogrel
c. Lidocaine, magnesium, and a calcium channel blocker
d. Nitroglycerin, a calcium channel blocker, and lidocaine

_____ 40. Nitroglycerin has been ordered for administration to this patient. Nitroglycerin:
a. Is contraindicated in hypotensive patients
b. Should be administered via the IV route for maximum benefit
c. Should be used with caution in patients with anterior infarction
d. Should be given every 15 to 20 minutes until chest discomfort is relieved

_____ 41. The patient's chest discomfort was unrelieved after the maximum recommended dosage of nitroglycerin tablets. Morphine sulfate was ordered and a 4 mg dose was given IV. The patient's blood pressure is now 80/60 and his skin is cool, moist, and pale. His breath sounds are clear. You should:
a. Prepare a lidocaine infusion at 1 to 4 mg/min
b. Prepare an epinephrine infusion at 2 mcg/min
c. Give a 250 mL IV fluid bolus of normal saline
d. Prepare a dopamine infusion at 2 to 10 mcg/kg/min

Questions 42 and 43 pertain to the following scenario:

A 65-year-old man is complaining of a sudden onset of chest pain. He is awake, alert, and diaphoretic. The patient states that his symptoms began 45 minutes ago while he was cleaning his garage. He denies nausea and has not vomited. The patient states that his discomfort is located in the center of his chest and radiates to his jaw. He rates the discomfort 10/10. His blood pressure is 108/50, ventilations 24. His SpO_2 on room air is 96%.

_____ 42. The cardiac monitor reveals the following rhythm (lead II):

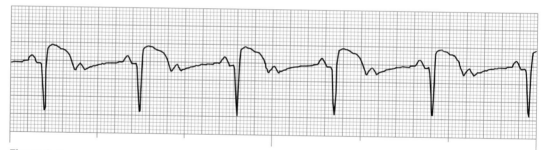

Figure 8-3

This rhythm is:
a. Junctional rhythm with ST elevation
b. Sinus bradycardia with ST elevation
c. Complete AV block with ST elevation
d. Second-degree AV block (2:1 AV block) with ST elevation

____ 43. An IV is in place. The patient's 12-lead ECG reveals ST segment elevation in leads II, III, and aVF. Which of the following statements is correct?

  a. The patient's 12-lead results are inconclusive. Additional testing is needed before treatment is begun.

  b. Since relief of pain is a priority in patients experiencing an acute coronary syndrome, nitroglycerin and morphine should be given without further delay.

  c. Because an anterior wall infarction is suspected and this patient is at extreme risk for heart failure and cardiogenic shock, furosemide should be given without delay.

  d. Because an inferior MI is suspected, right chest leads should be quickly used to rule out right ventricular infarction before giving medications for pain relief.

Questions 44 through 46 pertain to the following scenario:

An 89-year-old man is complaining of a "racing heart." He states his symptoms began while he was playing a card game with friends. He had an MI 15 years ago and a coronary artery bypass graft 5 years ago. His blood pressure is 140/90, ventilatory rate 16. Breath sounds are clear and his tidal volume is adequate. His SpO_2 on room air is 90%.

____ 44. Based on the information provided, supplemental oxygen:

  a. Is unnecessary at this time

  b. Is indicated and should be delivered using a nasal cannula at 4 L/min

  c. Is indicated and should be delivered using positive pressure ventilation

  d. Should ideally be administered only after placement of an advanced airway

____ 45. You have started an IV and placed the patient on the cardiac monitor, which reveals the following rhythm:

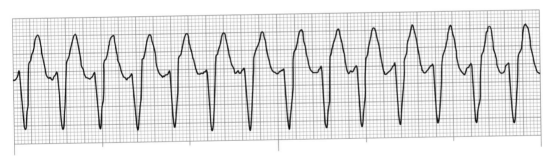

Figure 8-4

This rhythm can best be described as a:

  a. Regular, polymorphic, wide-QRS tachycardia

  b. Regular, monomorphic, wide-QRS tachycardia

  c. Irregular, polymorphic, wide-QRS tachycardia

  d. Irregular, monomorphic, wide-QRS tachycardia

____ 46. Which of the following statements is true regarding the management of this patient?

  a. The patient is unstable. Sedate the patient and defibrillate as quickly as possible.

  b. The patient is stable. Administration of IV verapamil is recommended for termination of the rhythm.

  c. The patient is stable. Administration of IV adenosine can be used as a therapeutic and diagnostic maneuver.

  d. The patient is unstable. Because there are recognizable QRS complexes on the monitor, synchronized cardioversion should be performed.

_____ 47. A 65-year-old woman experienced a cardiac arrest from which she was successfully resuscitated minutes ago. She is awake and knows her name, but is unaware of the date, where she is, or how she got there. Her blood pressure is 112/84. As you prepare to transfer the patient to the intensive care unit for further care, she abruptly informs you that her heart is "pounding." You observe the following rhythm on the cardiac monitor:

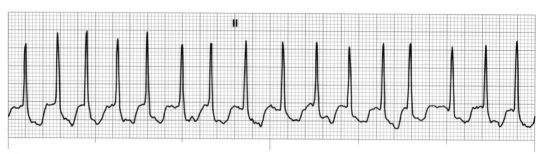

Figure 8-5

Your best course of action will be to:
a. Obtain a 12-lead ECG and seek expert consultation.
b. Prepare a lidocaine infusion and infuse at 2 mg/min.
c. Prepare a dopamine infusion and infuse at 5 mcg/kg/min.
d. Prepare an epinephrine infusion and infuse at 10 mcg/min.

_____ 48. An 81-year-old man is in cardiac arrest. High-quality CPR is in progress and a biphasic defibrillator is available. The cardiac monitor initially revealed asystole. Epinephrine was administered IV and 2 minutes later, the following rhythm is observed on the monitor:

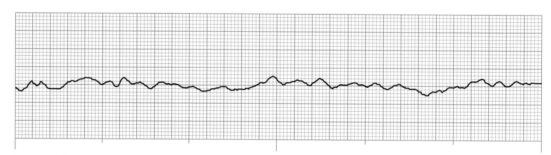

Figure 8-6

You should now:
a. Begin transcutaneous pacing.
b. Insert an advanced airway and then defibrillate using 360 J.
c. Defibrillate once using the manufacturer's recommended energy settings.
d. Defibrillate immediately using three stacked shocks of 200 J, 300 J, and 360 J.

Questions 49 and 50 pertain to the following scenario:

A 72-year-old woman presented with a sudden onset of shortness of breath and collapsed. After confirming the patient was unresponsive, apneic, and pulseless, CPR was begun.

_____ 49.   The cardiac monitor shows the following rhythm:

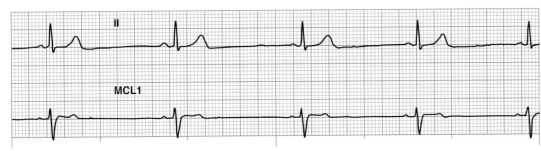

Figure 8-7

Which of the following ACLS treatment guidelines should be used in the initial treatment of this patient?
a. Symptomatic bradycardia
b. Narrow-QRS tachycardia
c. Pulseless electrical activity (PEA)
d. ACSs

_____ 50.   An IV has been established and the patient is being ventilated with a bag-mask device. You observe gentle bilateral chest rise with ventilations. Your next action should be to:
a. Defibrillate immediately.
b. Give 1 mg of atropine IV.
c. Give 1 mg of epinephrine IV.
d. Begin transcutaneous pacing.

ANSWER APPENDIX

PRETEST ANSWERS

Multiple Choice

1. a. Oral airways are available in a variety of sizes ranging from 0 for neonates up to 6 for large adults. The size of the airway is based on the distance, in millimeters, from the flange to the distal tip. Correct size is determined by selecting an oral airway that extends from the corner of the mouth to tip of the earlobe or the angle of the jaw. An oral airway should only be used in unresponsive patients who have no cough or gag reflex because it may stimulate vomiting or laryngospasm in responsive or semi-responsive patients. If the airway is too long, it may press the epiglottis against the entrance of the larynx resulting in a complete airway obstruction. If the airway is too short, it will not displace the tongue and may advance out of the mouth. A petroleum-based lubricant should never be used because it may damage the airway device and cause tissue inflammation. Objective: Discuss the indications, contraindications, advantages, and disadvantages of oral and nasal airways.

2. b. If patient findings are consistent with a possible or definite acute coronary syndrome (ACS), a targeted history and physical examination and initial 12-lead electrocardiogram (ECG) should be performed within 10 minutes of patient contact (prehospital) or arrival in the emergency department. Objective: Describe the initial management of a patient experiencing an ACS.

3. c. It has been estimated that cardiac output is approximately 25% to 33% of normal during CPR.[1] Therefore the quality of chest compressions is an important factor in the effectiveness of CPR. During cardiac arrest, the adult sternum should be depressed *at least* 2 inches (5 cm); "push hard." Do not spend more than 10 seconds checking for a pulse. If you do not feel a pulse or are unsure if you feel a pulse, begin CPR. Coronary perfusion declines rapidly if chest compressions are stopped for even a few seconds. When caring for a patient in cardiac arrest, it is *essential* that interruptions to analyze the ECG, charge the defibrillator, place an advanced airway, check a pulse, or other procedures be kept to a minimum. Compressors should rotate positions every 2 minutes to avoid tiring. Objective: Describe the links in the Chain of Survival.

4. b. From the information presented, it appears this patient is probably experiencing an ACS. Appropriate interventions in the management of this patient would include oxygen (not indicated in this patient), IV access, aspirin (if no contraindications), sublingual nitroglycerin, and morphine. The memory aid "MONA" (morphine, oxygen [if indicated], nitroglycerin, and aspirin) is used to help recall the immediate general treatment measures that should be considered for a patient experiencing an ACS. Supplemental oxygen administration is indicated if the patient is cyanotic, having difficulty breathing, has obvious signs of heart failure or shock, or if the patient's oxygen saturation level declines to less than 94%.[2] Atropine is used to treat a symptomatic bradycardia and is not indicated in this situation. The patient does not have hypotension that would warrant consideration of a fluid challenge. Although the patient is tachycardic, adenosine is not indicated for a sinus tachycardia. Objective: Given a patient situation, describe the ECG characteristics and initial emergency care for each of the following situations, including mechanical, pharmacological (i.e., indications, contraindications, doses, and route of administration of applicable medications), and electrical therapy, where applicable: too-fast rhythms, too-slow rhythms, and cardiac arrest rhythms.

5. d. There are four cardiac arrest rhythms: (1) Ventricular fibrillation (VF); (2) ventricular tachycardia (VT); (3) asystole, and (4) pulseless electrical activity (PEA). Shockable cardiac arrest rhythms include VF and VT. Defibrillation is not indicated for asystole or PEA. Objective: Differentiate between shockable and nonshockable cardiac arrest rhythms.

6. b. At an oxygen flow rate of 0.25 to 8 L/min, a nasal cannula can deliver about 22% to 45% oxygen. The use of a nasal cannula at 6 L/min or more is often irritating to the patient's nasal passages. Objective: Describe the advantages, disadvantages, oxygen liter flow per minute, and estimated oxygen percentage delivered for each of the following devices: Nasal cannula, simple face mask, partial nonrebreather mask, and nonrebreather mask.

7. c. Ventilation does not require interruption (or even pausing) of chest compressions once an advanced airway is in place. The patient should be ventilated at a rate of 1 breath about every 6 to 8 seconds (about 8 to 10 breaths per minute). Current resuscitation guidelines do not recommend bag-mask ventilation by a single rescuer during CPR. Instead, the single rescuer is encouraged to use the mouth-to-mouth or mouth-to-mask methods of ventilation because they are more efficient.[3] There is a knowledge gap (i.e., a lack of published research) regarding use of bag-mask ventilation by both inexperienced and experienced providers. Bag-mask ventilation should be a two-rescuer operation. With two rescuers, one is assigned the responsibility of opening and maintaining the airway while creating a good seal with the mask. The correct ratio of compressions to ventilations in adult CPR is 30:2. Objective: Describe methods used to confirm the correct placement of an advanced airway and describe the ventilation of a patient who has an advanced airway in place.

8. c. The primary survey focuses on basic life support assessment and intervention. The secondary survey focuses on advanced life support assessment and interventions. Thus establishing vascular access is part of "C" (Circulation) in the secondary survey. Objective: List the purpose and components of the primary and secondary surveys.

9. a. The tracheal route of medication administration has been greatly deemphasized. The intravenous or intraosseous routes are preferred because they provide more predictable drug delivery and pharmacologic effect.[3] Studies have shown that naloxone, atropine, vasopressin, epinephrine, and lidocaine are absorbed via the trachea. Although the optimal tracheal dose of most drugs is unknown, the typical dose given by the tracheal route is 2 to 2.5 times the recommended IV dose. Dilute the recommended dose in 5 to 10 mL of sterile water or normal saline and administer. Objective: Given a patient situation, describe the ECG characteristics and initial emergency care for each of the following situations, including mechanical, pharmacological (i.e., indications, contraindications, doses, and route of administration of applicable medications), and electrical therapy, where applicable: too-fast rhythms, too-slow rhythms, and cardiac arrest rhythms.

10. c. For pharmacologic termination of a stable wide-QRS tachycardia that is most likely VT, procainamide, amiodarone, or sotalol may be used. These medications are considered first-line antiarrhythmics for monomorphic VT and have complex mechanisms of action. They are used for both atrial and ventricular dysrhythmias. Although lidocaine is a ventricular antiarrhythmic, it is considered a second-line antiarrhythmic in the management of monomorphic VT because it is reported to be less effective than the first-line agents in terminating VT. If the decision is made to administer procainamide, amiodarone, or sotalol, it is recommended that expert consultation be sought before administering another. Adenosine, diltiazem, and verapamil may be used in the management of *narrow*-QRS tachycardias. Adenosine may also be used to assist in diagnosis when the origin of a wide-QRS tachycardia is unclear. Atropine and isoproterenol are used in the management of symptomatic bradycardias. Objective: Given a patient situation, describe the ECG characteristics and initial emergency care for each of the following situations, including mechanical, pharmacological (i.e., indications, contraindications, doses, and route of administration of applicable medications), and electrical therapy, where applicable: too-fast rhythms, too-slow rhythms, and cardiac arrest rhythms.

11. b. Mouth-to-mask breathing combined with supplemental oxygen at a minimum flow rate of 10 L/min can deliver an oxygen concentration of approximately 50%. Objective: Describe the oxygen liter flow per minute and estimated inspired oxygen concentration delivered for a pocket mask and bag-mask device.

12. a. The first *antiarrhythmic* administered in the management of the patient in pulseless VT or VF is amiodarone (or lidocaine if amiodarone is unavailable). Epinephrine and vasopressin are *vasopressors*, not antiarrhythmics. Procainamide is an antiarrhythmic but it is not used in cardiac arrest. Objective: Given a patient situation, describe the ECG characteristics and initial emergency care for each of the following situations, including mechanical, pharmacological (i.e., indications, contraindications, doses, and route of administration of applicable medications), and electrical therapy, where applicable: too-fast rhythms, too-slow rhythms, and cardiac arrest rhythms.

13. a. Hyperventilation is a common cause of excessive intrathoracic pressure during CPR. It is important to ventilate a patient in cardiac arrest at an age-appropriate rate and with just enough volume

to see the patient's chest rise gently. Ventilating a cardiac arrest patient too fast or with too much volume results in excessive intrathoracic pressure, which results in decreased venous return into the chest, decreased coronary and cerebral perfusion pressures, diminished cardiac output, and decreased rates of survival. Objective: Describe the phases of cardiopulmonary resuscitation.

14. b. Supplemental oxygen administration is indicated if the patient is hypoxic, cyanotic, having difficulty breathing, has obvious signs of heart failure or shock, or if her oxygen saturation declines to less than 94%. Titrate oxygen therapy to maintain the patient's SpO_2 at 94% or greater. Since 2004, the American College of Cardiology/American Heart Association guidelines have indicated that there appears to be little justification for continuing the routine use of oxygen beyond 6 hours in cases of uncomplicated ACSs. Objective: Discuss the evaluation of oxygenation and ventilation using pulse oximetry and capnography.

15. a. If breath sounds are absent on both sides of the chest after placing a tracheal tube, assume esophageal intubation. Deflate the tracheal tube cuff and remove the tube. If breath sounds are diminished on the left after intubation but present on the right, assume right primary bronchus intubation. Deflate the tracheal tube cuff, pull back the tube slightly, reinflate the cuff, and reevaluate breath sounds. Once placement is confirmed, note and record the depth (centimeter marking) of the tube at the patient's teeth and secure the tube in place. The presence of a mucus plug in the tracheal tube would likely result in increased resistance during positive pressure ventilation. Objective: Describe methods used to confirm the correct placement of an advanced airway and describe the ventilation of a patient who has an advanced airway in place.

16. c. Transcutaneous pacing (TCP) is a reasonable temporizing measure that may be useful in the treatment of symptomatic bradycardia. Because transcutaneous and transvenous pacing in cardiac arrest do not improve the likelihood of return of spontaneous circulation or survival outcome, pacing is not recommended in pulseless patients. Two randomized adult trials comparing TCP to drug therapy showed no difference in survival for patients who had a symptomatic bradycardia with a pulse. TCP is painful in conscious patients, particularly with the use of 50 mA or more, and typically requires the use of sedation or analgesia to manage patient discomfort. Objective: Given a patient situation, describe the ECG characteristics and initial emergency care for each of the following situations, including mechanical, pharmacological (i.e., indications, contraindications, doses, and route of administration of applicable medications), and electrical therapy, where applicable: too-fast rhythms, too-slow rhythms, and cardiac arrest rhythms.

17. a. Drugs given during cardiac arrest that constrict blood vessels (vasopressors such as epinephrine) may improve perfusion pressures. Drugs given that dilate blood vessels (vasodilators) decrease perfusion pressures. Objective: Describe the phases of cardiopulmonary resuscitation.

18. c. The AVPU acronym is used to quickly assess a patient's level of responsiveness. AVPU–**A**lert, responds to **V**erbal stimuli, responds to **P**ainful stimuli, **U**nresponsive. ABCD are components of the primary and secondary surveys. OPQRST is an acronym used when evaluating a patient's complaint of pain. CAB is an acronym new to the 2010 resuscitation guidelines that emphasizes the importance of performing chest compressions first, followed by opening the airway and assessing breathing, in victims of cardiac arrest. Objective: List the purpose and components of the primary and secondary surveys.

19. d. Remember that an open airway does not ensure adequate ventilation. This patient's breathing is inadequate as evidenced by his rate and depth of ventilations. The patient with inadequate breathing requires positive pressure ventilation with supplemental oxygen. Of the choices listed, the only device that can provide positive pressure ventilation is the bag-mask. If readily available, an oral airway should be inserted before beginning bag-mask ventilation (if the patient does not have a gag or cough reflex). Objective: Describe indications for positive pressure ventilation and demonstrate how to provide positive pressure ventilation with a barrier device and pocket mask.

20. b. In acute stroke management, the phrase **time is brain** reflects the need for rapid assessment and intervention because delays in diagnosis and treatment may leave the patient neurologically impaired and disabled. Objective: Describe the initial emergency care for acute ischemic stroke.

21. b. If defibrillation eliminates pulseless VT/VF and then it recurs, defibrillate at the last successful energy setting. Beginning at a lower setting may cost valuable time and lead to increased impedance to electrical flow. Objective: Explain defibrillation, its indications, proper pad or paddle placement, relevant precautions, and the steps required to perform this procedure with a manual defibrillator and an automated external defibrillator.

22. d. Hypotension that results from nitroglycerin or morphine administration usually responds to supine positioning and administration of IV fluids. Based on the information provided, it is reasonable to give a fluid challenge of 250 to 500 mL of normal saline and reassess. Because the patient is clearly hypotensive, additional doses of nitroglycerin are contraindicated. Vagal maneuvers, adenosine, and synchronized cardioversion are not warranted for a sinus tachycardia. Objective: Describe the initial management of a patient experiencing an ACS.

23. b. In addition to clinical assessment, continuous quantitative waveform capnography is recommended as the most reliable method for confirmation and monitoring of tracheal tube placement. If waveform capnography is not available, an esophageal detector device or nonwaveform exhaled CO_2 monitor in addition to clinical assessment is considered reasonable. Gastric insufflation sounds should not be heard over the stomach if the tracheal tube is in the trachea. The presence of water vapor in the tube is not a completely reliable sign of proper tracheal tube placement. Oxygen saturation levels can be assessed with a pulse oximeter if the patient has a perfusing rhythm; however, it is not the preferred method for confirming tracheal tube position. Objective: Describe methods used to confirm the correct placement of an advanced airway and describe the ventilation of a patient who has an advanced airway in place.

24. a. The initial treatment of any patient with a symptomatic bradycardia should focus on support of airway and breathing. Assess the patient's oxygen saturation and determine if signs of increased work of breathing are present such as retractions, tachypnea, or paradoxical abdominal breathing. Give supplemental oxygen if oxygenation or ventilation is inadequate. If serious signs and symptoms are present because of the slow rate, start an IV, and prepare to administer IV atropine. Although atropine is recommended as the first-line drug for symptomatic bradycardia, it is important to recognize that some bradycardias are unlikely to respond to atropine (e.g., complete atrioventricular [AV] blocks, wide-QRS AV blocks). Other interventions that may be used in the treatment of symptomatic bradycardia include epinephrine, dopamine, or isoproterenol IV infusions and TCP. Objective: Given a patient situation, describe the ECG characteristics and initial emergency care for each of the following situations, including mechanical, pharmacologic (i.e., indications, contraindications, doses, and route of administration of applicable medications), and electrical therapy, where applicable: too-fast rhythms, too-slow rhythms, and cardiac arrest rhythms.

25. b. Because no drugs used in cardiac arrest have been shown to improve survival to hospital discharge, the priorities of care in a cardiac arrest are CPR and defibrillation (if indicated). Objective: Discuss the phase response of code organization.

26. c. One dose of vasopressin 40 U IV/IO bolus may replace either the first or second dose of epinephrine in the treatment of pulseless arrest. Objective: Given a patient situation, describe the ECG characteristics and initial emergency care for each of the following situations, including mechanical, pharmacologic (i.e., indications, contraindications, doses, and route of administration of applicable medications), and electrical therapy, where applicable: too-fast rhythms, too-slow rhythms, and cardiac arrest rhythms.

27. b. The incidence of dysrhythmias, such as VF, is highest during the first 4 hours after onset of symptoms and remains an important contributing factor to death in the first 24 hours after ST elevation myocardial infarction (STEMI). Objective: Identify the most common complications of an acute myocardial infarction (MI).

28. d.

TYPE OF SHOCK	RHYTHM	RECOMMENDED ENERGY LEVELS
Defibrillation*	Pulseless VT/VF Sustained polymorphic VT	Varies depending on the device used: • The biphasic defibrillator effective dose is typically 120 J to 200 J • If the effective dose range of the defibrillator is unknown, consider using at the maximal dose • If using a monophasic defibrillator, use 360 J for all shocks
Synchronized cardioversion*	Unstable narrow-QRS tachycardia	The biphasic dose is typically 50 J to 100 J initially, increase in a stepwise fashion if the initial shock fails

Continued

TYPE OF SHOCK	RHYTHM	RECOMMENDED ENERGY LEVELS
	Unstable atrial flutter	The biphasic dose is typically 50 J to 100 J initially, increase in a stepwise fashion if the initial shock fails
	Unstable atrial fibrillation	The biphasic dose is typically 120 J to 200 J initially; increase in a stepwise fashion if the initial shock fails; begin with 200 J if using monophasic energy and increase if unsuccessful
	Unstable monomorphic VT	The biphasic dose is typically 100 J initially; it is reasonable to increase in a stepwise fashion if the initial shock fails

*Use energy levels recommended by the device manufacturer.

Objective: For each of the following rhythms, identify the energy levels that are currentlyrecommended and indicate if the shock delivered should be a synchronized or unsynchronized countershock: pulseless VT/VF, monomorphic VT, polymorphic VT, narrow-QRS tachycardia, atrial fibrillation with a rapid ventricular response, and atrial flutter with a rapid ventricular response.

29. c. For a patient with symptoms of stroke on awakening, the time of onset is assumed to be the time the patient was last known to be symptom-free before retiring (last known well time). If a patient had mild impairments but then had worsening over the subsequent hours, the time the first symptom began is assumed to be the time of onset. Objective: Describe the initial emergency care for acute ischemic stroke.

30. b. Hypotension and bradycardia are the most common adverse effects of amiodarone administration. Objective: Given a patient situation, describe the ECG characteristics and initial emergency care for each of the following situations, including mechanical, pharmacologic (i.e., indications, contraindications, doses, and route of administration of applicable medications), and electrical therapy, where applicable: too-fast rhythms, too-slow rhythms, and cardiac arrest rhythms.

31. b. If peripheral IV access is unsuccessful during cardiac arrest, consider an intraosseous infusion before considering placement of a central line. Objective: Given a patient situation, describe the ECG characteristics and initial emergency care for each of the following situations, including mechanical, pharmacologic (i.e., indications, contraindications, doses, and route of administration of applicable medications), and electrical therapy, where applicable: too-fast rhythms, too-slow rhythms, and cardiac arrest rhythms.

32. d. Clopidogrel (Plavix) is an antiplatelet agent that helps prevent platelets from sticking together and forming clots. Several studies have documented its efficacy for patients with non-ST-elevation myocardial infarction (NSTEMI) and those with STEMI. In patients younger than 75 years of age, an oral loading dose of 300 to 600 mg is recommended for NSTEMI and STEMI regardless of whether the patient undergoes reperfusion with fibrinolytic therapy or does not receive reperfusion therapy.[2] In the emergency department, a 300-mg oral dose is recommended for the patient with a suspected ACS who is unable to take aspirin because of hypersensitivity or major gastrointestinal intolerance. An oral dose of 300 mg should be administered in the emergency department to STEMI patients up to 75 years of age who receive aspirin, heparin, and fibrinolysis. Objective: Desribe the initial management of a patient experiencing an ACS.

33. a. A clot (thrombus) is the most common cause of stroke. In a thrombotic stroke, atherosclerosis of large vessels in the brain causes progressive narrowing and platelet clumping. Platelet clumping results in the development of blood clots within the brain artery itself (cerebral thrombosis). When the blood clots are of sufficient size to block blood flow through the artery, the area previously supplied by that artery becomes ischemic. Ischemia occurs because the tissue supplied by the blocked artery does not receive oxygen and the essential nutrients needed for normal brain function. The patient's signs and symptoms depend on the location of the artery affected and the areas of brain ischemia. Objective: Describe the two major types of stroke.

34. c. When TCP is used to treat a symptomatic bradycardia, the rate is set at a nonbradycardiac rate, generally between 60 and 80 pulses per minute (ppm). After the rate has been regulated, set the stimulating current. Increase the current slowly but steadily until capture is achieved. Sedation and/or analgesia may be needed to minimize patient discomfort. Objective: Discuss the procedure for TCP as well as its indications and possible complication.

Matching

35. o	44. j
36. d	45. f
37. b	46. k
38. n	47. a
39. e	48. h
40. l	49. p
41. i	50. c
42. g	
43. m	

CHAPTER 1 STOP AND REVIEW ANSWERS

Matching

1. b	17. c	33. a
2. a	18. b	34. x
3. b	19. c	35. k
4. a	20. a	36. d
5. c	21. b	37. q
6. b	22. c	38. r
7. a	23. p	39. n
8. c	24. l	40. g
9. b	25. h	41. u
10. b	26. s	42. e
11. c	27. w	43. b
12. a	28. j	44. f
13. b	29. v	45. m
14. c	30. i	46. c
15. c	31. t	
16. a	32. o	

CHAPTER 2 STOP AND REVIEW ANSWERS

True/False

1. F. The laryngeal mask airway is available in many sizes and is used in infants, children, and adults. Objective: Describe methods used to confirm the correct placement of an advanced airway and describe the ventilation of a patient who has an advanced airway in place.
2. F. A colorimetric capnometer is placed between a tracheal tube or advanced airway device, and a bag-mask device. The presence of CO_2 (evidenced by a color change on the pH-sensitive litmus paper housed in the detector) suggests placement of the tube in the trachea. This type of capnometer simply shows the presence of CO_2. It has no ability to provide an actual CO_2 reading or indicate the presence of hypercarbia, and it provides no opportunity for ongoing monitoring to ensure the tube remains in the trachea.
3. T. If a good seal is maintained between the patient's mouth and the mask, you can deliver a greater tidal volume to the patient with mouth-to-mask ventilation than with a bag-mask device because both of your hands can be used to secure the mask in place while simultaneously maintaining proper head position. Your vital capacity can also compensate for leaks between the mask and the patient's face, resulting in greater lung ventilation. Objective: Describe how to provide positive pressure ventilation with a barrier device and pocket face mask.
4. F. Pulse oximetry provides important information about oxygenation, but does not provide information about the effectiveness of a patient's ventilation. Capnography provides information about

the effectiveness of ventilation, but does not measure oxygenation. Objective: Discuss the evaluation of oxygenation and ventilation using pulse oximetry and capnography.

5. T. A bag-mask device can be used to assist ventilations in a spontaneously breathing patient as well as a nonbreathing patient. Objective: Describe how to ventilate a patient with a bag-mask and two rescuers.

6. T. Healthcare professionals who have been trained to use a supraglottic airway (e.g., Combitube, laryngeal tube, laryngeal mask airway) can use it as an acceptable alternative to bag-mask ventilation or a tracheal tube for airway management in cardiac arrest. Objective: Describe methods used to confirm the correct placement of an advanced airway and describe the ventilation of a patient who has an advanced airway in place.

Multiple Choice

7. d. It is estimated that airway bleeding can occur in up to 30% of patients after insertion of a nasal airway. Because of the possibility of intracranial placement in patients who have a basilar skull fracture, nasal airways should be avoided in patients with severe craniofacial trauma. Use of an oral airway is preferred if the patient has a bleeding disorder or in the presence of a known or suspected basal skull fracture. Objective: Discuss the indications, contraindications, advantages, and disadvantages of oral and nasal airways.

8. a. Esophageal trauma, including lacerations, bruising, and subcutaneous emphysema, are possible complications of Combitube use. A Combitube is inserted blindly (i.e., does not require visualization of the vocal cords). Ventilation begins with the esophageal tube because of the high probability of esophageal placement after blind insertion. Combitubes are available in two sizes. The 37-French (Fr) diameter size is used for patients between 4 and 5 feet tall. The 41-Fr size is used for patients taller than 5 feet. Objective: Describe methods used to confirm the correct placement of an advanced airway and describe the ventilation of a patient who has an advanced airway in place.

9. a. An oral airway should only be used in unresponsive patients who have no cough or gag reflex because it may stimulate vomiting or laryngospasm in responsive or semi-responsive patients. If the airway is too long, it may press the epiglottis against the entrance of the larynx resulting in a complete airway obstruction. If the airway is too short, it will not displace the tongue and may advance out of the mouth. A petroleum-based lubricant should never be used because it may damage the airway device and cause tissue inflammation. A nasal airway (not an oral airway) may inadvertently enter the cranial vault if it inserted into the nose of a patient who has sustained a craniofacial injury. Objective: Discuss the indications, contraindications, advantages, and disadvantages of oral and nasal airways.

10. b. Common internal diameters of tracheal tubes for adults typically range from 7.5 mm (adult females) to 9 mm (adult males). Because of the size variation in adults, several sizes of tubes should be on hand. At a minimum, have available a tracheal tube that is 0.5 mm smaller and 0.5 mm larger than the estimated tube size. Objective: Describe methods used to confirm the correct placement of an advanced airway and describe the ventilation of a patient who has an advanced airway in place.

11. c. Tracheal intubation should be preceded by attempts to ventilate by another method. Tracheal intubation is indicated in situations where the patient is unable to protect his/her own airway. Tracheal intubation reduces (but does not eliminate) the risk of aspiration of gastric contents and, when attempted, should be performed in less than 30 seconds. Objective: Describe methods used to confirm the correct placement of an advanced airway and describe the ventilation of a patient who has an advanced airway in place.

12. b. Because the air in the esophagus normally has very low levels of CO_2, a lack of carbon dioxide on an end-tidal CO_2 detector generally means the tracheal tube is improperly positioned in the esophagus. Objective: Describe methods used to confirm the correct placement of an advanced airway and describe the ventilation of a patient who has an advanced airway in place.

13. d. If not already attached, connect a one-way valve to the ventilation port on the pocket face mask and connect oxygen tubing to the oxygen inlet on the mask. Set the oxygen flow rate at 10 to 12 L/min. Objective: Describe the oxygen liter flow per minute and estimated inspired oxygen concentration delivered for a pocket face mask and bag-mask device.

14. c. When giving rescue breaths, you are more likely to get dizzy or lightheaded if you take deep breaths before each delivering each rescue breath. Take a normal breath before each ventilation

and ventilate at a rate of 10 to 12 breaths/min (1 breath every 5 to 6 seconds). Objective: Describe how to provide positive pressure ventilation with a barrier device and pocket face mask.

Completion

15. When suctioning, apply intermittent suction while <u>withdrawing</u> the catheter. Objective: Describe the procedure for suctioning the upper airway and possible complications associated with this procedure. Describe the procedure for suctioning the lower airway and possible complications associated with this procedure.

16. A bag-mask used with supplemental oxygen set at a flow rate of 15 L/min with no reservoir will deliver approximately <u>40%</u> to <u>60%</u> oxygen to the patient. Objective: Describe the oxygen liter flow per minute and estimated inspired oxygen concentration delivered for a pocket face mask and bag-mask device.

Matching

17. h
18. j
19. n
20. o
21. f
22. i
23. a
24. k

25. c
26. g
27. l
28. e
29. d
30. b
31. m

Short Answer

32. Soft suction catheters are also called *whistle tip*, *flexible*, or *French* catheters. They are long, narrow, flexible pieces of plastic primarily used to clear blood or mucus from a tracheal tube or the nasopharynx. A soft suction catheter can be inserted into the nares, oropharynx, or nasopharynx; through an oral or nasal airway; or through a tracheal tube or tracheostomy tube. Caution: Insertion of a suction catheter into the nares may result in bleeding because of trauma to the nasal passages. Objective: Describe the procedure for suctioning the lower airway and possible complications associated with this procedure.

33. Align the nasal airway on the side of the patient's face. Proper size is determined by selecting a device that extends from the tip of the nose to the angle of the jaw or the tip of the ear. Objective: Describe how to correctly size and insert an oral airway and nasal airway.

34.

DEVICE	APPROXIMATE INSPIRED OXYGEN CONCENTRATION	LITER FLOW (LITERS/MINUTE)
Nasal Cannula	**22% to 45%**	**0.25 to 8**
Simple Face Mask	**35% to 60%**	**5 to 10**
Partial Rebreather Mask	35% to 60%	Typically 6 to 10 to prevent bag collapse on inspiration
Nonrebreather Mask	**60% to 100%**	**Typically 10 or higher to prevent bag collapse on inspiration**

Objective: Describe the advantages, disadvantages, oxygen liter flow per minute, and estimated oxygen percentage delivered for each of the following devices: Nasal cannula, simple face mask, partial nonrebreather mask, and nonrebreather mask.

35. The most frequent problems with bag-mask ventilation are the inability to deliver adequate ventilatory volumes and gastric inflation. Objective: Describe the signs of adequate and inadequate bag-mask ventilation.

36. If resistance is encountered, a gentle back-and-forth rotation of the device between your fingers may ease insertion. If resistance continues, withdraw the nasal airway, reapply lubricant, and

attempt insertion in the patient's other nostril. Objective: Describe how to correctly size and insert an oral airway and nasal airway.

37. Hold the device against the side of the patient's face and select an airway that extends from the corner of the mouth to the tip of the earlobe or the angle of the jaw. Objective: Describe how to correctly size and insert an oral airway and nasal airway.

CHAPTER 3 STOP AND REVIEW ANSWERS

True/False

1. T. During a resuscitation effort, team members should frequently reassess the patient and inform the team leader of any changes in the patient's vital signs or condition. Patient reassessment and communication with the team leader should occur at least every 3 to 5 minutes through the resuscitation effort. Objective: Describe the role of each member of the resuscitation team.

2. F. Avoid calcium channel blockers in patients with wide-QRS tachycardia (may precipitate ventricular fibrillation). Objective: Given a patient situation, describe the ECG characteristics and initial emergency care for each of the following situations, including mechanical, pharmacologic (i.e., indications, contraindications, doses, and route of administration of applicable medications), and electrical therapy, where applicable: too-fast rhythms, too-slow rhythms, and cardiac arrest rhythms.

3. T. Delta waves are produced with accessory pathways that insert directly into ventricular muscle. A delta wave is the initial slurred deflection at the beginning of the QRS complex. It results from initial activation of the QRS by conduction over the accessory pathway, as in Wolff-Parkinson-White syndrome. Objective: Given a patient situation, describe the ECG characteristics and initial emergency care for each of the following situations, including mechanical, pharmacologic (i.e., indications, contraindications, doses, and route of administration of applicable medications), and electrical therapy, where applicable: too-fast rhythms, too-slow rhythms, and cardiac arrest rhythms.

4. T. During cardiac arrest, interruptions in CPR should be as brief as possible and only as necessary to assess rhythm, shock VF/VT, perform a pulse check when an organized rhythm is detected, or place an advanced airway. Objective: Given a patient situation, describe the ECG characteristics and initial emergency care for each of the following situations, including mechanical, pharmacologic (i.e., indications, contraindications, doses, and route of administration of applicable medications), and electrical therapy, where applicable: too-fast rhythms, too-slow rhythms, and cardiac arrest rhythms.

Multiple Choice

5. b. The heart's pacemaker cells have a built-in (i.e., intrinsic) rate that becomes slower and slower from the SA node down to the end of the His-Purkinje system. The intrinsic rate of the SA node is 60 to 100 beats/min. The AV junction has pacemaker cells that have an intrinsic rate of 40 to 60 beats/min. The Purkinje fibers have pacemaker cells that have an intrinsic rate of 20 to 40 beats/min.

6. c. Examples of irregular tachycardias include atrial fibrillation, atrial flutter, and polymorphic VT. Asystole, accelerated idioventricular rhythm, and accelerated junctional rhythm are not tachycardias. Objective: Given a patient situation, describe the ECG characteristics and initial emergency care for each of the following situations, including mechanical, pharmacologic (i.e., indications, contraindications, doses, and route of administration of applicable medications), and electrical therapy, where applicable: too-fast rhythms, too-slow rhythms, and cardiac arrest rhythms.

7. a. The QRS complex consists of the Q wave, R wave, and S wave and represents the spread of the electrical impulse through the ventricles (ventricular depolarization). The QRS complex begins as a downward deflection, the Q wave. A Q wave is *always* a negative waveform. The QRS complex continues as a large, upright, triangular waveform called the R wave. The S wave is the negative waveform following the R wave. An R wave is *always* positive and an S wave is *always* negative. Thus, the R wave is the first positive deflection after the P wave on the ECG.

8. d. Atrial tachycardia, AV nodal reentrant tachycardia (AVNRT), and AV reentrant tachycardia (AVRT) are types of supraventricular tachycardia. The most common type of paroxysmal supraventricular tachycardia is AVNRT. The next most common is AVRT. A ventricular escape rhythm is a bradycardia (20 to 40 beats/min), not a tachycardia and it is a ventricular (not a supraventricular) rhythm. Objective: Given a patient situation, describe the ECG characteristics and initial emergency care for each of the following situations, including mechanical, pharmacologic (i.e., indications, contraindications, doses, and route of administration of applicable medications), and electrical therapy, where applicable: too-fast rhythms, too-slow rhythms, and cardiac arrest rhythms.

9. d. The circumflex and anterior descending are the main branches of the left coronary artery.

10. d. When peripheral IV cannulation is unsuccessful or is taking too long, an intraosseous (IO) infusion is an alternative method of gaining access to the vascular system and should be considered before considering placement of a central line. To improve flow rates during an IO infusion, the use of a pressure bag or infusion pump may be necessary. If IV or IO access cannot be achieved to give drugs during a cardiac arrest, the tracheal route can be used to give selected medications. The tracheal route of drug administration is not preferred because multiple studies have shown that giving resuscitation drugs tracheally results in lower blood concentrations than the same dose given IV. Objective: Identify a patient experiencing a cardiac dysrhythmia as asymptomatic, symptomatic but stable, symptomatic but unstable, or pulseless. Given a patient situation, describe the ECG characteristics and initial emergency care for each of the following situations, including mechanical, pharmacologic (i.e., indications, contraindications, doses, and route of administration of applicable medications), and electrical therapy, where applicable: too-fast rhythms, too-slow rhythms, and cardiac arrest rhythms.

11. c. Three or more PVCs occurring in a row at a rate of more than 100/min is called a salvo, burst, or run of VT.

12. a. When using vagal maneuvers, make sure oxygen, suction, a defibrillator, and emergency medications are available before attempting the procedure. Continuous monitoring of the patient's ECG is essential and a 12-lead ECG recording is desirable. Carotid sinus pressure should be avoided in older patients and in patients with carotid artery bruits. Simultaneous, bilateral carotid pressure should *never* be performed. Objective: Given a patient situation, describe the ECG characteristics and initial emergency care for each of the following situations, including mechanical, pharmacologic (i.e., indications, contraindications, doses, and route of administration of applicable medications), and electrical therapy, where applicable: too-fast rhythms, too-slow rhythms, and cardiac arrest rhythms.

13. b. Second-degree AV block type II is often associated with anteroseptal MI and may progress rapidly to a third-degree AV block. Objective: Given a patient situation, describe the ECG characteristics and initial emergency care for each of the following situations, including mechanical, pharmacologic (i.e., indications, contraindications, doses, and route of administration of applicable medications), and electrical therapy, where applicable: too-fast rhythms, too-slow rhythms, and cardiac arrest rhythms.

14. c. In adults, the normal duration of the QRS complex is 0.11 second or less.

15. a. The cardiac monitor displays a second degree AV block, type I. A second-degree AV block type I is usually associated with a narrow-QRS. Atropine is often effective in increasing the heart rate in symptomatic narrow-QRS bradycardias. Because atropine will likely result in an increase in heart rate, the resulting increased rate will also increase myocardial oxygen demand. This must be considered when giving atropine to a patient who may be experiencing an acute MI. Adenosine is used to slow the heart rate in symptomatic narrow-QRS tachycardias. Because this patient has a bradycardia, adenosine is not indicated. Sublingual nitroglycerin (NTG) should not be given at this time because the patient's heart rate is less than 50 beats/min and his blood pressure is low. Nitrates are contraindicated in patients with hypotension (systolic blood pressure less than 90 mm Hg or 30 mm Hg or more below baseline), extreme bradycardia (slower than 50 beats/min), or tachycardia in the absence of heart failure (faster than 100 beats/min) and in patients with right ventricular infarction (RVI). Although morphine is used to relieve pain, the patient's blood pressure is very low. Since the patient's breath sounds are clear, consider a 250 mL IV fluid challenge of normal saline to try to increase the patient's blood pressure. Give NTG and morphine as needed for pain relief if the patient's systolic blood pressure rises above 90 to 100 mm Hg (check your local protocols) and the heart rate increases to more than 50 beats/min (but less than 100). Objective: Given a patient situation, describe the

ECG characteristics and initial emergency care for each of the following situations, including mechanical, pharmacologic (i.e., indications, contraindications, doses, and route of administration of applicable medications), and electrical therapy, where applicable: too-fast rhythms, too-slow rhythms, and cardiac arrest rhythms.

16. c. An IV bolus of epinephrine is indicated in cardiac arrest. Cardiac arrest rhythms include PEA, asystole, pulseless VT and VF. Epinephrine is not given IV bolus to patients who have a pulse. Although epinephrine may be given to patients for symptomatic bradycardia, it is given as an IV infusion, not an IV bolus. Objective: Given a patient situation, describe the ECG characteristics and initial emergency care for each of the following situations, including mechanical, pharmacologic (i.e., indications, contraindications, doses, and route of administration of applicable medications), and electrical therapy, where applicable: too-fast rhythms, too-slow rhythms, and cardiac arrest rhythms.

17. d. The cardiac monitor shows monomorphic VT. Objective: Given a patient situation, describe the ECG characteristics and initial emergency care for each of the following situations, including mechanical, pharmacologic (i.e., indications, contraindications, doses, and route of administration of applicable medications), and electrical therapy, where applicable: too-fast rhythms, too-slow rhythms, and cardiac arrest rhythms.

18. c. Based on the information presented, the patient appears to be stable. Because the patient has a pulse, CPR, defibrillation, and vasopressin are not indicated. The patient denies chest pain so NTG is not indicated. The drug of choice for a stable patient in monomorphic VT is procainamide. Alternative drugs include amiodarone and sotalol. Objective: Identify a patient experiencing a cardiac dysrhythmia as asymptomatic, symptomatic but stable, symptomatic but unstable, or pulseless. Given a patient situation, describe the ECG characteristics and initial emergency care for each of the following situations, including mechanical, pharmacologic (i.e., indications, contraindications, doses, and route of administration of applicable medications), and electrical therapy, where applicable: too-fast rhythms, too-slow rhythms, and cardiac arrest rhythms.

19. b. The cardiac monitor displays a regular narrow-QRS tachycardia at a rate of about 210 beats/min. This patient is unstable (chest discomfort, altered level of consciousness, hypotension, difficulty breathing). Consider sedation, perform synchronized cardioversion, and reassess the patient. NTG is contraindicated because of the patient's rapid heart rate and low blood pressure. Adenosine and verapamil may be used for *stable* patients who are symptomatic with a narrow-QRS tachycardia. Objective: Identify a patient experiencing a cardiac dysrhythmia as asymptomatic, symptomatic but stable, symptomatic but unstable, or pulseless. Given a patient situation, describe the ECG characteristics and initial emergency care for each of the following situations, including mechanical, pharmacologic (i.e., indications, contraindications, doses, and route of administration of applicable medications), and electrical therapy, where applicable: too-fast rhythms, too-slow rhythms, and cardiac arrest rhythms.

20. d. The cardiac monitor displays a sinus tachycardia. Despite the presence of an organized rhythm on the cardiac monitor, the patient is pulseless. The clinical situation is PEA. Begin CPR immediately, establish vascular access, give epinephrine, and search for a reversible cause of the arrest. TCP is not indicated in cardiac arrest. Defibrillation is not indicated for PEA. Objective: Identify a patient experiencing a cardiac dysrhythmia as asymptomatic, symptomatic but stable, symptomatic but unstable, or pulseless. Given a patient situation, describe the ECG characteristics and initial emergency care for each of the following situations, including mechanical, pharmacologic (i.e., indications, contraindications, doses, and route of administration of applicable medications), and electrical therapy, where applicable: too-fast rhythms, too-slow rhythms, and cardiac arrest rhythms.

21. c. A rapid, wide-QRS rhythm associated with pulselessness, shock, or heart failure should be presumed to be VT until proven otherwise. Objective: Given a patient situation, describe the ECG characteristics and initial emergency care for each of the following situations, including mechanical, pharmacologic (i.e., indications, contraindications, doses, and route of administration of applicable medications), and electrical therapy, where applicable: too-fast rhythms, too-slow rhythms, and cardiac arrest rhythms.

22. c. The AV node is normally the only electrical connection between the atria and ventricles. Pre-excitation is a term used to describe rhythms that originate from above the ventricles but in which the impulse travels via a pathway other than the AV node and bundle of His. Thus the supraventricular impulse excites the ventricles earlier than would be expected if the impulse traveled by way of the normal conduction system. Patients with pre-excitation syndromes are prone to AV

reentrant tachycardia. When the AV junction is bypassed by an abnormal pathway, the abnormal route is called an accessory pathway. An accessory pathway is an extra bundle of working myocardial tissue that forms a connection between the atria and ventricles outside the normal conduction system. The term bypass tract is used when one end of an accessory pathway is attached to normal conductive tissue.

23. b. When atropine is used to treat a symptomatic bradycardia, the correct dose is 0.5 mg IV every 3 to 5 minutes to a maximum dose of 3 mg. Objective: Given a patient situation, describe the ECG characteristics and initial emergency care for each of the following situations, including mechanical, pharmacologic (i.e., indications, contraindications, doses, and route of administration of applicable medications), and electrical therapy, where applicable: too-fast rhythms, too-slow rhythms, and cardiac arrest rhythms.

24. d. Although amiodarone is the preferred antiarrhythmic in cardiac arrest due to pulseless VT/VF, lidocaine may be considered if amiodarone is not available. The initial dose is 1 to 1.5 mg/kg IV push. Repeat doses of 0.5 to 0.75 mg/kg IV push may be given at 5- to 10-minute intervals, to a maximum dose of 3 mg/kg. Objective: Given a patient situation, describe the ECG characteristics and initial emergency care for each of the following situations, including mechanical, pharmacologic (i.e., indications, contraindications, doses, and route of administration of applicable medications), and electrical therapy, where applicable: too-fast rhythms, too-slow rhythms, and cardiac arrest rhythms.

25. c. The cardiac monitor shows atrial fibrillation with a rapid ventricular response. Objective: Identify a patient experiencing a cardiac dysrhythmia as asymptomatic, symptomatic but stable, symptomatic but unstable, or pulseless. Given a patient situation, describe the ECG characteristics and initial emergency care for each of the following situations, including mechanical, pharmacologic (i.e., indications, contraindications, doses, and route of administration of applicable medications), and electrical therapy, where applicable: too-fast rhythms, too-slow rhythms, and cardiac arrest rhythms.

26. c. This patient is unstable (e.g., sudden altered mental status, hypotension, chest pain). The patient should be sedated and then synchronized cardioversion should be performed. Defibrillation is not indicated for AFib. Although dopamine will increase blood pressure, it usually increases heart rate as well. A better course of action would be to treat the rate problem with synchronized cardioversion and then reassess the patient's blood pressure. By correcting the rate problem, it is likely the patient's blood pressure will improve. TCP is used to increase heart rate. Since the patient is tachycardic, it is not indicated in this situation. Adenosine is used for narrow-QRS tachycardias that use the AV node to perpetuate the rhythm. When adenosine is given, it is administered as a rapid IV push over 1 to 3 seconds (not a slow IV push). Drugs that slow conduction through the AV node will not generally convert AFib (or atrial flutter) to a sinus rhythm because the reentry circuit is located in the atria (not the AV node) and is not affected. In AFib, the AV node does not play a part in the maintenance of the tachycardia. The AV node serves only to passively conduct the supraventricular rhythm into the ventricles. Objective: Identify a patient experiencing a cardiac dysrhythmia as asymptomatic, symptomatic but stable, symptomatic but unstable, or pulseless. Given a patient situation, describe the ECG characteristics and initial emergency care for each of the following situations, including mechanical, pharmacologic (i.e., indications, contraindications, doses, and route of administration of applicable medications), and electrical therapy, where applicable: too-fast rhythms, too-slow rhythms, and cardiac arrest rhythms.

27. c. The rhythm shown is polymorphic VT. The patient is unstable (e.g., acute altered mental status, hypotension). Consider sedation and defibrillate immediately. Although synchronized cardioversion is an appropriate treatment for unstable patients with a tachycardia, it is used for tachycardias that have a relatively uniform amplitude. Because the amplitude of the waveforms in polymorphic VT varies, defibrillation should be used instead. Adenosine and diltiazem are not indicated. Objective: Identify a patient experiencing a cardiac dysrhythmia as asymptomatic, symptomatic but stable, symptomatic but unstable, or pulseless. Given a patient situation, describe the ECG characteristics and initial emergency care for each of the following situations, including mechanical, pharmacologic (i.e., indications, contraindications, doses, and route of administration of applicable medications), and electrical therapy, where applicable: too-fast rhythms, too-slow rhythms, and cardiac arrest rhythms.

28. b. The rhythm shown is asystole. Appropriate emergency care includes performing high-quality CPR, providing positive pressure ventilation, establishing vascular access, giving epinephrine, and

considering possible reversible causes of the arrest. Vasopressin can be used in place of the first or second dose of epinephrine. Although amiodarone is used in the management of many atrial and ventricular dysrhythmias, it is not indicated in the treatment of asystole. Defibrillation is not indicated in the treatment of asystole. Isoproterenol can be used in the management of a symptomatic bradycardia (when the patient has a pulse). It is not indicated in asystole. Objective: Identify a patient experiencing a cardiac dysrhythmia as asymptomatic, symptomatic but stable, symptomatic but unstable, or pulseless. Given a patient situation, describe the ECG characteristics and initial emergency care for each of the following situations, including mechanical, pharmacologic (i.e., indications, contraindications, doses, and route of administration of applicable medications), and electrical therapy, where applicable: too-fast rhythms, too-slow rhythms, and cardiac arrest rhythms.

29. c. The initial dose of procainamide is 20 to 50 mg/min IV. The maximum dose is 17 mg/kg and the maintenance infusion dose is 1 to 4 mg/min. Objective: Given a patient situation, describe the ECG characteristics and initial emergency care for each of the following situations, including mechanical, pharmacologic (i.e., indications, contraindications, doses, and route of administration of applicable medications), and electrical therapy, where applicable: too-fast rhythms, too-slow rhythms, and cardiac arrest rhythms.

Completion

30. One hundred percent ventricular paced rhythm. Objective: Given a patient situation, describe the ECG characteristics and initial emergency care for each of the following situations, including mechanical, pharmacologic (i.e., indications, contraindications, doses, and route of administration of applicable medications), and electrical therapy, where applicable: too-fast rhythms, too-slow rhythms, and cardiac arrest rhythms.

31. 2:1 AV block with ST-segment depression. Objective: Given a patient situation, describe the ECG characteristics and initial emergency care for each of the following situations, including mechanical, pharmacologic (i.e., indications, contraindications, doses, and route of administration of applicable medications), and electrical therapy, where applicable: too-fast rhythms, too-slow rhythms, and cardiac arrest rhythms.

32. Atrial fibrillation (controlled ventricular response). Objective: Given a patient situation, describe the ECG characteristics and initial emergency care for each of the following situations, including mechanical, pharmacologic (i.e., indications, contraindications, doses, and route of administration of applicable medications), and electrical therapy, where applicable: too-fast rhythms, too-slow rhythms, and cardiac arrest rhythms.

33. Sinus bradycardia at 58 beats/min with borderline first-degree AV block. Objective: Given a patient situation, describe the ECG characteristics and initial emergency care for each of the following situations, including mechanical, pharmacologic (i.e., indications, contraindications, doses, and route of administration of applicable medications), and electrical therapy, where applicable: too-fast rhythms, too-slow rhythms, and cardiac arrest rhythms.

34. Narrow-QRS tachycardia with ST-segment depression. Objective: Given a patient situation, describe the ECG characteristics and initial emergency care for each of the following situations, including mechanical, pharmacologic (i.e., indications, contraindications, doses, and route of administration of applicable medications), and electrical therapy, where applicable: too-fast rhythms, too-slow rhythms, and cardiac arrest rhythms.

35. Sinus rhythm with first-degree AV block. Objective: Given a patient situation, describe the ECG characteristics and initial emergency care for each of the following situations, including mechanical, pharmacologic (i.e., indications, contraindications, doses, and route of administration of applicable medications), and electrical therapy, where applicable: too-fast rhythms, too-slow rhythms, and cardiac arrest rhythms.

36. Sinus rhythm at 65 beats/min with ST-segment elevation. Objective: Given a patient situation, describe the ECG characteristics and initial emergency care for each of the following situations, including mechanical, pharmacologic (i.e., indications, contraindications, doses, and route of administration of applicable medications), and electrical therapy, where applicable: too-fast rhythms, too-slow rhythms, and cardiac arrest rhythms.

37. Third-degree (complete) AV block at 29 beats/min with ST-segment elevation. Objective: Given a patient situation, describe the ECG characteristics and initial emergency care for each of the

following situations, including mechanical, pharmacologic (i.e., indications, contraindications, doses, and route of administration of applicable medications), and electrical therapy, where applicable: too-fast rhythms, too-slow rhythms, and cardiac arrest rhythms.

38. Junctional bradycardia at 30 beats/min to sinus rhythm at 75 beats/min. Objective: Given a patient situation, describe the ECG characteristics and initial emergency care for each of the following situations, including mechanical, pharmacologic (i.e., indications, contraindications, doses, and route of administration of applicable medications), and electrical therapy, where applicable: too-fast rhythms, too-slow rhythms, and cardiac arrest rhythms.

39. Atrial flutter at 55 beats/min. Objective: Given a patient situation, describe the ECG characteristics and initial emergency care for each of the following situations, including mechanical, pharmacologic (i.e., indications, contraindications, doses, and route of administration of applicable medications), and electrical therapy, where applicable: too-fast rhythms, too-slow rhythms, and cardiac arrest rhythms.

40. Sinus tachycardia at 115 beats/min with ST-segment elevation. Objective: Given a patient situation, describe the ECG characteristics and initial emergency care for each of the following situations, including mechanical, pharmacologic (i.e., indications, contraindications, doses, and route of administration of applicable medications), and electrical therapy, where applicable: too-fast rhythms, too-slow rhythms, and cardiac arrest rhythms.

41. Sinus rhythm at 75 beats/min with uniform premature ventricular complexes. Objective: Given a patient situation, describe the ECG characteristics and initial emergency care for each of the following situations, including mechanical, pharmacologic (i.e., indications, contraindications, doses, and route of administration of applicable medications), and electrical therapy, where applicable: too-fast rhythms, too-slow rhythms, and cardiac arrest rhythms.

42. One hundred percent ventricular paced rhythm. Objective: Given a patient situation, describe the ECG characteristics and initial emergency care for each of the following situations, including mechanical, pharmacologic (i.e., indications, contraindications, doses, and route of administration of applicable medications), and electrical therapy, where applicable: too-fast rhythms, too-slow rhythms, and cardiac arrest rhythms.

43. Narrow-QRS tachycardia at 233 beats/min with ST-segment depression. Objective: Given a patient situation, describe the ECG characteristics and initial emergency care for each of the following situations, including mechanical, pharmacologic (i.e., indications, contraindications, doses, and route of administration of applicable medications), and electrical therapy, where applicable: too-fast rhythms, too-slow rhythms, and cardiac arrest rhythms.

44. Coarse ventricular fibrillation. Objective: Given a patient situation, describe the ECG characteristics and initial emergency care for each of the following situations, including mechanical, pharmacologic (i.e., indications, contraindications, doses, and route of administration of applicable medications), and electrical therapy, where applicable: too-fast rhythms, too-slow rhythms, and cardiac arrest rhythms.

45. Second-degree AV block type II at 37 beats/min. Objective: Given a patient situation, describe the ECG characteristics and initial emergency care for each of the following situations, including mechanical, pharmacologic (i.e., indications, contraindications, doses, and route of administration of applicable medications), and electrical therapy, where applicable: too-fast rhythms, too-slow rhythms, and cardiac arrest rhythms.

Matching

46. d	52. c	58. d
47. h	53. i	59. k
48. f	54. b	60. f
49. g	55. j	61. a
50. a	56. g	62. c
51. e	57. h	63. i

64. e	69. j	74. a
65. b	70. c	75. l
66. e	71. i	76. h
67. k	72. m	77. b
68. d	73. f	78. g

Short Answer

79. Cardiac rhythms can be classified into four main groups: normal, absent/pulseless (cardiac arrest rhythms), slower than normal for age (bradycardia), or faster than normal for age (tachycardia).
80. No. Depolarization is an electrical event. Contraction is a mechanical event.
81.

LEAD	HEART SURFACE VIEWED	LEAD	HEART SURFACE VIEWED
Lead I	Lateral	V_1	Septum
Lead II	Inferior	V_2	Septum
Lead III	Inferior	V_3	Anterior
aVR	None	V_4	Anterior
aVL	Lateral	V_5	Lateral
aVF	Inferior	V_6	Lateral

82.

PARAMETER	SINUS BRADYCARDIA	JUNCTIONAL RHYTHM	VENTRICULAR ESCAPE RHYTHM
Rate	Less than 60 beats/min	40 to 60 beats/min	20 to 40 beats/min
Rhythm	Regular	Regular	Essentially regular
P Waves (lead II)	Upright	May occur before, during, or after the QRS. If visible, the P wave is inverted in leads II, III, and aVF.	Usually absent or, with retrograde conduction to the atria, may appear after the QRS (usually upright in the ST-segment or T wave)
PR Interval	0.12 to 0.20 sec	If a P wave is present before the QRS, usually less than or equal to 0.12 sec. If no P wave occurs before the QRS, there will be no PR interval.	None
QRS	0.11 sec or less unless an intraventricular conduction delay exists.	0.11 sec or less unless an intraventricular conduction delay exists.	0.12 sec or more

83. During circulatory collapse or cardiac arrest, the preferred vascular access site is the largest, most accessible vein that does not require the interruption of resuscitation efforts. If no IV is in place before the arrest, establish IV access using a peripheral vein–preferably the antecubital or external jugular vein.
84. Alpha$_1$ receptor sites are located in vascular smooth muscle, beta$_1$ receptor sites are located in the heart and kidneys, beta$_2$ receptor sites are located in the smooth muscle of the bronchi and skeletal blood vessels.

CHAPTER 4 STOP AND REVIEW ANSWERS

True/False

1. F. Studies have shown that the anterolateral, anteroposterior, anterior-left infrascapular, and anterior-right infrascapular paddle or pad positions are equally effective to treat atrial or ventricular dysrhythmias. Objective: Explain defibrillation, its indications, proper pad or paddle placement, relevant precautions, and the steps required to perform this procedure with a manual defibrillator and an AED.

2. T. When using hand-held paddles, the use of gels, pastes, or pregelled defibrillation pads aids the passage of current at the interface between the defibrillator paddles/electrodes and the body surface. Failure to use conductive material results in increased transthoracic impedance, a lack of penetration of current, and burns to the skin surface. Combination pads are pregelled and do not require the application of additional gel to the patient's chest. Objective: Explain defibrillation, its indications, proper pad or paddle placement, relevant precautions, and the steps required to perform this procedure with a manual defibrillator and an AED.

Multiple Choice

3. a. After confirming that the patient is unresponsive, not breathing, and has no pulse, CPR should be performed while the AED is being readied for use. Turn on the power to the AED, apply the pads to the patient's chest, and then analyze the patient's rhythm. All movement around the patient must stop when the AED is analyzing the patient's rhythm. For example, positive pressure ventilation, chest compressions, and vehicle movement must temporarily stop during rhythm analysis. If movement is detected, the AED will stop analyzing the rhythm. This is a safety feature because movement can cause distortion of the patient's cardiac rhythm. Distortion can cause a nonshockable rhythm to look like a shockable rhythm, and a shockable rhythm to look like a nonshockable rhythm. Objective: Explain defibrillation, its indications, proper pad or paddle placement, relevant precautions, and the steps required to perform this procedure with a manual defibrillator and an AED.

4. b. Synchronized cardioversion is the timed delivery of a shock during the QRS complex. It is indicated in the management of a patient who is exhibiting serious signs and symptoms related to a tachycardia. It is used to treat rhythms that have a clearly identifiable QRS complex and a rapid ventricular rate (such as some narrow-QRS tachycardias and VT). Objective: Explain synchronized cardioversion, describe its indications, and list the steps required to perform this procedure.

5. d. Coughing, burns, and failure to recognize that the pacemaker is not capturing are possible complications of TCP. Once pacing has begun, it is important to reassess the patient and his or her cardiac rhythm often. Because burns are possible with prolonged pacing, check the condition of the patient's skin at the site of pacing pads at least every 30 minutes. Flail chest is a possible contraindication for TCP. Objective: Discuss the procedure for TCP as well as its indications and possible complications.

6. c. Defibrillation is indicated in the management of pulseless VT and VF. It is not indicated in the management of PEA. Remember that defibrillation is performed in order to depolarize the myocardial cells at one time and provide an opportunity for one of the heart's natural pacemakers to take over. In PEA, an organized rhythm is present on the monitor. Thus, pacemaker activity is already present but there is inadequate cardiac output and no pulse. PEA is not shocked because a shock could disrupt the organized rhythm and cause chaos (e.g., VF). Defibrillation is not indicated in asystole. Objective: Explain defibrillation, its indications, proper pad or paddle placement, relevant precautions, and the steps required to perform this procedure with a manual defibrillator and an AED.

7. d. The patient's chest pain, decreasing level of responsiveness, and hypotension indicate that he is clearly unstable. Your best course of action will be to administer sedation and perform synchronized cardioversion with 50 J. Transcutaneous pacing is not indicated. Defibrillation with an initial shock of 360 J is warranted for pulseless VT, VF, and unstable (sustained) polymorphic VT (when using a monophasic defibrillator). Objective: For each of the following rhythms, identify the energy

levels that are currently recommended and indicate if the shock delivered should be a synchronized or unsynchronized countershock: Pulseless VT/VF, monomorphic VT, polymorphic VT, narrow-QRS tachycardia, atrial fibrillation, and atrial flutter.

8. d. TCP may be useful for symptomatic bradycardias when the patient's signs and symptoms are due to the slow heart rate. TCP is not indicated for any of the other rhythms listed. Objective: Discuss the procedure for transcutaneous pacing as well as its indications and possible complications.

9. a. CPR and defibrillation are the most important treatments for the patient in cardiac arrest due to pulseless VT or VF. Insertion of advanced airways and administration of resuscitation medications are of secondary importance. Although synchronized cardioversion may be used in the treatment of an unstable patient in monomorphic VT with a pulse, it is not indicated for pulseless VT. Objective: Explain defibrillation, its indications, proper pad or paddle placement, relevant precautions, and the steps required to perform this procedure with a manual defibrillator and an AED.

10. c. Although an organized rhythm is present on the monitor, the patient has no pulse. This clinical situation is PEA. You should begin CPR immediately, ventilate the patient with a bag-mask device, and give epinephrine 1 mg IV. TCP, defibrillation, and atropine administration are not indicated for PEA. Objective: Explain defibrillation, its indications, proper pad or paddle placement, relevant precautions, and the steps required to perform this procedure with a manual defibrillator and an AED.

11. c. The patient's chest discomfort and hypotension indicate that her condition is unstable. You should administer sedation and perform synchronized cardioversion with 100 J. TCP and CPR are not indicated. Defibrillation is warranted for pulseless VT, VF, and unstable (sustained) polymorphic VT. Objective: Explain synchronized cardioversion, describe its indications, and list the steps required to perform this procedure.

Matching

12. f	18. l	24. j
13. m	19. e	25. b
14. i	20. p	26. k
15. h	21. a	27. g
16. n	22. o	
17. c	23. d	

Short Answer

28. The purpose of defibrillation (i.e., unsynchronized countershock) is to deliver a uniform electrical current of sufficient intensity to depolarize myocardial cells (including fibrillating cells) at the same time, briefly "stunning" the heart. This provides an opportunity for the heart's natural pacemakers to resume normal activity. When the cells repolarize, the pacemaker with the highest degree of automaticity should assume responsibility for pacing the heart. Objective: Explain defibrillation, its indications, proper pad or paddle placement, relevant precautions, and the steps required to perform this procedure with a manual defibrillator and an AED.

29. Defibrillation is indicated for sustained polymorphic VT, pulseless VT, and VF. Objective: Explain defibrillation, its indications, proper pad or paddle placement, relevant precautions, and the steps required to perform this procedure with a manual defibrillator and an AED.

30. Manual defibrillation refers to the placement of paddles or pads on a patient's chest, interpretation of the patient's cardiac rhythm by a trained healthcare professional, and the healthcare professional's decision to deliver a shock (if indicated). Automated external defibrillation refers to the placement of paddles or pads on a patient's chest and interpretation of the patient's cardiac rhythm by the defibrillator's computerized analysis system. Depending on the type of automated external defibrillator used, the machine will deliver a shock (if a shockable rhythm is detected) or instruct the operator to deliver a shock. Objective: Explain defibrillation, its indications, proper pad or paddle placement, relevant precautions, and the steps required to perform this procedure with a manual defibrillator and an AED.

31. Possibilities include no power, loose leads, true asystole, unplugged cables, no connection to the patient, and no connection to the defibrillator/monitor.

32. An implantable cardioverter-defibrillator (ICD) is usually located subcutaneously in the left upper quadrant of the patient's abdomen or the left pectoral region. Objective: Explain defibrillation, its indications, proper pad or paddle placement, relevant precautions, and the steps required to perform this procedure with a manual defibrillator and an AED.

33. When defibrillating (or cardioverting) a patient with a permanent (implanted) pacemaker or ICD, be careful not to place the defibrillator paddles or combination pads directly over the device. Although placement of paddles or pads should not delay defibrillation, defibrillator paddles or combination pads should ideally be placed at least 3 inches (8 cm) from the pulse generator (i.e., bulge under the patient's skin). Objective: Explain defibrillation, its indications, proper pad or paddle placement, relevant precautions, and the steps required to perform this procedure with a manual defibrillator and an AED.

34. Turn on the power
    Attach the device
    Analyze the rhythm
    Deliver a shock if indicated and safe
    Objective: Explain defibrillation, its indications, proper pad or paddle placement, relevant precautions, and the steps required to perform this procedure with a manual defibrillator and an AED.

35. If the rhythm changes to VF after synchronized cardioversion, confirm that the patient has no pulse while another team member quickly verifies that all electrodes and cable connections are secure, turn off the sync control, and defibrillate. Objective: Explain defibrillation, its indications, proper pad or paddle placement, relevant precautions, and the steps required to perform this procedure with a manual defibrillator and an AED.

CHAPTER 5 STOP AND REVIEW ANSWERS

True/False

1. T. Ischemia prolonged more than just a few minutes results in myocardial injury. Myocardial injury refers to myocardial tissue that has been cut off from or experienced a severe reduction in its blood and oxygen supply. Injured myocardial cells are still alive but will die (infarct) if the ischemia is not quickly corrected. Objective: Explain the pathophysiology of ACSs.

2. F. Currently, fibrinolytic therapy is not indicated for patients with unstable angina/non-ST elevation myocardial infarction (UA/NSTEMI) except for those with a true posterior myocardial infarction (MI) evidenced as ST-segment depression in two contiguous anterior chest leads and/or isolated ST-segment elevation in posterior chest leads. Objective: Describe the initial management of a patient experiencing an ACS.

3. T. During their initial presentation, patients with unstable angina often cannot be distinguished from those with an acute MI because their clinical presentations and ECG findings may be identical. Early assessment, including a focused history, and intervention are essential to prevent worsening ischemia. Serial ECGs and continuous ECG monitoring should be performed. Objective: Describe the forms of ACSs.

4. T. Not all patients experiencing an ACS present similarly. Atypical presentation refers to uncharacteristic signs and symptoms perceived by some patients. Atypical chest discomfort is localized to the chest area but may have musculoskeletal, positional, or pleuritic features. Objective: Explain atypical presentation and its significance in ACSs.

5. F. Glycoprotein IIb/IIIa inhibitors (abciximab [ReoPro], eptifibatide [Integrilin], tirofiban [Aggrastat]) prevent fibrinogen binding and platelet aggregation. At this time, there is insufficient data to support the routine use of GP IIb/IIIa inhibitors in patients with ST elevation myocardial infarction (STEMI) or non-ST elevation ACSs in the prehospital or emergency department settings. For selected high-risk patients with non-ST elevation ACSs, abciximab, eptifibatide, or tirofiban administration may be acceptable, provided percutaneous coronary intervention (PCI) is planned. Objective: Describe the initial management of a patient experiencing an ACS.

6. F. Decisions regarding the care of a patient experiencing an ACS are primarily based on his or her assessment findings and symptoms, history, presence of risk factors, serial 12-lead ECG results,

laboratory test results (e.g., cardiac biomarkers), and other diagnostic tests. Objective: Describe the initial management of a patient experiencing an ACS.

7. F. Angiotensin-converting enzyme (ACE) inhibitors produce vasodilation by blocking the conversion of angiotensin I to angiotensin II. Because angiotensin is a potent vasoconstrictor, limiting its production decreases peripheral vascular resistance, reducing the pressure the heart must pump against, and decreasing myocardial workload. ACE inhibitors also increase renal blood flow, which helps rid the body of excess sodium and fluid accumulation. Beta-blockers act on $beta_1$ and $beta_2$ receptors to slow sinus rate, depress AV conduction, and reduce blood pressure. Objective: Describe the initial management of a patient experiencing an ACS.

Multiple Choice

8. b. Ischemia affects the heart's cells responsible for contraction as well as those responsible for generation and conduction of electrical impulses. Because ischemia affects repolarization, its effects can be viewed on the ECG as brief changes in ST-segments and T waves in the leads facing the affected area of the ventricle. ST-segment depression of more than 0.5 mm in leads V_2 and V_3 and more than 1 mm in all other leads is suggestive of myocardial ischemia when viewed in two or more anatomically contiguous leads. Negative (inverted) T waves may also be present. Objective: Identify the ECG changes associated with myocardial ischemia, injury, and infarction.

9. a. Inhibition of $beta_1$ adrenergic receptor sites reduces myocardial contractility, sinoatrial node rate, and AV node conduction velocity, decreasing cardiac work and reducing myocardial oxygen demand. Objective: Describe the initial management of a patient experiencing an ACS.

10. c. Aspirin should be chewed by patients who have not taken aspirin before presentation with an ACS. The initial dose should be 162 mg to 325 mg and continued indefinitely at a daily dose of 75 to 162 mg (assuming there are no contraindications to its use). Objective: Describe the initial management of a patient experiencing an ACS.

11. b. Dopamine increases heart rate and cardiac contractility directly by stimulating $beta_1$ receptors on the myocardium and indirectly by causing the release of norepinephrine from storage sites in sympathetic nerve endings. Dopamine is not an analgesic; therefore, it is not useful in relieving pain or discomfort. Dopamine is not an antiarrhythmic; therefore, it does not suppress ventricular ectopy. Dopamine does not affect the width of the QRS complex. Objective: Describe the initial management of a patient experiencing an ACS.

12. a. The incidence of VF is highest during the first 4 hours after onset of symptoms and remains an important contributing factor to death in the first 24 hours after STEMI. Objective: Identify the most common complications of an acute MI.

13. c. Electrical complications of an acute MI include bradydysrhythmias (sinus bradycardia is most common), tachydysrhythmias, AV blocks, bundle branch and fascicular blocks, and sudden cardiac death. Ventricular aneurysm, papillary muscle disorders, and left ventricular failure are examples of mechanical complications of an acute MI. Pericarditis is an inflammatory complication. Acute stroke and pulmonary embolism are embolic complications. Objective: Identify the most common complications of an acute MI.

14. b. Morphine is the preferred analgesic for patients with STEMI who experience persistent chest discomfort unresponsive to nitrates. Other narcotics may be considered in patients allergic to morphine. Objective: Describe the initial management of a patient experiencing an ACS.

15. c. Acute pericarditis is an inflammatory process, often with fluid accumulation, involving the pericardium that results in a clinical syndrome with the triad of chest pain, pericardial friction rub, and ECG changes. The cause is viral or unknown in 90% of cases. The pain of pericarditis can often be localized with one finger and is usually worse with inspiration, intensified when lying supine, and lessened by sitting forward. Objective: Identify the most common complications of an acute MI.

16. a. Initial management of a patient experiencing an ACS should include primary and secondary surveys, oxygen (if indicated), IV, monitor, vital signs, aspirin if not already given (and no contraindications) and a 12-lead ECG within 10 minutes of patient contact or patient arrival in the emergency department. Thus far, we have no idea what the patient's cardiac rhythm is so preparations for defibrillation and TCP are not warranted. A fluid challenge is not routinely given to a patient experiencing an ACS. Furthermore, we do not yet know the patient's vital signs or the status of his lung sounds. Objective: Describe the initial management of a patient experiencing an ACS.

17. d. The sinus tachycardia seen on the cardiac monitor is most likely associated with the discomfort and ACS the patient is experiencing. The treatment for a sinus tachycardia is treatment of the underlying cause. In this case, the patient should be given medications to relieve his discomfort as soon as possible. A tachycardia is a concern in a patient experiencing an ACS because it results in decreased ventricular filling time and decreased coronary perfusion pressure. Vagal maneuvers and adenosine are not appropriate interventions for a sinus tachycardia. These interventions are used for stable patients who are symptomatic because of a narrow-QRS tachycardia such as AVNRT. Synchronized cardioversion is not appropriate for a sinus tachycardia. It is used to treat unstable patients who have a rhythm with a clearly identifiable QRS complex and a rapid ventricular rate (e.g., some narrow-QRS tachycardias, VT). Objective: Describe the initial management of a patient experiencing an ACS.

18. b. A 12-lead ECG is essential to decision making in the emergency care of a patient with an ACS and should be obtained with 10 minutes of patient contact (prehospital) or arrival in the emergency department. Objective: Explain the importance of the 12-lead ECG for the patient with an ACS.

19. c. NTG relaxes smooth muscle, thereby dilating peripheral arteries and veins. This causes a pooling of venous blood and decreased venous return to the heart, which decreases preload. NTG also dilates normal and atherosclerotic epicardial coronary arteries, and reduces left ventricular systolic wall tension, which decreases afterload. Aspirin (not NTG) blocks the formation of thromboxane A_2 (thromboxane A_2 causes platelets to clump and arteries to constrict). Objective: Describe the initial management of a patient experiencing an ACS.

20. b. Before giving NTG, assess the degree of the patient's pain or discomfort using a 0-to-10 scale. Also asses and record the pain's duration, time of onset, the activity that was being done, and the pain quality. Reassess and document the patient's vital signs and level of discomfort after each dose.

    Make sure that the patient has not used a phosphodiesterase inhibitor such as sildenafil (e.g., Viagra) within 24 hours or tadalafil (e.g., Cialis) within 48 hours before NTG administration. The combination of a phosphodiesterase inhibitor and nitrates may result in severe hypotension.

    Nitrates should not be administered to patients with a systolic blood pressure lower than 90 mm Hg or 30 mm Hg or more below baseline, severe bradycardia (slower than 50 beats/min), tachycardia in the absence of heart failure (faster than 100 beats/min), or suspected RVI. Objective: Describe the initial management of a patient experiencing an ACS.

21. b. Patients with ongoing ischemic discomfort should receive sublingual NTG (0.4 mg) every 3 to 5 minutes for a total of three doses, after which an assessment should be made about the need for IV NTG. IV NTG is indicated for relief of ongoing ischemic discomfort, control of hypertension, or management of pulmonary congestion. Unless contraindicated by hypotension or intolerance, morphine may be administered with intravenous NTG, with careful blood pressure monitoring. Objective: Describe the initial management of a patient experiencing an ACS.

22. b. Once the 12-lead ECG has been obtained, it should be reviewed carefully. Look at each lead for the presence of ST segment displacement (elevation or depression). If ST segment elevation is present, note its elevation in millimeters. Examine the T waves for any changes in orientation, shape, and size. Examine each lead for the presence of a Q wave. If a Q wave is present, measure its duration. Assess the areas of ischemia or injury by assessing lead groupings. Remember that ECG evidence must be found in at least two contiguous leads. Objective: Identify the ECG changes associated with myocardial ischemia, injury, and infarction.

23. b. When viewing the ECG of a patient experiencing an ACS, the presence of ST-segment elevation in the leads facing the affected area suggests myocardial injury. Objective: Identify the ECG changes associated with myocardial ischemia, injury, and infarction.

24. a. Leads V_1 and V_2 view the septum. Leads V_3 and V_4 view the anterior surface of the left ventricle. ST-segment elevation in these leads suggests an anteroseptal MI. Objective: Identify the ECG leads that view the anterior wall, inferior wall, lateral wall, septum, inferobasal wall, and right ventricle.

25. d. Relief of pain is a priority in the management of a patient experiencing an ACS. Relief of pain decreases anxiety, myocardial oxygen demand, and the risk of cardiac dysrhythmias. When treating a patient with an ACS, it is not enough to simply reduce the patient's degree of pain or discomfort. The goal is to ensure that the patient is free of pain, while closely monitoring his or her vital signs. Before giving morphine, assess the degree of the patient's pain or discomfort using a 0-to-10 scale. Also assess and record the pain's duration, time of onset, the activity that was being done, and the pain quality. Give morphine (generally in 2 mg increments) slow IV push. Give additional doses

at 5- to 15-minute intervals while closely monitoring his or her vital signs. Reassess and document the patient's vital signs and level of discomfort after each morphine dose. Objective: Describe the initial management of a patient experiencing an ACS.

26. b. Blockage of the midportion of the left anterior descending (LAD) coronary artery results in an anterior infarction. However, an infarction involving the anterior wall is usually not localized only to this area. For example, proximal occlusion of the LAD may become an anteroseptal infarction if the septal branch is involved or an anterolateral infarction if the marginal branch is involved. If the blockage occurs proximal to both the septal and diagonal branches, an extensive anterior infarction (anteroseptal-lateral MI) will result.

Because the LAD supplies approximately 40% of the heart's blood and a critical section of the left ventricle, a blockage in this area can lead to complications such as left ventricular dysfunction, including heart failure and cardiogenic shock. Increased sympathetic nervous system activity is common with anterior MIs with resulting sinus tachycardia and/or high blood pressure. An anterior wall MI may cause dysrhythmias including PVCs, atrial flutter, or AFib. Although some portions of the bundle branches are supplied by the right coronary artery (RCA), the left coronary artery supplies most of the bundle branch tissue. Thus bundle branch blocks may occur if the left coronary artery is blocked. Objective: Identify the most common complications of an acute MI.

Completion

27. Ischemia is a decreased supply of oxygenated blood to a body part or organ. Objective: Explain the pathophysiology of ACSs.

28. In an ACS, the zone of injury produces ST-segment elevation in the leads facing the affected area due to abnormal repolarization. Objective: Identify the ECG changes associated with myocardial ischemia, injury, and infarction.

29. Fibrinolytic therapy is one reperfusion option for patients with ST elevation MI. Objective: Describe the initial management of a patient experiencing an ACS.

30. A positive inotropic effect refers to an increase in myocardial contractility. Objective: Describe the initial management of a patient experiencing an ACS.

31. Unfractionated heparin (UFH) is an anticoagulant that indirectly inhibits thrombin, acting at multiple sites in the normal coagulation system. Objective: Describe the initial management of a patient experiencing an ACS.

Matching

32. f
33. k
34. h
35. m
36. p
37. b
38. i
39. q
40. d
41. c
42. j

43. r
44. n
45. e
46. t
47. l
48. u
49. a
50. o
51. s
52. g

Short Answer

53. 1. ST segment elevation (or new left bundle branch block).
2. ST segment depression or transient ST-segment/T-wave changes.
3. Normal/nondiagnostic ECG.
   Objective: Discuss the three groups used when categorizing the 12-lead ECG findings of the patient experiencing an ACS.

54. Unstable angina, which is also known as preinfarction angina, is a condition of intermediate severity between stable angina and acute MI. It occurs most often in men and women 60 to 80 years of age who have one or more of the major risk factors for coronary artery disease.

Unstable angina is characterized by one or more of the following:
- Symptoms that occur at rest and usually last more than 20 minutes
- Symptoms that are severe and/or of new onset (i.e., within 2 months)
- Symptoms that are increasing in intensity, duration, and/or frequency in a patient with a history of stable angina
Objectiv.e: Describe the forms of ACSs.

55. Injured myocardial cells are still alive but will die (i.e., infarct) if the ischemia is not quickly corrected. If the blocked vessel can be quickly opened, restoring blood flow and oxygen to the injured area, no tissue death occurs. An MI occurs when blood flow to the heart muscle stops or is suddenly decreased long enough to cause cell death. Objective: Describe the forms of ACSs.

56. Anginal equivalent symptoms are symptoms of myocardial ischemia other than chest pain or discomfort. Objective: Explain and give examples of anginal equivalents.

57. Two leads are contiguous if they look at the same or adjacent areas of the heart or if they are numerically consecutive chest leads. Objective: Explain the importance of the 12-lead ECG for a patient with an ACS.

58. In the standard 12-lead ECG, three leads (i.e., II, III, and aVF) "look" at tissue supplied by the RCA. Objective: Identify the ECG leads that view the anterior wall, inferior wall, lateral wall, septum, inferobasal wall, and right ventricle.

59. Examples of anginal equivalents include the following:
- Difficulty breathing
- Dizziness
- Dysrhythmias
- Excessive sweating
- Fatigue
- Generalized weakness
- Isolated arm or jaw pain
- Palpitations
- Syncope or near-syncope
- Unexplained nausea or vomiting
Objective: Explain and give examples of anginal equivalents.

CHAPTER 6 STOP AND REVIEW ANSWERS

True/False

1. F. Stroke kills more than twice as many American women every year as breast cancer.
2. F. A hemorrhagic stroke is caused by either rupture of an artery with bleeding into the spaces surrounding the brain (i.e., subarachnoid hemorrhage) or bleeding into the brain tissue (1.e., intracerebral hemorrhage). Objective: Describe the two major types of stroke.
3. F. The National Institutes of Health Stroke Scale (NIHSS) aids in localizing a stroke lesion and determining stroke severity. The NIHSS is an 11-item, 42-point scale that assesses the patient's level of alertness and comprehension as well as motor, sensory, visual, and language function. Objective: Describe the initial emergency care for acute ischemic stroke.
4. T. A noncontrast brain computed tomography (CT) scan or brain magnetic resonance imaging (MRI) study should be obtained in all patients with suspected acute ischemic stroke. In addition, blood should be drawn and laboratory tests including serum glucose, complete blood count (including platelet count), electrolytes, cardiac biomarkers, renal function, prothrombin and partial thromboplastin times, done immediately. Objective: Describe the initial emergency care for acute ischemic stroke.

Multiple Choice

5. b. Recognition of stroke signs and symptoms by the patient, family, or bystanders is critical. "For the purposes of treatment, the onset is assumed as the time that the patient was last known to be symptom-free. Because ischemic stroke is often painless, most patients are not awakened by its occurrence. Thus, for a patient with symptoms of stroke on awakening, the time of onset is

assumed to be the time the patient was last known to be symptom-free before retiring. If a patient had mild impairments but then had worsening over the subsequent hours, the time the first symptom began is assumed to be the time of onset. In contrast, if a patient has symptoms that completely resolved (transient ischemic attack [TIA]) and then has a second event, the time of onset of the new symptoms is used."[4] Objective: Describe the initial emergency care for acute ischemic stroke.

6. b. Most strokes are the result of blockages due to blood clots that develop within the brain artery itself (i.e., cerebral thrombosis) or clots that arise elsewhere in the body and then migrate to the brain (i.e., cerebral embolism). Objective: Describe the two major types of stroke.

7. b. The middle cerebral artery is the most commonly blocked vessel in a stroke. It is the largest branch of the internal carotid artery. Objective: Describe the two major types of stroke.

8. b. Current stroke protocols recommend that a possible stroke patient presenting to the emergency department be seen by a physician within 10 minutes of his or her arrival. A noncontrast CT scan of the brain should be completed within 25 minutes and read within 45 minutes of the patient's arrival. Objective: Describe the initial emergency care for acute ischemic stroke.

9. c. Patients experiencing AFib may develop intra-atrial emboli because the atria are not contracting and blood stagnates in the atrial chambers. This predisposes the patient to systemic emboli, particularly stroke, if the clots dislodge spontaneously or because of conversion to a sinus rhythm. Objective: Describe the two major types of stroke.

10. b. Currently, the window of opportunity to use IV recombinant form of tissue plasminogen activator (rtPA) to treat most ischemic stroke patients is 3 hours. To be evaluated and receive treatment, patients need to be at a hospital within 60 minutes of symptom onset. Studies have demonstrated clinical improvement when IV rtPA was administered to a carefully selected group of patients who met eligibility criteria and presented within a 3- and 4.5-hour window after the onset of stroke symptoms. The American Heart Association states that administration of IV rtPA to patients with acute ischemic stroke who meet specific eligibility criteria is recommended if rtPA is administered by physicians in the setting of a clearly defined protocol, a knowledgeable team, and institutional commitment.[5] Objective: Describe the initial emergency care for acute ischemic stroke.

11. a. The three areas measured with the Glasgow Coma Scale (GCS) are eye opening, verbal response, and motor response. The GCS measures impairment but is of limited use in an intubated patient, a patient with orbital trauma, or a patient with previous neurologic impairment. Objective: Describe the initial emergency care for acute ischemic stroke.

12. d. The American Heart Association Stroke Council recommends withholding antihypertensive agents unless the systolic blood pressure is greater than 220 mm Hg or the diastolic blood pressure is greater than 120 mm Hg in an acute ischemic stroke patient who is not treated with fibrinolytics.[6] If blood pressure lowering is indicated, it should be instituted cautiously to avoid hypotension. Any treatment given should be based on multiple blood pressure measurements taken at least 5 minutes apart. Objective: Describe the initial emergency care for acute ischemic stroke.

13. d. The patient's history of a cholecystectomy 2 weeks ago is a contraindication for fibrinolytic therapy. Objective: Describe the initial emergency care for acute ischemic stroke.

14. b. A TIA is a brief episode of neurologic dysfunction caused by focal brain or retinal ischemia, with clinical symptoms typically lasting less than one hour, and without evidence of acute infarction. This definition is tissue-based rather than time-based because some patients with traditionally defined transient ischemic attacks have, in fact, had a stroke. Some studies have shown positive MRI findings of stroke in up to two thirds of patients with a clinical TIA diagnosis. The longer the duration of symptoms, the more likely that the MRI result is positive. A TIA should be treated with the same urgency as a completed stroke. Objective: Describe the initial emergency care for acute ischemic stroke.

Short Answer

15. There are two major types of stroke: ischemic and hemorrhagic. An ischemic stroke occurs when a blood vessel supplying the brain is blocked. It can be life threatening, but rarely leads to death within the first hour. A hemorrhagic stroke occurs when a cerebral artery bursts. It can be fatal at onset. Objective: Describe the two major types of stroke.

16. The two main areas of injury in an ischemic stroke are as follows: (1) the zone of ischemia and (2) the ischemic penumbra (transitional zone). Objective: Describe the two major types of stroke.

17. The serum glucose level should be determined during the initial management of a possible stroke patient because hypoglycemia can mimic the signs and symptoms of a stroke. The glucose test is performed to rule out hypoglycemia before proceeding with stroke treatment. Objective: Describe the initial emergency care for acute ischemic stroke.

18. The Cincinnati Prehospital Stroke Scale (CPSS) is taught as the three Ds of "**D**rift (arm), **D**roop (facial weakness), and **D**ysarthria (slurred speech)" under the acronym "FAST" for **F**acial droop, **A**rm drift, and **S**peech (dysarthria and aphasia) with *T* for onset **T**ime. Objective: Describe the initial emergency care for acute ischemic stroke.

POSTTEST ANSWERS

Multiple Choice

1. c. After forming a general impression, you should approach the patient and assess her level of responsiveness. If the patient is unresponsive, quickly determine if the patient is not breathing (or only gasping) and then check for a pulse for up to 10 seconds. If there is no pulse, begin chest compressions. Objective: Describe the links in the Chain of Survival.

2. c. The compression-to-ventilation ratio for adults is 30:2. When possible, the switch of compressor and ventilator roles should occur in 5 seconds or less to minimize interruption of chest compressions. An adult should be given 10 to 12 ventilations/min (1 ventilation every 5 to 6 seconds) and compressions at a rate of at least 100/min. Chest compressions are the initial action performed when starting CPR in victims of cardiac arrest. Objective: Describe the links in the Chain of Survival.

3. a. Vagal maneuvers are methods used to stimulate baroreceptors located in the internal carotid arteries and the aortic arch. Stimulation of these receptors results in reflex stimulation of the vagus nerve and release of acetylcholine. Acetylcholine slows conduction through the AV node, resulting in slowing of the heart rate. Vagal maneuvers can be attempted as an initial action in a stable patient with a narrow-QRS tachycardia. Synchronized cardioversion is not indicated in the management of a stable patient. Diltiazem and verapamil are calcium channel blockers that are used in the treatment of stable, narrow-QRS tachycardias if the rhythm remains uncontrolled or unconverted by adenosine or vagal maneuvers or if tachycardia is recurrent. Objective: Given a patient situation, describe the ECG characteristics and initial emergency care for each of the following situations, including mechanical, pharmacological (i.e., indications, contraindications, doses, and route of administration of applicable medications), and electrical therapy, where applicable: too-fast rhythms, too-slow rhythms, and cardiac arrest rhythms.

4. b. When administering epinephrine in cardiac arrest, it is given as an IV bolus using the 1:10,000 solution. Give the drug as quickly as possible, follow it with a 20 mL flush of IV solution, and raise the affected extremity to help speed the delivery of the drug to the central circulation. Objective: Given a patient situation, describe the ECG characteristics and initial emergency care for each of the following situations, including mechanical, pharmacological (i.e., indications, contraindications, doses, and route of administration of applicable medications), and electrical therapy, where applicable: too-fast rhythms, too-slow rhythms, and cardiac arrest rhythms.

5. a. To prevent fires during defibrillation attempts, remove supplemental oxygen sources from the area of the patient's bed before defibrillation and cardioversion attempts and place them at least 3.5 to 4 feet away from the patient's chest. Be sure to use defibrillator paddles or pads of the appropriate size. Studies have shown that adult paddles or pads should be used for patients weighing more than 10 kg (22 lb) (older than 1 year). Use pediatric paddles or pads for infants and children weighing less than 10 kg (22 lb) or those whose chests are too small to accommodate standard paddles or pads. When applying combination pads to a patient's bare chest, press from one edge of the pad across the entire surface to remove all air. Do not use gels or pastes that are not specifically made for defibrillation (e.g., ultrasound gel). Use of improper pastes, creams, gels, or pads can cause burns or sparks and pose a risk of fire in an oxygen-enriched environment. Objective: Explain defibrillation, its indications, proper pad or paddle placement, relevant precautions, and the steps required to perform this procedure with a manual defibrillator and an AED.

6. b. The dose of adenosine should be decreased in patients on dipyridamole (Persantine), carbamazepine (Tegretol), those with transplanted hearts, or if given via a central IV line. Consider increasing the dose in patients on theophylline, caffeine, or theobromine. Objective: Given a patient situation, describe the ECG characteristics and initial emergency care for each of the following situations, including mechanical, pharmacologic (i.e., indications, contraindications, doses, and route of administration of applicable medications), and electrical therapy, where applicable: too-fast rhythms, too-slow rhythms, and cardiac arrest rhythms.

7. c. Absence of chest wall expansion and gurgling heard over the epigastrium indicate misplacement of the tracheal tube into the esophagus. If breath sounds were present bilaterally with bag-mask ventilation before placement of a tracheal tube, the presence of breath sounds on only one side of the chest after placement of the tube suggests right primary bronchus intubation. Objective: Describe methods used to confirm the correct placement of an advanced airway and describe the ventilation of a patient who has an advanced airway in place.

8. a. Your next course of action would include a dopamine infusion at 2 to 10 mcg/kg/min. Epinephrine is given by continuous IV infusion (not IV bolus) in the treatment of a symptomatic bradycardia. Isoproterenol (given as an IV infusion) is an alternative medication that can be considered in the management of a symptomatic bradycardia. Amiodarone and lidocaine are not indicated. Objective: Given a patient situation, describe the ECG characteristics and initial emergency care for each of the following situations, including mechanical, pharmacologic (i.e., indications, contraindications, doses, and route of administration of applicable medications), and electrical therapy, where applicable: too-fast rhythms, too-slow rhythms, and cardiac arrest rhythms.

9. c. Epinephrine and vasopressin are potent vasoconstrictors. Drugs given during cardiac arrest that constrict blood vessels (vasopressors) may improve coronary perfusion pressure. Objective: Given a patient situation, describe the ECG characteristics and initial emergency care for each of the following situations, including mechanical, pharmacologic (i.e., indications, contraindications, doses, and route of administration of applicable medications), and electrical therapy, where applicable: too-fast rhythms, too-slow rhythms, and cardiac arrest rhythms.

10. d. From the information provided, the patient appears to be clinically stable at this time. Procainamide would be appropriate to consider in this situation. Acceptable alternatives include amiodarone and sotalol. Dopamine increases the force of myocardial contraction, heart rate, and blood pressure. Since this patient is not hypotensive and he has a rapid heart rate, dopamine is not indicated. Nitroglycerin is a vasodilator. The patient has no complaint of chest pain so NTG is not indicated. Furosemide (Lasix) is also not indicated since there are no signs of pulmonary congestion. Atropine is not indicated because the patient has a tachycardia, not a symptomatic bradycardia. Objective: Given a patient situation, describe the ECG characteristics and initial emergency care for each of the following situations, including mechanical, pharmacologic (i.e., indications, contraindications, doses, and route of administration of applicable medications), and electrical therapy, where applicable: too-fast rhythms, too-slow rhythms, and cardiac arrest rhythms.

11. a. Most resuscitation efforts do not result in a return of spontaneous circulation. Surveys have revealed that most relatives of patients requiring CPR would like to be offered the possibility of being in the resuscitation room. A resuscitation team member should be assigned to the family to answer questions, clarify information, and provide comfort throughout the resuscitation effort. Pastoral care, social workers, and other support staff should be sought for assistance as needed. In a survey of family members of patients who had died, the most important features of delivering bad news were determined to be the attitude of the news-giver and the clarity of the message. The news-giver's attire and knowledge and ability to answer questions were less important. Objective: Discuss the phase response of code organization.

12. c. Parasympathetic nervous system hyperactivity is common with inferior wall myocardial infarctions, resulting in bradydysrhythmias. Ischemia of the AV node can result in first-degree or second-degree type 1 AV block. These dysrhythmias are relatively common with an inferior infarction, usually transient (resolving within 2 to 3 days), generally do not warrant treatment, and have a low mortality rate unless associated with hypotension and/or heart failure. Objective: Identify the most common complications of an acute MI.

13. a. Although IV or IO administration of drugs is preferred, vasopressin, epinephrine, and lidocaine can be given tracheally during cardiac arrest if vascular access is delayed or cannot be achieved. Objective: Given a patient situation, describe the ECG characteristics and initial emergency care

for each of the following situations, including mechanical, pharmacologic (i.e., indications, contraindications, doses, and route of administration of applicable medications), and electrical therapy, where applicable: too-fast rhythms, too-slow rhythms, and cardiac arrest rhythms.

14. c. When defibrillating (or cardioverting) a patient with a permanent pacemaker or ICD, be careful not to place the defibrillator paddles or combination pads directly over the device. Although placement of paddles or pads should not delay defibrillation, paddles or pads should ideally be placed at least 3 inches (8 cm) from the pulse generator (i.e., the bulge under the patient's skin). The anterior-posterior and anterolateral paddle or pad positions are considered acceptable in these patients. Because some of the defibrillation current flows down the pacemaker leads, a patient who has a permanent pacemaker or ICD should have the device checked to ensure proper function after defibrillation. Objective: Explain defibrillation, its indications, proper pad or paddle placement, relevant precautions, and the steps required to perform this procedure with a manual defibrillator and an AED.

15. c. The recommended dose of epinephrine, when administered via a tracheal tube, is 2 to 2.5 times the IV dose. Since the recommended IV dose is 1 mg, the tracheal dose would be 2 to 2.5 mg. Objective: Given a patient situation, describe the ECG characteristics and initial emergency care for each of the following situations, including mechanical, pharmacologic (i.e., indications, contraindications, doses, and route of administration of applicable medications), and electrical therapy, where applicable: too-fast rhythms, too-slow rhythms, and cardiac arrest rhythms.

16. a. ST-segment depression of more than 0.5 mm in leads V_2 and V_3 and more than 1 mm in all other leads is suggestive of myocardial ischemia when viewed in two or more anatomically contiguous leads. Objective: Identify the ECG changes associated with myocardial ischemia, injury, and infarction.

17. b. After an advanced airway is inserted in a cardiac arrest, the rate of ventilations should be decreased from 10 to 12 breaths/min to 8 to 10 breaths/min (1 ventilation every 6 to 8 seconds). Compressions should be performed at a rate of at least 100/min and should not be interrupted for ventilations unless ventilation is inadequate when compressions are not paused.

18. a. Currently, the window of opportunity to use IV rtPA to treat ischemic stroke patients is 3 hours. The window for intra-arterial fibrinolytics is about 6 hours. The time from onset of stroke symptoms until treatment is a key factor for success of any therapy. The earlier the treatment for stroke, the more favorable the results are likely to be. Blood flow needs to be restored to the affected area as quickly as possible. Objective: Describe the initial emergency care for acute ischemic stroke.

19. b. Synchronized cardioversion is a type of electrical therapy in which a shock is timed or programmed for delivery during ventricular depolarization (i.e., the QRS complex). It is indicated in the management of a patient who is exhibiting serious signs and symptoms related to a tachycardia. Because the machine must be able to detect a QRS complex in order to "sync," synchronized cardioversion is used to treat rhythms that have a clearly identifiable QRS complex and a rapid ventricular rate, such as some narrow-QRS tachycardias and VT. Objective: Explain synchronized cardioversion, describe its indications, and list the steps required to perform this procedure.

20. a. Appropriate care at this time includes immediate defibrillation. Transcutaneous pacing can be used in the management of symptomatic bradycardia. It is not used for cardiac arrest rhythms such as VF. Synchronized cardioversion is not used to treat disorganized rhythms (such as polymorphic VT) or those that do not have a clearly identifiable QRS complex (such as VF). Objective: Explain defibrillation, its indications, proper pad or paddle placement, relevant precautions, and the steps required to perform this procedure with a manual defibrillator and an AED.

21. a. Administration of magnesium sulfate IV can be used to aid in the termination of torsades de pointes (TdP) (an irregular polymorphic VT associated with a prolonged QT interval), including cardiac arrest associated with TdP. When magnesium is given in cardiac arrest associated with TdP it is administered as an IV/IO bolus at a dose of 1 to 2 g diluted in 10 mL dextrose 5% in water (D_5W). Magnesium sulfate is not indicated in the management of asystole, symptomatic bradycardia, or monomorphic VT. Objective: Given a patient situation, describe the ECG characteristics and initial emergency care for each of the following situations, including mechanical, pharmacologic (i.e., indications, contraindications, doses, and route of administration of applicable medications), and electrical therapy, where applicable: too-fast rhythms, too-slow rhythms, and cardiac arrest rhythms.

22. a. Gasping breathing is not effective breathing. After recognizing that the patient is unresponsive and is not breathing normally, activate the emergency response system and check for a pulse for

no more than 10 seconds. If you do not feel a pulse or unsure if you feel a pulse during that period, begin chest compressions. Objective: Describe the links in the Chain of Survival.

23. c. If an unstable patient with a narrow-QRS tachycardia requires electrical therapy and a biphasic defibrillator is available, perform synchronized cardioversion using 50 J to 100 J initially, increasing in stepwise fashion if the initial shock fails. For example, if the initial synchronized shock was delivered using 50 J and failed, reasonable energy levels to use for the second and subsequent shocks would be 100 J, then 200 J, 300 J, and 360 J (assuming the rhythm failed to convert with each shock). Objective: Given a patient situation, describe the ECG characteristics and initial emergency care for each of the following situations, including mechanical, pharmacologic (i.e., indications, contra-indications, doses, and route of administration of applicable medications), and electrical therapy, where applicable: too-fast rhythms, too-slow rhythms, and cardiac arrest rhythms.

24. d. The use of cricoid pressure in adult cardiac arrest is not recommended. Studies suggest that cricoid pressure is frequently applied incorrectly. In some studies participants applied too little pressure, placing patients at risk of regurgitation, and in others excessive pressure was used. Although some studies have not found cricoid pressure to cause a barrier to advanced airway insertion, most have shown that cricoid pressure impedes placement, impairs the rate of successful ventilation, and hinders ventilation. Aspiration can occur despite application of pressure. Compli-cations of cricoid pressure include laryngeal trauma when excessive force is applied and esophageal rupture from unrelieved high gastric pressures. Excessive pressure may obstruct the trachea in small children. Objective: Describe how to ventilate a patient with a bag-mask and two rescuers.

25. a. Patients experiencing an ACS who are most likely to present atypically include older adults, diabetic individuals, women, patients with prior cardiac surgery, and patients in the immediate postoperative period of noncardiac surgery. Objective: Explain atypical presentation and its sig-nificance in ACSs.

26. d. No drugs used in cardiac arrest have been shown to improve survival to hospital discharge. Amiodarone, an antiarrhythmic, has reportedly been demonstrated to improve the rate of return of spontaneous circulation and hospital admission in adults with refractory pulseless VT/VF. In cardiac arrest due to pulseless VT/VF, a vasopressor (e.g., epinephrine, vasopressin) should be given if the rhythm persists after delivery of one or two shocks and CPR. Amiodarone can be admin-istered if the rhythm persists after two to three shocks, CPR, and administration of a vasopressor. Lidocaine can be considered if amiodarone is not available. Amiodarone (and lidocaine) is not indicated in all cardiac arrests. For example, it may be used in cardiac arrest due to pulseless VT or VF but it is not indicated in cardiac arrest due to asystole or PEA. Objective: Given a patient situation, describe the ECG characteristics and initial emergency care for each of the following situations, including mechanical, pharmacologic (i.e., indications, contraindications, doses, and route of administration of applicable medications), and electrical therapy, where applicable: too-fast rhythms, too-slow rhythms, and cardiac arrest rhythms.

27. b. A suspected tension pneumothorax should be treated with needle decompression (not pericar-diocentesis). Acute myocardial ischemia or infarction should be considered as a possible cause of refractory pulseless VT/VF cardiac arrest. Fibrinolytic therapy may be considered if pulmonary embolism is presumed or known to be the cause of the arrest. Cardiac arrest associated with severe blood volume loss may benefit from administration of crystalloid IV/IO infusion. Objective: Given a patient situation, describe the ECG characteristics and initial emergency care for each of the following situations, including mechanical, pharmacologic (i.e., indications, contraindications, doses, and route of administration of applicable medications), and electrical therapy, where appli-cable: too-fast rhythms, too-slow rhythms, and cardiac arrest rhythms.

28. a. Although atropine is considered a first-line agent for symptomatic bradycardia, atropine usually is ineffective for wide-QRS bradycardias. A reasonable course of action will be to administer atropine while preparing for immediate TCP or while preparing a dopamine or epinephrine infu-sion. Although epinephrine can be used in the management of a symptomatic bradycardia, it is given as a continuous IV infusion, *not* as an IV bolus. Objective: Given a patient situation, describe the ECG characteristics and initial emergency care for each of the following situations, including mechanical, pharmacologic (i.e., indications, contraindications, doses, and route of administration of applicable medications), and electrical therapy, where applicable: too-fast rhythms, too-slow rhythms, and cardiac arrest rhythms.

29. b. Adenosine is the first drug used for most forms of narrow-QRS tachycardia. Adenosine slows conduction time through AV node and can interrupt reentry pathways through the AV node.

Objective: Given a patient situation, describe the ECG characteristics and initial emergency care for each of the following situations, including mechanical, pharmacologic (i.e., indications, contraindications, doses, and route of administration of applicable medications), and electrical therapy, where applicable: too-fast rhythms, too-slow rhythms, and cardiac arrest rhythms.

30. b. The three major physical findings evaluated with the Cincinnati Prehospital Stroke Scale are facial droop, arm drift, and speech abnormalities. If any one of these signs is abnormal, the stroke probability is about 72%. Objective: Describe the initial emergency care for acute ischemic stroke.

31. c. Intravenous fluid boluses can be considered if the patient is hypotensive after the return of spontaneous circulation. If therapeutic hypothermia is planned, cold fluids may be given. Vasopressor IV infusions such as epinephrine, dopamine, or norepinephrine may be started if necessary and titrated to achieve a minimum systolic blood pressure of less than 90 mm Hg. Isoproterenol is an alternative agent that is primarily used to increase heart rate in a patient with a symptomatic bradycardia. Because it is not a vasopressor, it is not used to treat hypotension. Procainamide is an antiarrhythmic used to treat many atrial and ventricular dysrhythmias. Procainamide is not a vasopressor and because an adverse effect of procainamide administration is hypotension, it would not be used to treat hypotension. Objective: Identify the most common complications of an acute MI.

32. b. The rhythm shown is a sinus rhythm at 65 beats/min with occasional premature complexes. ST elevation is present in leads V_2 through V_5. An anterior STEMI is suspected. ST depression is present in leads III and aVF. T waves are inverted in lead III. Objective: Identify the ECG changes associated with myocardial ischemia, injury, and infarction.

33. a. Immediate management of a patient who is experiencing a possible ACS includes monitoring ABCs, giving supplemental oxygen if the patient is hypoxemic (i.e., oxygen saturation level of less than 94%), having difficulty breathing, or has signs of heart failure; starting an IV, and giving aspirin as soon as possible if there are no contraindications. The cardiac monitor shows a sinus rhythm at 75 beats/min. Since atropine is used to increase heart rate, it is not indicated in this situation. Adenosine is used for symptomatic narrow-QRS tachycardias such as AVNRT. Amiodarone may be used to treat many atrial and ventricular dysrhythmias, but it is not used for sinus rhythm or sinus dysrhythmias. Objective: Describe the initial management of a patient experiencing an ACS.

34. d. The patient's initial 12-lead ECG should be reviewed and the patient classified into one of three categories: ST-segment elevation, ST-segment depression, normal/nondiagnostic ECG. Objective: Discuss the three groups used when categorizing the 12-lead ECG findings of the patient experiencing an ACS.

35. d. The patient's 12-lead ECG shows ST-segment elevation in leads I, aVL, V_2, V_3, V_4, and V_5. Q waves are present in leads aVL and V_2 through V_4. Objective: Identify the ECG leads that view the anterior wall, inferior wall, lateral wall, septum, inferobasal wall, and right ventricle.

36. b. Two leads are contiguous if they look at the same or adjacent areas of the heart or they are numerically consecutive chest leads. V_2, V_3, and V_4 are numerically consecutive chest leads. Objective: Identify the ECG changes associated with myocardial ischemia, injury, and infarction.

37. b. ECG evidence of myocardial injury in progress can be seen on the ECG as ST-segment elevation in the leads facing the affected area. For men 40 years of age and older, the threshold value for abnormal J-point elevation is 2 mm in leads V_2 and V_3 and 1 mm in all other leads. For men younger than 40 years of age, the threshold value for abnormal J-point elevation in leads V_2 and V_3 is 2.5 mm. For women, the threshold value for abnormal J-point elevation is 1.5 mm in leads V_2 and V_3 and greater than 1 mm in all other leads. Objective: Identify the ECG changes associated with myocardial ischemia, injury, and infarction.

38. b. The patient's 12-lead ECG shows ST-segment elevation in lead I, aVL, and V_2 through V_5. Because these leads view the lateral and anterior surfaces of the left ventricle, an anterolateral infarction is suspected. Objective: Identify the ECG changes associated with myocardial ischemia, injury, and infarction.

39. a. Aspirin should be administered as soon as possible after symptom onset to patients with suspected ACSs, if there are no contraindications. Nitroglycerin relaxes vascular smooth muscle and decreases myocardial oxygen consumption. Morphine decreases anxiety, pain, and myocardial oxygen requirements and is the preferred analgesic for patients with STEMI who have persistent chest discomfort unrelieved by nitrates. An oral beta-blocker should be started within the first 24 hours after hospitalization in the absence of contraindications to beta blockade. IV administration may be warranted at the time of presentation to patients who have severe hypertension or

tachydysrhythmias in the setting of ACS and who do not have contraindications to beta blockade. Clopidogrel (Plavix) is an antiplatelet agent that is typically administered in the emergency department and is useful for patients younger than 75 years with NSTEMI and those with STEMI. Calcium channel blockers have not been shown to reduce mortality after acute MI and may be harmful in some patients with cardiovascular disease. Prophylactic administration of lidocaine to prevent VT or VF is not recommended. Routine administration of magnesium to patients with acute MI is not recommended. Objective: Describe the initial management of a patient experiencing an ACS.

40. a. Patients with ischemic discomfort should receive up to three doses of sublingual nitroglycerin tablets or spray at 3- to 5-minute intervals until chest discomfort is relieved or hypotension limits its use. Nitrates are contraindicated in patients with hypotension (systolic blood pressure below 90 mm Hg or 30 mm Hg or more below baseline), extreme bradycardia (slower than 50 beats/min), or tachycardia in the absence of heart failure (faster than 100 beats/min), and in patients with RVI. Nitrates should be used with caution in patients with known inferior infarction. Research has not demonstrated conclusive evidence supporting the routine use of IV, oral, or topical nitrates in patients with acute MI. Objective: Describe the initial management of a patient experiencing an ACS.

41. c. Your best course of action will be to place the patient supine and give a 250 mL IV fluid bolus of normal saline. Reassess his blood pressure, other vital signs, and breath sounds after administration. Objective: Given a patient situation, describe the ECG characteristics and initial emergency care for each of the following situations, including mechanical, pharmacologic (i.e., indications, contraindications, doses, and route of administration of applicable medications), and electrical therapy, where applicable: too-fast rhythms, too-slow rhythms, and cardiac arrest rhythms.

42. d. The rhythm shown is second-degree AV block (2:1 AV block) at 55 beats/min, with ST-segment elevation. Objective: Given a patient situation, describe the ECG characteristics and initial emergency care for each of the following situations, including mechanical, pharmacologic (i.e., indications, contraindications, doses, and route of administration of applicable medications), and electrical therapy, where applicable: too-fast rhythms, too-slow rhythms, and cardiac arrest rhythms.

43. d. Leads II, III, and aVF view the inferior wall of the left ventricle. Because an inferior MI is suspected, right chest leads should be quickly used to rule out RVI before giving medications for pain relief. Morphine and nitroglycerin are vasodilators, and thus they reduce preload. This reduction in preload, while usually beneficial, can be undesirable in the setting of RVI and may cause profound hypotension. Therefore caution must be exercised when giving nitroglycerin and morphine to patients experiencing RVI. Objective: Describe the initial management of a patient experiencing an ACS.

44. b. Administer supplemental oxygen as needed to maintain the patient's oxygen saturation level at 94% or higher. Because it is generally better tolerated than a mask, a nasal cannula is reasonable to use. If the patient's oxygen saturation level does not adequately improve with the use of the cannula, it may be necessary to switch to oxygen delivery by mask. Because the patient's breathing is adequate, advanced airway placement and positive pressure ventilation is not necessary at this time. However, if the patient becomes unresponsive or his breathing becomes inadequate, administer oxygen by positive pressure ventilation. Objective: Describe the advantages, disadvantages, oxygen liter flow per minute, and estimated oxygen percentage delivered for each of the following devices: Nasal cannula, simple face mask, partial nonrebreather mask, and nonrebreather mask.

45. b. *Monomorphic* is a term used to describe QRS complexes that are of the same shape and amplitude. When the QRS complexes vary in shape and amplitude from beat to beat, the term *polymorphic* is used. The rhythm shown is a regular, monomorphic, wide-QRS tachycardia. A 12-lead ECG should be obtained to help determine the origin of the rhythm. It is wise to seek expert consultation when treating a patient with a wide-QRS tachycardia. Objective: Given a patient situation, describe the ECG characteristics and initial emergency care for each of the following situations, including mechanical, pharmacologic (i.e., indications, contraindications, doses, and route of administration of applicable medications), and electrical therapy, where applicable: too-fast rhythms, too-slow rhythms, and cardiac arrest rhythms.

46. c. Based on the information provided, the patient is stable at this time. Administration of IV adenosine can be used as a therapeutic and diagnostic maneuver. Verapamil is a calcium channel blocker and should only be given to patients with narrow-QRS tachycardias (regular or irregular). It should not be given to patients with a wide-complex tachycardia. Because electrical therapy is

used for *unstable* patients, neither synchronized cardioversion nor defibrillation is indicated for this patient. *If* he were unstable, synchronized cardioversion would be used because the patient has a pulse and there are recognizable QRS complexes on the monitor. Defibrillation would be performed if the rhythm observed was polymorphic VT, pulseless monomorphic VT, or VF. Objective: Given a patient situation, describe the ECG characteristics and initial emergency care for each of the following situations, including mechanical, pharmacologic (i.e., indications, contraindications, doses, and route of administration of applicable medications), and electrical therapy, where applicable: too-fast rhythms, too-slow rhythms, and cardiac arrest rhythms.

47. a. The cardiac monitor shows atrial fibrillation with a rapid ventricular response of 125-200 beats/min. Because the management of irregular tachycardia is often complex, your best course of action will be to obtain a 12-lead ECG and seek expert consultation. Lidocaine, epinephrine, and dopamine are not indicated. Objective: Given a patient situation, describe the ECG characteristics and initial emergency care for each of the following situations, including mechanical, pharmacologic (i.e., indications, contraindications, doses, and route of administration of applicable medications), and electrical therapy, where applicable: too-fast rhythms, too-slow rhythms, and cardiac arrest rhythms.

48. c. Remember that during a cardiac arrest, your two most important priorities are CPR and, if a shockable rhythm is present, defibrillation. Giving drugs and inserting an advanced airway are of secondary importance. Although the monitor initially showed asystole (a nonshockable rhythm), ventricular fibrillation is now visible on the monitor and should be defibrillated using the defibrillator manufacturer's recommended energy settings. An initial shock of 360 J for VF is recommended when using a *monophasic* defibrillator. Defibrillation is performed using *one* shock, and then CPR is immediately resumed, beginning with chest compressions. Stacked (also called sequential) shocks were recommended before 2005 but are no longer recommended. Transcutaneous pacing is not indicated for VF or any other cardiac arrest rhythm. Objective: Given a patient situation, describe the ECG characteristics and initial emergency care for each of the following situations, including mechanical, pharmacologic (i.e., indications, contraindications, doses, and route of administration of applicable medications), and electrical therapy, where applicable: too-fast rhythms, too-slow rhythms, and cardiac arrest rhythms.

49. c. Despite the presence of an organized rhythm on the monitor, the patient has no pulse. This situation is PEA. Objective: Given a patient situation, describe the ECG characteristics and initial emergency care for each of the following situations, including mechanical, pharmacologic (i.e., indications, contraindications, doses, and route of administration of applicable medications), and electrical therapy, where applicable: too-fast rhythms, too-slow rhythms, and cardiac arrest rhythms.

50. c. Give 1 mg of 1:10,000 epinephrine IV. Defibrillation attempts to deliver a uniform electrical current of sufficient intensity to depolarize myocardial cells (including fibrillating cells) at the same time, briefly "stunning" the heart. This provides an opportunity for the heart's natural pacemakers to resume normal activity. In this situation, organized electrical activity is already present on the cardiac monitor; therefore, defibrillation is contraindicated. Atropine, although once used for asystole and bradycardic pulseless electrical activity, is no longer recommended. Transcutaneous pacing is not indicated in cardiac arrest. Objective: Given a patient situation, describe the ECG characteristics and initial emergency care for each of the following situations, including mechanical, pharmacologic (i.e., indications, contraindications, doses, and route of administration of applicable medications), and electrical therapy, where applicable: too-fast rhythms, too-slow rhythms, and cardiac arrest rhythms.

REFERENCES

1. Berg RA, Hemphill R, Abella BS, et al: Part 5: adult basic life support: 2010 American Heart Association guidelines for cardiopulmonary resuscitation and emergency cardiovascular care, *Circulation* 122(Suppl 3):S685–S705, 2010.

2. O'Connor RE, Brady W, Brooks SC, et al: Part 10: acute coronary syndromes: 2010 American Heart Association guidelines for cardiopulmonary resuscitation and emergency cardiovascular care, *Circulation* 122(Suppl 3):S787–S817, 2010.

3. Neumar RW, Otto CW, Link MS, et al: Part 8: adult advanced cardiovascular life support: 2010 American Heart Association guidelines for cardiopulmonary resuscitation and emergency cardiovascular care, *Circulation* 122(Suppl 3):S729–S767, 2010.

4. Adams HP Jr, Adams RJ, Brott T, et al: Stroke Council of the American Stroke Association. Guidelines for the early management of patients with ischemic stroke: a scientific statement from the Stroke Council of the American Stroke Association, *Stroke* 34(4):1056–1083, 2003 Apr.

5. Jauch EC, Cucchiara B, Adeoye O, et al: Part 11: adult stroke: 2010 American Heart Association guidelines for cardiopulmonary resuscitation and emergency cardiovascular care, *Circulation* 122(Suppl 3):S818–S828, 2010.

6. Adams HP Jr, del Zoppo G, Alberts MJ, et al: Guidelines for the early management of adults with ischemic stroke: a guideline from the American Heart Association/American Stroke Association Stroke Council, Clinical Cardiology Council, Cardiovascular Radiology and Intervention Council, and the Atherosclerotic Peripheral Vascular Disease and Quality of Care Outcomes in Research Interdisciplinary Working Groups [published corrections appear in Stroke. 2007;38:e38 and Stroke. 2007;38:e96], *Stroke* 38:1655–1711, 2007.

GLOSSARY

Absolute bradycardia A heart rate of less than 60 beats/min.

Absolute refractory period Corresponds with the onset of the QRS complex to approximately the peak of the T wave on the electrocardiogram; cardiac cells cannot be stimulated to conduct an electrical impulse, no matter how strong the stimulus.

Accelerated idioventricular rhythm (AIVR) Dysrhythmia originating in the ventricles with a rate between 41 and 100 beats/min.

Accessory pathway An extra bundle of working myocardial tissue that forms a connection between the atria and ventricles outside the normal conduction system.

Action potential A five-phase cycle that reflects the difference in the concentration of charged particles across the cell membrane at any given time.

Acute coronary syndrome (ACS) A term used to refer to distinct conditions caused by a similar sequence of pathologic events and that involve a temporary or permanent blockage of a coronary artery; ACSs consist of three major syndromes: unstable angina (UA), non–ST-segment elevation myocardial infarction (NSTEMI), and ST-segment elevation myocardial infarction (STEMI).

Angina pectoris Chest discomfort or other related symptoms of sudden onset that may occur because the increased oxygen demand of the heart temporarily exceeds the blood supply (myocardial ischemia).

Anginal equivalent Symptom of myocardial ischemia other than chest pain or discomfort.

Arteriosclerosis A chronic disease of the arterial system characterized by abnormal thickening and hardening of the vessel walls.

Atherosclerosis A form of arteriosclerosis in which the thickening and hardening of the vessel walls are caused by a buildup of fat-like deposits in the inner lining, specifically of large and middle-sized muscular arteries.

Atypical presentation Uncharacteristic signs and symptoms perceived by some patients.

Automated external defibrillation The placement of paddles or pads on a patient's chest and interpretation of the patient's cardiac rhythm by the defibrillator's computerized analysis system. Depending on the type of automated external defibrillator (AED) used, the machine will deliver a shock (if a shockable rhythm is detected) or instruct the operator to deliver a shock.

Automated external defibrillator (AED) A machine with a sophisticated computer system that analyzes a patient's heart rhythm using an algorithm to distinguish shockable rhythms from nonshockable rhythms and providing visual and auditory instructions to the rescuer to deliver an electrical shock, if a shock is indicated.

Automaticity The ability of cardiac pacemaker cells to create an electrical impulse without being stimulated from another source.

AV junction AV node and the bundle of His.

AV node Specialized cells located in the lower portion of the right atrium; delays the electrical impulse in order to allow the atria to contract and complete filling of the ventricles.

Bundle of His Fibers located in the upper portion of the interventricular septum that conduct an electrical impulse through the heart.

Capacitor A device for storing an electrical charge.

Capnography The continuous analysis and recording of carbon dioxide concentrations in respiratory gases.

Cardiopulmonary (cardiac) arrest The absence of cardiac mechanical activity, which is confirmed by the absence of a detectable pulse, unresponsiveness, and apnea or agonal, gasping breathing.

Cardiovascular collapse A sudden loss of effective blood flow caused by cardiac and/or peripheral vascular factors that may reverse spontaneously (e.g., syncope) or only with interventions (e.g., cardiac arrest).

Cardiovascular disease (CVD) A collection of conditions that involve the circulatory system, which contains the heart (cardio) and blood vessels (vascular), including congenital cardiovascular diseases.

Carina The point where the trachea divides into the right and left primary bronchi.

Chain of Survival The ideal series of events that should take place immediately after the recognition of the onset of sudden illness.

Conduction system A system of pathways in the heart composed of specialized electrical (pacemaker) cells.

Conductivity The ability of a cardiac cell to receive an electrical impulse and conduct it to an adjoining cardiac cell.

Contractility The ability of myocardial cells to shorten in response to an impulse, resulting in contraction.

Coronary artery disease (CAD) Disease affecting the arteries that supply the heart muscle with blood.

Coronary heart disease (CHD) Disease of the coronary arteries and their resulting complications, such as angina pectoris or acute myocardial infarction.

Cricothyroid membrane A fibrous membrane located between the cricoid and thyroid cartilages.

Defibrillation Delivery of an electrical current across the heart muscle over a very brief period to terminate an abnormal heart rhythm; also called unsynchronized countershock or asynchronous countershock because the delivery of current has no relationship to the cardiac cycle.

Defibrillator A device used to administer an electrical shock at a preset energy level to terminate a cardiac dysrhythmia.

Delta wave Slurring of the beginning portion of the QRS complex, caused by pre-excitation.

Depolarization Movement of ions across a cell membrane, causing the inside of the cell to become more positive; an electrical event expected to result in contraction.

Electrocardiogram (ECG) A recording of the heart's electrical activity that appears on ECG paper as specific waveforms and complexes.

Electrode Adhesive pad that contains a conductive gel and is applied at a specific location on the patient's chest wall and extremities and is connected by cables to an ECG machine.

Electrolyte An element or compound that breaks into charged particles (ions) when melted or dissolved in water or another solvent.

End-tidal (exhaled) carbon dioxide detector A capnometer that provides a noninvasive estimate of alveolar ventilation, the concentration of exhaled carbon dioxide from the lungs, and arterial carbon dioxide content.

Epiglottis A small, leaf-shaped cartilage located at the top of the larynx that prevents foreign material from entering the trachea during swallowing.

Excitability The ability of cardiac muscle cells to respond to an outside stimulus.

Failure to capture The inability of a pacemaker stimulus to depolarize the myocardium.

Failure to pace A pacemaker malfunction that occurs when the pacemaker fails to deliver an electrical stimulus or when it fails to deliver the correct number of electrical stimulations per minute; also referred to as failure to fire.

Fascicle Small bundle of nerve fibers.

Fibrinolysis The breakdown of fibrin, the main component of blood clots.

Glottis The true vocal cords and the space between them.

Hard palate Bony portion of the roof of the mouth that forms the floor of the nasal cavity.

Heart disease A broad term that refers to conditions affecting the heart.

Impedance Resistance to the flow of current. Transthoracic impedance (resistance) refers to the resistance of the chest wall to current.

Interval On the ECG, a waveform and a segment.

Ion Electrically charged particle.

Ischemia A decreased supply of oxygenated blood to a body part or organ.

Joule The basic unit of energy; equivalent to watt-seconds.

Lead Electrical connection attached to the body to record electrical activity.

Lown-Ganong-Levine (LGL)syndrome Type of preexcitation syndrome in which part or all of the AV conduction system is bypassed by an abnormal AV connection from the atrial muscle to the bundle of His; characterized by a short PR interval (usually less than 0.12 second) and a normal QRS duration.

Manual defibrillation The placement of paddles or pads on a patient's chest, interpretation of the patient's cardiac rhythm by a trained healthcare professional, and the healthcare professional's decision to deliver a shock (if indicated).

Membrane potential Difference in electrical charge across the cell membrane.

Minute volume The amount of air moved in and out of the lungs in 1 minute; it is determined by multiplying the tidal volume by the ventilatory rate (breaths/min).

Myocardial cells Working cells of the myocardium that contain contractile filaments and form the muscular layer of the atrial walls and the thicker muscular layer of the ventricular walls.

Nasal cannula A piece of plastic tubing with two soft prongs that project from the tubing; used to delivery supplemental oxygen to a spontaneously breathing patient.

Ohm The basic unit of measurement of resistance.

Oxygenation The process of getting oxygen into the body and to its tissues for metabolism.

Pacemaker cells Specialized cells of the heart's electrical conduction system, capable of spontaneously generating and conducting electrical impulses.

Paroxysmal supraventricular tachycardia (PSVT) A regular, narrow-QRS tachycardia that starts or ends suddenly.

Periarrest period One hour before and 1 hour after a cardiac arrest.

Permeability Ability of a cell membrane channel to allow passage of electrolytes once it is open.

Polarized state Period after repolarization of a myocardial cell (also called the resting state) when the outside of the cell is positive and the interior of the cell is negative.

Prearrest period The interval preceding a cardiac arrest.

Pre-excitation Term used to describe rhythms that originate from above the ventricles but in which the impulse travels by a pathway other than the AV node and bundle of His; thus the supraventricular impulse excites the ventricles earlier than normal.

Public access defibrillation Defibrillation performed by citizens (such as flight attendants, casino security officers, athletic or golf club employees, and ushers at sporting events) at the scene using an automated external defibrillator.

Pulse oximetry A noninvasive method of measuring oxygen saturation of functional hemoglobin.

Pulseless electrical activity (PEA) Organized electrical activity observed on a cardiac monitor (other than ventricular tachycardia) without the patient having a palpable pulse.

Purkinje fibers Fibers found in both ventricles that conduct an electrical impulse through the heart.

Refractoriness A term used to describe the period of recovery that cells need after being discharged before they are able to respond to a stimulus.

Relative bradycardia A term that refers to a situation in which a patient's heart rate may be more than 60 beats/min but, physiologically, the patient needs a tachycardia (as in hypovolemia) and is unable to increase his or her heart rate due to sinoatrial node disease, beta-blockers, or other medications.

Relative refractory period Corresponds with the downslope of the T wave on the ECG; cardiac cells can be stimulated to depolarize if the stimulus is strong enough.

Repolarization Movement of ions across a cell membrane in which the inside of the cell is restored to its negative charge.

Respiration The exchange of oxygen and carbon dioxide during cellular metabolism.

Risk factors Traits and lifestyle habits that may increase a person's chance of developing a disease.

Simple face mask An oxygen delivery device that consists of a plastic reservoir that fits over a patient's nose and mouth and a small diameter tube connected to the base of the mask through which oxygen is delivered; also called a standard mask.

Soft palate The back part of the roof of the mouth that is made up of mucous membrane, muscular fibers, and mucous glands.

Stroke A sudden change in neurologic function caused by a change in cerebral blood flow.

Stylet A relatively stiff but flexible metal rod covered by plastic and inserted into a tracheal tube that is used for maintaining the shape of the relatively pliant tracheal tube and "steering" it into position.

Sudden cardiac death (SCD) A natural death of cardiac cause that is preceded by an abrupt loss of consciousness within 1 hour of the onset of an acute change in cardiac status.

Supranormal period Period during the cardiac cycle when a weaker than normal stimulus can cause cardiac cells to depolarize; extends from the end of phase 3 to the beginning of phase 4 of the cardiac action potential.

Supraventricular Originating from a site above the bifurcation of the bundle of His, such as the sinoatrial node, atria, or AV junction.

Supraventricular arrhythmias (SVA) Rhythms that begin in the SA node, atrial tissue, or the AV junction.

Synchronized cardioversion The timed delivery of a shock during the QRS complex.

Tidal volume The volume of air moved into or out of the lungs during a normal breath.

Tracheal intubation An advanced airway procedure in which a tube is placed directly into the trachea for a variety of reasons including the delivery of anesthesia, assisting a patient's breathing with positive pressure ventilation, and protection of the patient's airway from aspiration.

Transient ischemic attack (TIA) A brief episode of neurologic dysfunction caused by focal brain or retinal ischemia, with clinical symptoms typically lasting less than 1 hour, and without evidence of acute infarction.

Transthoracic impedance (resistance) The resistance of the chest wall to current.

Uvula Fleshy tissue that hangs down from the soft palate and into the posterior portion of the oral cavity.

Vallecula The space or "pocket" between the base of the tongue and the epiglottis.

Ventilation The mechanical movement of gas or air into and out of the lungs.

Voltage Difference in electrical charge between two points; the electrical pressure that drives current through a defibrillator circuit (such as the chest).

Wolff-Parkinson-White syndrome Type of pre-excitation syndrome, characterized by a slurred upstroke of the QRS complex (delta wave) and wide QRS.

ILLUSTRATION CREDITS

Chapter 1

1-1 From Libby: Braunwald's Heart Disease: A Textbook of Cardiovascular Medicine, ed 8, 2007, Saunders.

1-2 From Chapleau W, Pons P: Emergency Medical Technician: Making the Difference, 2006, St. Louis: Mosby.

1-3 From Berg RA, Hemphill R, Abella BS, et al. Part 5: Adult Basic Life Support: 2010 American Heart Association Guidelines for Cardiopulmonary Resuscitation and Emergency Cardiovascular Care. *Circulation.* 2010;122(Suppl 3):S685-S705.

1-4 From Henry M, Stapleton E: EMT Prehospital Care, ed 4, 2008, St. Louis: Mosby.

1-5 From Chapleau W: Emergency First Responder: Making the Difference, 2004, St. Louis: Mosby.

1-6 From Henry M, Stapleton E: EMT Prehospital Care, ed 4, 2008, St. Louis: Mosby.

Chapter 2

2-1 From Hicks GH: Cardiopulmonary Anatomy and Physiology, Philadelphia, 2000, WB Saunders.

2-2 From Thibodeau G, Patton K: Anatomy and Physiology, ed 7, St. Louis, 2010, Mosby.

2-3 Modified from Aehlert B: Paramedic Practice Today, St. Louis, 2010, Mosby.

2-4 From Thibodeau G, Patton K: Anatomy and Physiology, ed 7, St. Louis, 2010, Mosby.

2-5 From Wilkins RL, Stoller JK, Kacmarek RM: Egan's Fundamentals of Respiratory Care, ed 9, St. Louis, 2009, Mosby.

2-6 From Herlihy B, Maebius N: The Human Body in Health and Illness, ed 4, Philadelphia, 2011, Saunders.

2-7 From Thibodeau GA, Patton KT: Structure and Function of the Body, ed 13, St. Louis, 2007, Mosby.

2-8 From Aehlert B: Paramedic Practice Today, St. Louis, 2010, Mosby.

2-9 Modified from Gardner RM: J Cardiovasc Nurs; 1:79, 1987, as found in Wilkins RL, Stoller JK, Kacmarek RM: Egan's Fundamentals of Respiratory Care, ed 9, St. Louis, 2009, Mosby.

2-10 Image used by permission from Nellcor Puritan Bennett LLC, Boulder, Colo., doing business as Covidien.

2-11, 2-12 From Aehlert B: Paramedic Practice Today, St. Louis, 2010, Mosby.

2-13 From Sole, ML, Klein DG, Moseley MJ: Introduction to Critical Care Nursing, ed 5, Philadelphia, 2008, Saunders.

2-14, 2-15 Modified from Shade BR, Collins TE, Wertz EM, et al: Mosby's EMT Intermediate Textbook for the 1999 National Standard Curriculum, ed 3, St. Louis, 2007, Mosby.

2-16 From Aehlert B: Paramedic Practice Today, St. Louis, 2010, Mosby.

2-17 From Shade BR, Collins TE, Wertz EM, et al: Mosby's EMT Intermediate Textbook for the 1999 National Standard Curriculum, ed 3, St. Louis, 2007, Mosby.

2-18, 2-19 From Aehlert B: Paramedic Practice Today, St. Louis, 2010, Mosby.

2-20 From Shade BR, Collins TE, Wertz EM, et al: Mosby's EMT Intermediate Textbook for the 1999 National Standard Curriculum, ed 3, St. Louis, 2007, Mosby.

2-21 From Stoy W, Platt T, Lejeune D: Mosby's EMT-Basic Textbook, ed 2, St. Louis, 2005, Mosby.

2-22 From Shade BR, Collins TE, Wertz EM, et al: Mosby's EMT Intermediate Textbook for the 1999 National Standard Curriculum, ed 3, St. Louis, 2007, Mosby.

2-23, 2-24, 2-25 From McSwain N, Paturas J: The Basic EMT, ed 2, St. Louis, 2003, Mosby.

2-26 From Stoy W, Platt T, Lejeune D: Mosby's EMT-Basic Textbook, ed 2, St. Louis, 2005, Mosby.

2-27, 2-28, 2-29, 2-30 From Shade BR, Collins TE, Wertz EM, et al: Mosby's EMT Intermediate Textbook for the 1999 National Standard Curriculum, ed 3, St. Louis, 2007, Mosby.

2-31 From Auerbach PS: Wilderness Medicine, ed 5, St. Louis, 2007, Mosby.

2-32 From Henry M, Stapleton E: EMT Prehospital Care, ed 4, St. Louis, 2009, Mosby.

2-33 From Shade BR, Collins TE, Wertz EM, et al: Mosby's EMT Intermediate Textbook for the 1999 National Standard Curriculum, ed 3, St. Louis, 2007, Mosby.

2-34 From Aehlert B: Paramedic Practice Today, St. Louis, 2010, Mosby.

2-35 Courtesy King Systems, Noblesville, Ind.

2-36, 2-37, 2-38 From Aehlert B: Paramedic Practice Today, St. Louis, 2010, Mosby.

2-39, 2-40, 2-41, 2-42 From Shade BR, Collins TE, Wertz EM, et al: Mosby's EMT Intermediate Textbook for the 1999 National Standard Curriculum, ed 3, St. Louis, 2007, Mosby.

2-43, 2-44, 2-45 From Aehlert B: Paramedic Practice Today, St. Louis, 2010, Mosby.

Skill 2-1

Steps 1-6 From Aehlert B: Paramedic Practice Today, St. Louis, 2010, Mosby.

Skill 2-2

Steps 1-5 From Aehlert B: Paramedic Practice Today, St. Louis, 2010, Mosby.

Skill 2-3

Steps 1-4 From Aehlert B: Paramedic Practice Today, St. Louis, 2010, Mosby.

Step 5 From Chapleau W, Pons P: Emergency Medical Responder: Making the Difference, St. Louis, 2007, Mosby.

Skill 2-4

Steps 1-4 From Chapleau W, Pons P: Emergency Medical Responder: Making the Difference, St. Louis, 2007, Mosby.

Skill 2-5

Steps 1-2 From Aehlert B: Paramedic Practice Today, St. Louis, 2010, Mosby.

Skill 2-6

Step 1 From Chapleau W, Pons P: Emergency Medical Responder: Making the Difference, St. Louis, 2007, Mosby.

Steps 2-3 from Aehlert B: Paramedic Practice Today, St. Louis, 2010, Mosby.

Skill 2-7

Steps 1-7 from Aehlert B: Paramedic Practice Today, St. Louis, 2010, Mosby.

Chapter 3

3-2 From Patton K, Thibodeau G: Anatomy & Physiology, ed 7, St. Louis, 2009, Mosby.

3-3, 3-4, 3-5 From Herlihy B: The Human Body in Health and Illness, St. Louis, 2010, Saunders.

3-6 From Huszar RJ: Basic Dysrhythmias: Interpretation and Management, ed 3, St. Louis, 2001, Mosby.

3-7 From Crawford MV, Spence MI: Commonsense Approach to Coronary Care, ed 6 revised, St. Louis, 1994, Mosby.

3-8 From Herlihy B: The Human Body in Health and Illness, St. Louis, 2010, Saunders.

3-9 From Aehlert B: ECGs Made Easy, ed 4, St. Louis, 2009, Mosby.

3-10 From Aehlert B: Paramedic Practice Today, St. Louis, 2010, Mosby.

3-11 From Goldberger A: Clinical Electrocardiography: A Simplified Approach, ed 6, St. Louis, 1999, Mosby.

3-12 From Aehlert B: ECGs Made Easy, ed 4, St. Louis, 2009, Mosby.

3-13 From Urden L, Stacy K, Lough M: Thelan's Critical Care Nursing: Diagnosis and Management, ed 5, St. Louis, 2006, Mosby.

3-14 From Goldberger A: Clinical Electrocardiography: A Simplified Approach, ed 6, St. Louis, 1999, Mosby.

3-15 From Urden L, Stacy K, Lough M: Thelan's Critical Care Nursing: Diagnosis and Management, ed 5, St. Louis, 2006, Mosby.

3-16 From Lounsbury P, Frye S: Cardiac Rhythm Disorders, A Nursing Approach, ed 2, St. Louis, 1992, Mosby.

3-17 From Phalen T, Aehlert A: The 12-Lead ECG in Acute Coronary Syndromes, ed 3, St. Louis, 2012, Mosby.

3-18 From Aehlert B: ECGs Made Easy, ed 4, St. Louis, 2009, Mosby.

3-19 From Patton K, Thibodeau G: Anatomy & Physiology, ed 7, St. Louis, 2009, Mosby.

3-20 From Aehlert B: ECGs Made Easy, ed 4, St. Louis, 2009, Mosby.

3-21 From Urden L, Stacy K, Lough M: Thelan's Critical Care Nursing: Diagnosis and Management, ed 5, St. Louis, 2006, Mosby.

3-22 From Goldberger A: Clinical Electrocardiography: A Simplified Approach, ed 6, St. Louis, 1999, Mosby.

3-23 Modified from Patton K, Thibodeau G: Anatomy & Physiology, ed 7, St. Louis, 2009, Mosby.

3-24, 3-25 From Aehlert B: ECGs Made Easy Study Cards, St. Louis, 2004, Mosby.

3-26 From Shade B, Rothenburg M, Wertz E, et al: Mosby's EMT-Intermediate Textbook, ed 2 revised, St. Louis, 2011, Mosby.

3-27 From Goldberger A: Clinical Electrocardiography: A Simplified Approach, ed 6, St. Louis, 1999, Mosby.

3-28 From Shade B, Rothenburg M, Wertz E, et al: Mosby's EMT-Intermediate Textbook, ed 2 revised, St. Louis, 2011, Mosby.

3-29 From Goldberger A: Clinical Electrocardiography: A Simplified Approach, ed 6, St. Louis, 1999, Mosby.

3-30, 3-31, 3-32, 3-33 From Guy, 2010.

3-34 From Conover MB: Understanding Electrocardiography, ed 8, St. Louis, 2003, Mosby.

3-35 From Goldman L, Braunwald E: Primary Cardiology, Philadelphia, 1998, Saunders.

3-36 From Aehlert B: ECGs Made Easy Study Cards, St. Louis, 2004, Mosby.

3-37 From Urden L, Stacy K, Lough M: Thelan's Critical Care Nursing: Diagnosis and Management, ed 5, St. Louis, 2006, Mosby.

3-38 From Crawford MV, Spence MI: Commonsense Approach to Coronary Care, ed 6 revised, St. Louis, 1994, Mosby.

3-39 From Surawics B, Knilans TK, Chou's Electrocardiography in Clinical Practice: Adult and Pediatric, ed 5, Philadelphia, 1996, Saunders.

3-40 From Andreoli TE, Benjamin I, Griggs RC, et al: Andreoli and Carpenter's Cecil Essentials of Medicine, ed 7, Philadelphia, 2007, Saunders.

3-41 From Aehlert B: ECGs Made Easy, ed 4, St. Louis, 2009, Mosby.

3-42 Reprinted with permission 2010 American Heart Association Guidelines for Cardiopulmonary Resuscitation and Emergency Cardiovascular Care, Part 4: CPR Overview. *Circulation* 2010;122[suppl 3]: S676-S684. ©2010 American Heart Association, Inc.

3-43 From Guy, 2010.

3-44 From Conover MB: Understanding Electrocardiography, ed 7, St. Louis, 1996, Mosby.

3-45, 3-46 From Phalen T, Aehlert B: The 12-Lead ECGS in Acute Coronary Syndromes, ed 3, St. Louis, 2012, Mosby.

3-47 From Aehlert B: ECGs Made Easy, ed 4, St. Louis, 2009, Mosby.

3-48 From Crawford MV, Spence MI: Commonsense Approach to Coronary Care, ed 6, St. Louis: 1995, Mosby-Year Book.

3-49 From Aehlert B: ECGs Made Easy Study Cards, St. Louis, 2004, Mosby.

3-50 From Aehlert B: ECGs Made Easy, ed 4, St. Louis, 2009, Mosby.

3-51 From Andreoli TE, Benjamin I, Griggs RC, et al: Andreoli and Carpenter's Cecil Essentials of Medicine, ed 7, Philadelphia, 2007, Saunders.

3-52 From Aehlert B: ECGs Made Easy Study Cards, St. Louis, 2004, Mosby.

3-53 From Goldberger A: Clinical Electrocardiography: A Simplified Approach, ed 6, St. Louis, 1999, Mosby.

3-54 From Grauer K: A Practical Guide to ECG Interpretation, ed 2, St. Louis, 1998, Mosby.

3-55 From Aehlert B: ECGs Made Easy Study Cards, St. Louis, 2004, Mosby.

3-56, 3-57 From Guy, 2010.

3-58 From Aehlert B: ECGs Made Easy, ed 4, St. Louis, 2009, Mosby.

3-59 From Shade B, Rothenburg M, Wertz E, et al: Mosby's EMT-Intermediate Textbook, ed 2 revised, St. Louis, 2011, Mosby.

3-60 From Guy, 2010.

3-61 From Aehlert, Paramedic Practice Today, St. Louis, 2010, Mosby.

3-62, 3-63 From Aehlert B: ECGs Made Easy, ed 4, St. Louis, 2009, Mosby.

3-64 From Shade B, Rothenburg M, Wertz E, et al: Mosby's EMT-Intermediate Textbook, ed 2 revised, St. Louis, 2011, Mosby.

3-65 From Aehlert B: ECGs Made Easy, ed 4, St. Louis, 2009, Mosby.

3-66 From Shade B, Rothenburg M, Wertz E, et al: Mosby's EMT-Intermediate Textbook, ed 2 revised, St. Louis, 2011, Mosby.

3-67 From Aehlert B: ECGs Made Easy, ed 4, St. Louis, 2009, Mosby.

3-68 From Shade B, Rothenburg M, Wertz E, et al: Mosby's EMT-Intermediate Textbook, ed 2 revised, St. Louis, 2011, Mosby.

3-69, 3-70, 3-71 From Aehlert B: ECGs Made Easy, ed 4, St. Louis, 2009, Mosby.

3-72 From Grauer K: A Practical Guide to ECG Interpretation, ed 2, St. Louis, 1998, Mosby.

3-73 From Shade B, Rothenburg M, Wertz E, et al: Mosby's EMT-Intermediate Textbook, ed 2 revised, St. Louis, 2011, Mosby.

3-74 From Aehlert B: ECGs Made Easy Study Cards, St. Louis, 2004, Mosby.

3-75 From Aehlert B: ECGs Made Easy, ed 4, St. Louis, 2009, Mosby.

3-76 Reprinted with permission 2010 American Heart Association Guidelines for Cardiopulmonary Resuscitation and Emergency Cardiovascular Care, Part 4: CPR Overview. *Circulation* 2010;122(Suppl 3): S676-S684. ©2010 American Heart Association, Inc.

3-77, 3-78 From Aehlert B: ECGs Made Easy Study Cards, St. Louis, 2004, Mosby.

3-79 From Guy, 2010.

3-80 From Aehlert B: ECGs Made Easy Study Cards, St. Louis, 2004, Mosby.

3-81 From Aehlert B: ECGs Made Easy, ed 4, St. Louis, 2009, Mosby.

3-82 From Aehlert B: ECGs Made Easy Study Cards, St. Louis, 2004, Mosby.

3-83 From Aehlert B: ECGs Made Easy, ed 4, St. Louis, 2009, Mosby.

3-84 A, B, Reprinted with permission 2010 American Heart Association Guidelines for Cardiopulmonary Resuscitation and Emergency Cardiovascular Care, Part 4: CPR Overview. *Circulation* 2010;122(suppl 3): S676-S684. ©2010 American Heart Association, Inc.

3-85 From Cummins R: ACLS Scenarios: Core Concepts for Case-Based Learning, St. Louis, 1996, Mosby.

3-86 From Aehlert B: ECGs Made Easy, ed 4, St. Louis, 2009, Mosby.

3-87 to 3-108 From Aehlert B: ECGs Made Easy Study Cards, St. Louis, 2004, Mosby.

Skill 3-1

Step 1 From Aehlert B: Paramedic Practice Today, St. Louis, 2010, Mosby.

Chapter 4

4-1 Courtesy Medtronic Emergency Response Systems.

4-2 A, B, Courtesy the Emergency Medical Services for Children and Services Administration, Maternal and Child Health Bureau. EMSC Slide Set (CD-ROM).

4-3, 4-4 From Aehlert B: ACLS Study Guide, ed 3, St. Louis, 2007, Mosby.

4-5 From Roberts JR, Hedges JR: Clinical Procedures in Emergency Medicine, ed 5, Philadelphia, 2009, Saunders.

4-6, 4-7 From Aehlert B: ACLS Study Guide, ed 3, St. Louis, 2007, Mosby.

4-8 From Shade B, Rothenberg M, Wertz E, et al: Mosby's EMT-Intermediate Textbook, 2011edition, St. Louis, 2012, Mosby.

4-9, 4-10, 4-11 From Aehlert B: Paramedic Practice Today, St. Louis, 2009, Mosby.

4-12 From Forbes CD, Jackson WF: Color Atlas and Text of Clinical Medicine, ed 3, London, Mosby, 2003

4-13 Courtesy Medtronic Inc., Minneapolis, MN.

4-14 Courtesy Philips Medical Systems.

4-15 From Chapleau W: Emergency First Responder: Making the Difference, St. Louis, 2004, Mosby.

4-16 to 4-26 From Aehlert B: Paramedic Practice Today, St. Louis, 2009, Mosby.

4-27 From Aehlert B: ECGs Made Easy, ed 3, St. Louis, 2006, Mosby.

4-28, 4-29 From Aehlert B: Paramedic Practice Today, St. Louis, 2009, Mosby.

4-30, 4-31 From Aehlert B: ECGs Made Easy, ed 3, St. Louis, 2006, Mosby.

Chapter 5

5-1, 5-2, 5-3 From Kumar V, Ramzi SC, Robbins SL: Robbins Basic Pathology, ed 8, Philadelphia, 2007, Saunders.

5-4 Falk A: Pathology of Atherosclerotic Plaque: Stable, Unstable, and Infarctional. In Roubin G, Califf R, O'Neill W (editors): Interventional Cardiovascular Medicine: Principles and Practice, New York, 1994, Churchill Livingstone.

5-5 From Goldman l, Braunwald E: Primary Cardiology, Philadelphia, 1998, Saunders.

5-6, 5-7 From Urden, LD, Stacey KM, Lough ME: Critical Care Nursing: Diagnosis and Management, ed 6, St. Louis, 2009, Mosby.

5-8 Modified from Huszar B: Basic Dysrhythmias: Interpretation and Management, ed 3, St. Louis 2006, Mosby.

5-9 Modified from Urden LD, Stacey KM, Lough ME: Critical Care Nursing: Diagnosis and Management, ed 6, St. Louis, 2010, Mosby.

5-10 From McCance KL, Heuther SE, Pathophysiology: The Biologic Basis for Disease in Adults and Children, ed 5, St. Louis, 2005, Mosby.

5-11 From Butler HA, Caplin M, McCaully E, et al (editors): Managing Major Diseases: Cardiac Disorders, vol 2, St. Louis, 1999, Mosby.

5-12 Modified from Grauer K: A Practical Guide to ECG Interpretation , ed 2, St. Louis, 1998, Mosby.

5-13 From Sanders MJ: Mosby's Paramedic Textbook , ed 3, St. Louis, 2005, Mosby.

5-14 From Grauer K: A Practical Guide to ECG Interpretation, ed 2, St. Louis, 1998, Mosby.

5-15 From Johnson R, Schwartz M: A Simplified Approach to Electrocardiography, Philadelphia, 1986, WB Saunders.

5-16, 5-17, 5-18, 5-19 From Phalen T, Aehlert B: The 12-Lead ECG in Acute Coronary Syndromes, ed 3, St. Louis, 2012, Mosby.

5-20 Goldberger A: Clinical Electrocardiography: A Simplified Approach, ed 6, St. Louis, 1999, Mosby.

5-21 From Phalen T, Aehlert B: The 12-Lead ECG in Acute Coronary Syndromes, ed 3, St. Louis, 2012, Mosby.

5-22 From Surawicz B, Knilans TK: Chou's Electrocardiography in Clinical Practice: Adult and Pediatric, ed 5, Philadelphia, 2001, WB Saunders.

5-23, 5-24, 5-25 From Phalen T, Aehlert B: The 12-Lead ECG in Acute Coronary Syndromes, ed3, St. Louis, 2012, Mosby.

5-26 From Grauer K: A Practical Guide to ECG Interpretation , ed 2, St. Louis, 1998, Mosby.

5-27 Modified from Kiney MP, Packa DR: Andreoli's Comprehensive Cardiac Care, ed 8, St. Louis, 1996, Mosby.

5-28 From Phalen T, Aehlert B: The 12-Lead ECG in Acute Coronary Syndromes, ed 3, St. Louis, 2012, Mosby.

5-29 From Urden LD, Stacey KM, Lough ME: Critical Care Nursing: Diagnosis and Management, ed 6, St. Louis, 2010, Mosby.

5-30 Reprinted with permission 2010 American Heart Association Guidelines for Cardiopulmonary Resuscitation and Emergency Cardiovascular Care, Part 4: CPR Overview Circulation.2010;122[suppl 3]: S676-S684. ©2010 American Heart Association, Inc.

5-31 Modified from Baim DS: Percutaneous Balloon Angioplasty and General Coronary Intervention. In Baim DS [ed]: Grossman's Cardiac Catheterization, Angiography, and Intervention, ed 7, Philadelphia, Lippincott Williams & Wilkins, 2005.

5-32 From Sole ML, Klein DG, Moseley MJ: Introduction to Critical Care Nursing, ed 5, Philadelphia, 2008, Saunders.

5-33, 5-34, 5-35 From Urden LD, Stacey KM, Lough ME: Critical Care Nursing: Diagnosis and Management, ed 6, St. Louis, 2010, Mosby.

5-36 Cleveland Clinic: Current Clinical Medicine 2009, Philadelphia, 2009, Saunders.

5-37, 5-38 From Gould BE: Pathophysiology for the Health Professions, ed 3, Philadelphia, 2006, Saunders.

5-39 From Marx J, Hockberger R, Walls R: Rosen's Emergency Medicine, ed 7, St. Louis, 2009, Mosby.

5-40 From Kumar V, Ramzi SC, Robbins SL: Robbins Basic Pathology, ed 8, Philadelphia, 2007, Saunders.

Chapter 6

6-1 From Thibodeau G, Patton K: Anatomy and Physiology, ed 5, St. Louis, 2003, Mosby.

6-2 From Aehlert B: ACLS Study Guide, ed 3, St. Louis, 2007, Mosby.

6-4 From Shade B, Rothenberg M, Wertz E, et al: Mosby's EMT-Intermediate Textbook, 2001 edition, St. Louis, 2012, Mosby.

6-5 Reprinted with permission 2010 American Heart Association Guidelines for Cardiopulmonary Resuscitation and Emergency Cardiovascular Care, Part 4: CPR Overview Circulation.2010;122[suppl 3]: S676-S684. ©2010 American Heart Association, Inc.

Case Studies

7-1 to 7-10 Aehlert B: ECGs Made Easy, ed 4, St. Louis, 2010, Mosby.

7-10 to 7-13 Aehlert B: ECG Made Easy Study Cards, St. Louis, 2004, Mosby.

7-14 Aehlert B: ECGs Made Easy, ed 4, St. Louis, 2010, Mosby.

Posttest

8-1 Phalen T, Aehlert B: The 12-Lead ECG in Acute Coronary Syndromes, ed 3, St. Louis 2012, Mosby.

8-2 Hampton J: The ECG in Practice , ed 5, Edinburgh, 2008, Churchill Livingstone.

8-3 Aehlert B: ECGs Made Easy, ed 4, St. Louis, 2010, Mosby.

8-4 Aehlert B: ECG Made Easy Study Cards, St. Louis, 2004, Mosby.

8-5 Aehlert B: ECGs Made Easy, ed 4, St. Louis, 2010, Mosby.

8-6, 8-7 Aehlert B: ECG Made Easy Study Cards, St. Louis, 2004, Mosby.

INDEX

Page numbers followed by f, t, or b indicate figures, tables, or boxed material, respectively.

P